MICROCIRCULATION AND INSULIN RESISTANCE

Editor:

Nicolas WIERNSPERGER, Ph.D.

CONTENTS

PREFACE

Insulin resistance (IR) is a common basis for many acute or long-term pathologies. Although it is best known in the area of cardiometabolic diseases because of the worldwide burden of obesity and diabetes, IR is observed in the vast majority of pathological situations. Very intensive research over the last 20 years has unravelled the defective mechanisms responsible for inadequate insulin receptor signaling and glucose transport and storage. However, the causal mechanisms producing IR are still elusive.

Many factors are known to lead to IR which, in view of the great variety of diseases exhibiting IR, suggests that they converge toward a common point from which tissue IR is initiated. The fact that by far not all IR states worsen toward diabetes indicates that this element may be only transiently disturbed by acute pathologies and repaired. Conceivably those patients unable to repair over a given period of time experience a delayed development of the deleterious consequences of IR such as cardiovascular diseases or metabolic syndrome or diabetes.

Since 1) a main physiological role of insulin is to supply the skeletal muscle cells with the excessive glucose in postprandial periods and 2) capillary flow is ultimately the key determinant of nutrient delivery to cells, we would like to expose and discuss a new concept stating that microcirculation and insulin sensitivity are linked such as to function both ways. In this book we describe many puzzling observations according to which IR and microvascular dysfunction are usually found concomitantly, well before cardiometabolic diseases are clinically observable; this parallel can even be seen in normal, healthy populations within a normal range of insulin sensitivity. This means that microvascular dysfunction could be a cause of IR and thus represent the guilty element underlying IR in so many clinical disorders.

Bouskela *et al.* present a concise but complete overview of the multiple specificities of micro-vs macrocirculation. It is shown how closely structure and regulation of microvessels correlate with the functions of individual typical segments of the microvascular tree (arterioles, capillaries, venules). In a complementary chapter, Kraemer-Aguiar and Bouskela detail and critically review the various techniques used to measure endothelial function and microvascular reactivity in humans. Indeed most informations are only partly or not at all derived from the microvasculature. These informations are of utmost importance for sorting the plethoric amount of published data in this field, as also thoroughly discussed in the first part of the last book chapter. Frisbee and Brock review data on microcirculation and IR by comparing IR in the presence vs absence of obesity in rodents. They give detailed information on the impact of IR on dilator and constrictor responses as well as capillary perfusion, and highlight the integrated way microcirculation functions. The clinical aspect of IR and microvascular dysfunction is the subject of the chapter by Serné et al, focusing on obesity and hypertension, two major components of the metabolic syndrome. In a very in-depth analysis of a broad series of consequent investigations, they delineate how microvascular and metabolic factors are linked and they shed particularly light on the links between adipose tissue and the microvasculature. Some selected mechanistic aspects are more specifically developed in a series of chapters because of their recognized importance for microcirculation in pathological circumstances. Adipose tissue being a major source of inflammatory factors, Singer and Granger deal with the impact cytokines may have on the microvasculature and how the subsequent defects underlie cardiovascular pathologies affecting obese patients. Low-grade inflammation is doubtless one main common denominator between the vast majority of diseases characterized by IR. The endothelium, playing such prominent roles in vasomotricity and nutrient transfer, is damaged by inflammation as well as by oxidative stress. Rösen and Rösen provide an overview on the origins, mechanisms and consequences of oxidative stress in microvessels. One typical defect characterizing endothelial damage is microalbuminuria; as developed by Haraldsson, microalbuminuria is not only a local renal phenomenon but reveals a more generalized endothelial dysfunction throughout the body, making this parameter an interesting early marker in clinical settings. Martinez and Andriantsitohaina present a very innovative aspect of microcirculation, namely the recently discovered existence of circulating microparticles. They have different origins and can induce deleterious as well as beneficial effects; although still relatively little is known about microparticles, we felt that this exciting new player was worth being developed in the present analysis. A cardinal feature in capillary perfusion is evidently the flow behaviour of blood, i.e. hemorheology. Hemorheology deals with aspects which have a major, but mostly very local importance, i.e. the physical properties of flowing blood such as viscosity (whole blood, plasma) and erythrocyte deformability/aggregation. While it is easily comprehensible that disturbed red blood cell behaviour impairs flow through tiny capillaries, it is less recognized that whole blood or plasma viscosity have major consequences too and, interestingly, they are also very early seen in these IR pathologies as exposed by Brun *et al.*

In the last chapter, divided in three distinct parts, Wiernsperger first critically describes the multiple confounding factors in epidemiological, hemodynamic and metabolic investigations which are likely to severely bias data interpretation; subsequently a broad description is given of the many different diseases characterized by microvascular defects. Of paramount interest are the many studies on healthy first degree relatives of parents with diabetes or cardiovascular diseases, as well as even normal healthy subjects in which the very early appearance of microvascular disturbances strongly suggests that they can be inherited.Part 2 addresses the specific emodynamic effects of insulin itself in the microcirculation and discusses the data under consideration of their physiological pertinence. In particular it is shown that very small increments in plasma insulin such as they occur at the very beginning of meals may be crucial to maximize opening of the microvascular bed in skeletal muscle for supply and storage of excess prandial glucose. Part 3 deals with an analysis of possible mechanisms whereby very early microvascular defects in life might impair proper microflow and thus interfere with the normal handling of glucose by insulin, i.e. induce IR.

This book is consciously prospective and proposes a concept based on physiological reasoning and established clinical and pathophysiological observations; by no means does this concept claim to be unique and valid for all situations. We are, however, convinced that there is sufficient available argumentation to deserve further fundamental and clinical research in order to definitively confirm or deny the correctness of what we believe is actually a "**solid hypothesis**", **namely that microvascular dysfunction can trigger insulin resistance**.

Nicolas Wiernsperger, *Ph.D.*
Editor

Eliete Bouskela, *M.D., Ph.D.*
L.Guilherme Kraemer-Aguiar, *M.D.*
Co-Editors

CONTRIBUTORS

Ramaroson Andriantsitohaina, PhD
INSERM U771, CNRS UMR 6214, Faculté de Médecine, Université d'Angers, France

Wineke Bakker, PhD
Laboratory for Physiology, Institute for cardiovascular research, VU medical Centre, Amsterdam, The Netherlands

Daniel Bottino, PhD
Laboratorio de Pesquisas em Microcirculaçao, Centro Biomedico, Uniersidade do Estado do Rio de Janeiro, Rio de Janeiro, Brazil

Eliete Bouskela, MD, PhD
Professor, Laboratorio de Pesquisas em Microcirculaçao, Centro Biomedico, Universidade do Estado do Rio de Janeiro, Rio de Janeiro, Brazil

Robert W. Brock, PhD
Dept of Physiology and Pharmacology, Center for Cardiovascular and Respiratory Sciences, West Virginia University Health Sciences Center, Morgantown, WV, USA

Jean-Frederic Brun, PhD
INSERM ERI25 Muscle et Pathologies, Service Central de Physiologie Clinique, CERAMM, CHU Lapeyronie, Montpellier, France

Michiel P. de Boer, MD
Dept of Internal Medicine, Institute for Cardiovascular Research, VU Medical Centre, Amsterdam, The Netherlands

Renate T. de Jongh, MD, PhD
Dept of Internal Medicine, Institute for Cardiovascular Research, VU Medical Centre, Amsterdam, The Netherlands

Etto C. Eringa, PhD
Laboratory for Physiology, Institute for cardiovascular research, VU medical Centre, Amsterdam, The Netherlands

Jefferson Frisbee, PhD
Dept of Physiology and Pharmacology, Center for Cardiovascular and Respiratory Sciences, West Virginia University Health Sciences Center, Morgantown, WV, USA

D. Neil Granger, PhD
Dept of Molecular and Cellular Physiology, LSU Health Sciences Center, Shreveport, LA, USA

Börje Haraldsson, PhD
Institute of Medicine, Dept of Molecular and Clinical Medicine,Nephrology, University of Gothenburg, Gothenburg, Sweden

Richard G. IJzerman, MD, PhD
Dept of Internal Medicine. Institute for Cardiovascular Research. VU Medical Centre.

L. Guilherme Kraemer-Aguiar, MD, PhD
Laboratorio de Pesquisas em Microcirculaçao, Centro Biomedico, Universidade do Estado do Rio de Janeiro, Rio de Janeiro, Brazil

Maria Carmen Martinez, PhD
INSERM U771, CNRS UMR 6214, Faculté de Médecine, Université d'Angers, France

Rick I. Meijer, MD
Dept of Internal Medicine, Institute for Cardiovascular Research, VU Medical Centre, Amsterdam, The Netherlands

Jacques Mercier, MD, PhD
INSERM ERI25 Muscle et Pathologies, Service Central de Physiologie Clinique, CERAMM, CHU Lapeyronie, Montpellier, France

Timothy I. Musch, PhD
Depts of Kinesiology, Anatomy and Physiology, Kansas State University, Manhattan, Kansas, USA

David C. Poole, PhD
Depts of Kinesiology, Anatomy and Physiology, Kansas State University, Manhattan, Kansas, USA

Eric Raynaud de Mauverger, PhD
INSERM ERI25 Muscle et Pathologies, Service Central de Physiologie Clinique, CERAMM, CHU Lapeyronie, Montpellier, France

Peter Rösen, PhD
German Diabetes Research Center, Dusseldorf, Germany

Renate Rösen, PhD
Institute of Pharmacology, University of Cologne, Germany

Mathieu Sardinoux, PhD
INSERM ERI25 Muscle et Pathologies, Service Central de Physiologie Clinique, CERAMM, CHU Lapeyronie, Montpellier, France

Eric H. Serné, MD, PhD
Dept of Internal Medicine, Institute for Cardiovascular Research, VU Medical Centre, Amsterdam, The Netherlands

Georg Singer, MD
Dept of Pediatric Surgery, Medical University of Graz, Graz, Austria

Emmanuelle Varlet-Marie, PhD
Laboratoire de Biophysique et Bioanalyses, Faculté de Pharmacie, Université de Montpellier I, Montpellier, France

Nicolas F. Wiernsperger, PhD
INSERM U870, INSA Lyon, Villeurbanne, France & Laboratorio de Pesquisas em Microcirculaçao, Centro Biomedico, Universidade do Estado do Rio de Janeiro, Rio de Janeiro Brazil

CHAPTER 1

Microcirculation: Structural and Functional Specificities

Eliete Bouskela[1], Daniel Bottino[1] and Nicolas Wiernsperger[1,2]

[1]*Laboratorio de Pesquisas em Microcirculaçao, Centro Biomedico, Universidade do estado do Rio de Janeiro, Pav.R.Haroldo Lisboa da Cunha, Rua Sao Francisco Xavier, 524, 20550-013, Rio de Janeiro (Brazil);* [2]*INSERM U870, INSA Lyon, Bat L. Pasteur, 11 avenue J. Capelle, F-69621 Villeurbanne Cedex (France); E-mail: eliete_bouskela@yahoo.com.br*

Abstract: Microcirculation is an « invisible » world, representing billions of smallest vessels and about $500m^2$ endothelium, the largest endocrine organ in human body. It is organized in a fractal fashion, in essentially three vessel subtypes: mid-and small sized arterioles (regulating vascular resistance), capillaries (<10μm) and venules which collect blood from tissues. Microvessel structure, effector mechanisms and their regulation are strictly adapted to function and fundamental differences exist between the microvessel segments, as well as between the microvascular and the macrovascular beds. This chapter aims at giving to the unaware reader a short but complete overview of these specificities for a better understanding of forthcoming chapters, which are devoted to describe our concept, namely that microcirculatory defects, eventually appearing very early in life, can cause and/or aggravate insulin resistance leading to diabetes and cardiovascular diseases some decades later.

1. INTRODUCTION

The vascular bed is an arborescence grossly divided into three main categories of vessel types: arterial vessels, microvessels and veins. Each category deserves defined functions, to which correspond specific structures and roles. Large and small arteries are mainly conduit vessels and are exposed to various physical strengths; thereby they have a relatively thick wall and are elastic. This part is responsible for at least 50% of the total vascular resistance [1]. Defects in these vessels typically lead to macroangiopathy, i.e. vascular accidents of atherosclerotic or hemorrhagic type. Veins are also large vessels, aimed at collecting blood having passed the tissues. They have relatively little tone and have a weak contracting capacity, being thereby prone to diseases typical of low venous return. The part of the vascular bed comprised between these two entities represents the immense network of microvessels; microcirculation is normally defined as the segments going from small arteries (<100μm) down to tiny capillaries (<10μm) and then to venules (<40μm). During the recent years, however, another more functional definition has been proposed stating that microvessels are those small vessels exhibiting myogenic tone.

2. HETEROGENEITY IS EVERYWHERE

Heterogeneity is a hallmark of the vascular bed. It is seen not only between large and small vessels but differs from one tissue to another and even along the same vessel differences exist. To name a few examples, conduit arteries differing in size exhibit different vascular functions [2,3]. Endothelium-dependent vasodilation was found to be present in high-oxidative - but not in low-oxidative- muscle fibres [4]. An excellent review about differences between arterial and venous endothelial cells has been recently issued [5]. On a more local basis, expression of matrix metalloproteinases in microvessels differs from that of macrovascular endothelial cells [6] as do endothelial microdomain signalling complexes [7].

The function of microcirculation is to deliver oxygen and nutrients to most remote tissue locations and to exchange waste products with interstitial fluid. Because the function of the microvascular bed is completely different from large vessels, the structures and controlling mechanisms differ accordingly. When arterioles branch into smaller ones the number of muscular layers decreases until a single layer of endothelial cells lying on a basement membrane forms the true capillaries. The myogenic tone increases with decreasing arteriolar diameter, thereby protecting the capillary bed against hyperperfusion and local hypertension [8,9]. Thus there is a great heterogeneity not only between large and smaller vessels but also within the microvascular bed. This heterogeneity is permitted via the fractal organization of the microvascular bed, which guarantees many levels of control [10].

This heterogeneity also concerns the tissue type: for example the permeability of venous capillaries is adapted to the function of the organ, being high in the splanchnic bed [fenestrated capillaries], moderate in skeletal muscle and very low in the brain. Another characteristic of microcirculation is that, despite deserving quite different tasks, arterioles and venules nevertheless communicate: venules are frequently apposed to arterioles, allowing transversal crosstalk; however even within the same vessel line arterioles receive feedback signals from downstream capillaries and venules via conducted signals. For example modification of ATP levels can dilate venules, a signal which is transmitted upstream to arterioles which subsequently dilate to increase capillary blood flow [11,12]. Finally heterogeneity is also observed within a microvascular unit, where blood flow is distributed unequally and varies greatly in time [13].

3. CAPILLARY BLOOD FLOW

Microcirculation is characterized by a myriad of microvascular units (or modules), where several capillaries are supplied by a single terminal arteriole [14], which controls the number of blood-perfused capillaries. This particular process is one of the most controversial points in microvascular research. Indeed an ongoing debate exists about the basal filling rate of the capillary bed. Because the capillary diameter is frequently below those of erythrocytes, these cells must adopt an elongated form, which also means that any defects in erythrocyte flexibility or in capillary entrance diameter or intracapillary endothelial/glycocalyx swelling will block red cells. Although little histological evidence could demonstrate the existence of true capillary sphincters, in situ observations by intravital capillaroscopy nevertheless shows an extreme heterogeneity of blood flow within a capillary unit or between units. This phenomenon is described as flowmotion (stop and go flow). At least for periods of some seconds, capillaries can be completely close [i.e. to both plasma and erythrocytes], partially close (only to erythrocytes) or fully open to whole blood.

The anatomical disposition varies greatly among organs; while in skeletal muscle capillaries largely run in parallel due to their disposition along and between muscle fibres, grey matter cerebral capillaries on the other hand form an extremely complicated 3D mesh, thereby leaving intercapillary distances very small because of the high oxygen demand of brain cells. The number of capillaries in skeletal muscle is directly adapted to the muscle fibre type, i.e. to its metabolic characteristics: thus up to 10 capillaries can be found around an individual red fibre, while only 2-3 may surround white fibres. Connections between capillaries also exist, allowing redistribution of flow in close vicinity. The fractal organization of microcirculation allows thereby extremely fine tuned flow adjustments to metabolic needs, by modification of the number and volume of capillaries as well as flow direction. In such a way, for example, two parallel running capillaries can exhibit countercurrent flow to avoid the occurrence of a hypoxic tissue zone.

Therefore it is easily understandable that capillary perfusion shows an ever-changing pattern which makes it somewhat difficult to quantify, even by direct visualization. It is thus not surprising that the filling rate of the capillary bed is subject to debate and its definition directly determines if capillary recruitment, estimated by the "functional capillary density", is possible or not. Increasing the absolute number of blood-perfused capillaries is considered as capillary recruitment, as can be an elevation in hematocrit in a poorly perfused capillary.

Injection of dyes supports at least the idea that all capillaries are permanently perfused with plasma [15]; in vivo direct observation of the microcirculation clearly shows great variations in the rate of blood-filled capillaries. Even the notion of capillary recruitment can be divided into a temporal component and a spatial component [16]. Redistribution of blood flow within the microvascular bed is undoubtedly a constant process in basal conditions, due to changes in the number of blood-perfused capillaries, in the amount of blood in the capillary tube and in the speed of passing blood, another determinant of oxygen supply [17]. In cases of increased metabolic demand, regional redistribution of blood can occur by closure of non-nutritive vessels, diverting blood towards nutritive microvessels [18]. Conversely impairment in microperfusion can occur if some vessels dilate too strongly, leading thereby to shunt flow and to hypoxic tissue areas [19].

Finally one should mention that under special conditions such as hypertriglyceridemia or obesity, perivascular fat accumulates at the level of arteriolar branches, which may contribute to impairment of flow regulation through local liberation of harmful cytokines such as TNFα or interleukins [20,21].

It is thus important to realize that microcirculation is under the simultaneous influence of anatomical, nervous, metabolic, hormonal and intrinsic myogenic factors, with many specific mechanisms which will be detailed below while still remaining under the influence of up-and downstream large vessels.

4. MICROVASCULAR SPECIFICITIES

4.1. Arteriolar Vasomotion

When blood flow is recorded continuously several types of waves of very different frequencies and amplitudes can be observed. They have various origins, some corresponding to respiration, some to heart rate, some to large and small vessel rythmicity. In arterioles an intrinsic rhythmic variation in microvessel diameter is observed under basal conditions, ranging from 1-20 cycles/min [22]. Under normal conditions mostly low-frequency vasomotion is seen and can be found in most intact tissues [23]; however it disappears or changes its characteristics in a number of situations (some anesthetics, ischemia, diabetes, etc..). Vasomotion is a highly debated topic because of very different rates of observations among research teams. Fig. (1) shows a schematic representation of arteriolar vasomotion and some factors impacting on its activity.

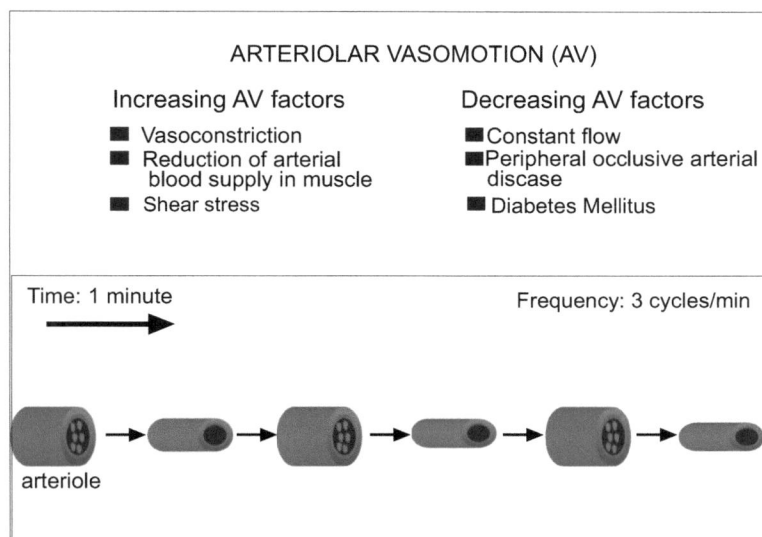

Figure 1: Schematic representation of arteriolar vasomotion and some regulatory factors

Direct visualization of small arterioles frequently shows cyclic diameter variations as well as transient apparent closures of terminal arterioles, stopping red blood cell (RBC) flow for some seconds. Transitory reversal of flow direction can also be observed. In a tissue like skeletal muscle, in situ videomicroscopy of a relatively simple microvascular bed shows a pattern of constantly changing, chaotic flow with highly variable hematocrit in capillaries. How vasomotion is initiated is currently unclear and may be some mixture of neurogenic and myogenic factors. While an intrinsic oscillator could not be conclusively demonstrated, there is now evidence that spontaneous, cyclic changes in arteriolar membrane potential occur [24]. Recently extensive investigations revealed that vasomotion is generated by the number of cells which become recruited, up to a point where synchronization occurs [25]. Calcium transients exist in localized areas of individual endothelial cells which can synchronize [26]. Subsequently calcium activates chloride channels which are cGMP sensitive [27,29]. Metabolites may affect vasomotion, in such a way that it might result from a mixture of sarcolemmal oscillator and a glycolytic metabolic oscillating signal [30,31]. Another point of inconsistency is whether vasomotion is induced by vessel constriction or dilation. Injection of acetylcholine, a NO-dependent dilator, reduced vasomotion while the NO-inhibitor L-NMMA stimulated vasomotion [32]. Acute glucose infusion in normal rats induced arteriolar constriction with concomitant activation of vasomotion in skeletal muscle [33]. Using a calcium agonist, vasoconstriction also led to vasomotion in glomerular afferent arterioles [34]. In favour of increased tone facilitating vasomotion is also the clinical observation that intermittent pneumatic compression restored it in patients with post-thrombotic venous insufficiency [35]. Vasomotion can also develop spontaneously in skeletal muscle-but not in skin- after reduction in arterial blood supply. The latter case could be interpreted as a tentative protective reaction, as suggested by data obtained in flap surgery [36]. Interestingly in the human situation neither inhibition of NO nor endothelin antagonism by bosentan affected vasomotion [36]. In muscle, therefore, most data suggest that vasomotion is triggered by an increased shear stress linked to moderate constriction, abolished by vasodilatation [Renaudin+NW]. Challenging this concept, it was recently proposed that insulin would improve glucose supply to muscle fibres by activating vasomotion. However this conclusion was a theoretical one and originated from data obtained with insulin in skin [37]. Interestingly, skin might behave differently from muscle since it was indeed found that in humans cutaneous vasomotion and vasodilatation were induced by iontophoretic application of insulin [38,39]. Skin vasomotion was found to be NO-dependent in humans [40] and NO is known to be involved in insulin-induced vasodilatation. In rat skeletal muscle, artificial elevation of plasma insulin in the presence of normal glycemia levels generated arteriolar vasomotion [33]; however this effect was blunted if the same insulin level was induced physiological by simultaneous hyperglycemia [33]. In humans hyperinsulinemia provoked by the artificial clamp procedure increased skeletal muscle vasomotion [41]. Differences in endothelium-dependency for vasodilatation have been reported according to muscle fibre types [4]. Whether these discrepancies are based on tissue differences [muscle vs skin], on mechanistic differences [NO dependence] or on species [rat vs human] is presently unclear. The fact that various types of low-frequency vasomotion apparently coexist [42] makes it difficult to compare data.

The relevance of arteriolar vasomotion is an open question because of the poor amount of available data. However a recent clinical study suggested that it might be a better indicator of microvascular disorders than blood flow [43, 44]. Mathematical models suggest that chaotic flow is more favourable for adequate tissue oxygenation than constant flow [45]. This notion is corroborated by observations in pathological situations, where vasomotion was found to protect adjacent tissues from capillary perfusion failure [46]. The physiological role of low frequency, high amplitude vasomotion has been suggested to spare blood in an economic way under basal conditions, leaving reserves for adaptive flow increases and further filling of the capillary bed upon higher demands such as physical exercise.

Precapillary vasomotion is blunted in peripheral occlusive arterial diseases [46, 47] as well as in diabetes [42,48-50,52]. Treatment of animals with the antidiabetic metformin showed that restoration of vasomotion was accompanied by increased functional capillary density, less leukocyte adhesion and survival of haemorrhaged animals [51, 52].

4.2. Arteriolar Constriction: The Venoarteriolar Reflex and the Myogenic Response

In order to prevent hyperperfusion and its detrimental consequences in the capillary bed of lower limbs in upright position, arterioles constrict reactively to the increase in transmural pressure [53]: this phenomenon is called venoarteriolar reflex and is based on the arteriolar myogenic response. The most powerful myogenic response is found in the smallest arterioles [54]. It is thus a component of the autoregulatory system of blood flow during alterations in blood pressure. The precise mechanisms have not been unravelled but it seems to be of local neurogenic origin [55], to which may add central neurogenic impacts as well as pure local myogenic components. The venoarteriolar reflex is deficient in peripheral vascular diseases, resulting in peripheral edema [56-58], as well as in diabetes [59-63]. This defect in venoarteriolar reflex is one self-speaking example of the importance of intact vasoconstricting capacity of small arterioles for correct vascular physiology [64].

4.3. Vascular Permeability

Although microvascular permeability is not the primary scope of this review, it represents nevertheless an extremely important property of the microvascular bed. Although arterioles exhibit some permeability [65], the main location of both physiological and pathophysiological vascular permeability is the venous capillary endothelium. Abnormally elevated capillary permeability results in microalbuminuria, an early indicator of generalized endothelial dysfunction. It is also responsible for oedema formation in arterial and venous peripheral diseases or retinopathy. Recently the role of glycocalyx has also been stressed out [66-68]. Permeability is increased in hypertensive patients with comorbid metabolic syndrome [69] as well as in insulin resistance and diabetes [70,71]. For more detailed information the reader is referred to a large review on permeability [72].

4.4. Hemorheology

Hemorheology encompasses the flow behaviour of whole blood as well as of its individual components, i.e. plasma and blood cells. Capillary pressure is low and the diameter of true capillaries is below the one of most blood cells, in particular red blood cells. Flow speed and tube hematocrit are important determinants of tissue oxygenation and nutrient exchange. Evidently any impairment in blood viscosity, in erythrocyte deformability, in reduction of capillary tube diameter or plugging by blood cells will be directly detrimental to the essential nutritive role of microcirculation. Whole blood viscosity depends both on plasma viscosity and on RBC viscosity. Whole blood viscosity correlates with metabolic syndrome [73] and it has been shown that plasma viscosity is increased in obese patients [74,75]. A detailed insight into this question can be found in this book [cf Brun].

RBCs have an axial diameter which is higher than the usual capillary internal diameter and, as a consequence, they must deform in order to cross these vessels; this is done by a conformational change resulting in a parachute-like configuration elongating the cell. The capacity of RBCs to deform depends closely on integrity of its cytoskeleton and membrane fluidity, properties which are easily affected by many intra-and extracellular factors [76,77]. To some extent RBCs regulate their own distribution within the microcirculation [78]. Impairment of RBC flow will modify shear stress and flow speed. Erythrocyte deformability is reduced in many diseases, including the metabolic syndrome where it correlates negatively with waist circumference [79]. Increased RBC adhesiveness to endothelium can also add to reduced deformability and hamper the passage through capillaries, for example in the presence of inflammatory factors and oxidative stress as is seen in insulin resistance [80-82]. RBCs are also subjected to aggregation, either as a consequence of low flow or of metabolic alterations. RBC aggregation can be reversible and slow down blood speed, or stable, in which case the aggregate will plug the capillary. Increased erythrocyte aggregation also relates to insulin resistance [80] and to metabolic syndrome where it is correlated with the number of components of the syndrome, more particularly with the lipid profile [83,84]. In obesity it was reported that RBC aggregation improved after weight loss [85].

Finally microflow behaviour is also dependent on hemostatic parameters, in particular fibrinolysis. Microvascular perfusion failure can be induced by microthrombi of less than 40μm [86]. Fibrinogen levels are increased in obese patients and do not improve after weight loss [75]. The main cause of reduction in fibrinolysis is an increase in PAI-1, which prevents normal fibrinolysis and promotes the formation of endothelial microparticles with procoagulant potential [87]. PAI-1 is considered to play a key role in insulin resistance and metabolic syndrome: it correlates strongly with these metabolic alterations [88-91] and is increased in prediabetic subjects such as offsprings of diabetic parents, independently of plasma insulin levels [92]. PAI-1 may represent an important link between insulin resistance, obesity and cardiovascular diseases [93,94].

4.5. Mechanisms of Microvascular Dilatation and Constriction

4.5.1. EDHF

The last decade has highlighted the key role played by NO in the dilatory action of many effectors of vessel dilation. In the microcirculation another factor is of great importance, however: endothelium-derived hyperpolarizing factor (EDHF), presently only poorly defined, may represent a whole family of factors able to add to-or substitute for- NO [95-97][for review see 98]. The relative importance of NO and EDHF changes with vessel size, so that EDHF becomes prominent with decreasing vessel diameter [99]. EDHF is present at sites where endothelial and smooth muscle cells are electrically coupled, such that an endothelial hyperpolarization spreads via myoendothelial gap junctions to induce relaxation of the vessel [100]. EDHF is reduced by interleukin-6, a cytokine strongly involved in insulin resistant states [101]. Thus, while large and mid-sized arteries and arterioles largely depend on NO for vasodilation, small terminal arterioles seem to depend essentially on EDHF, again illustrating the heterogeneity of the vascular bed.

4.5.2. Ion Channels

As seen above microvascular constriction is also very important physiologically, for induction of the myogenic response or vasomotion. In this context ion channels play a prominent role as effectors [102] and for the subject of interest of this chapter we would like to highlight chloride channels more particularly [103,104]. It is important to recall here the eminent role played by some subtypes of chloride channels for the induction of arteriolar constriction [27,105].

5. PHARMACOLOGY OF MICROCIRCULATION

In sharp contrast to macrocirculation, very few drugs have been shown convincingly to have direct actions on the microvascular bed. The main reason may be found in the fact that little specific drug development has been oriented towards this field, excepting tentatives for blocking venular permeability. The lack of awareness of the importance of microvascular disorders and the technical difficulties inherent to the poor accessibility of microvessels in situ may largely explain this situation. Therefore this paragraph will focus on only two substances which have been extensively studied for their microvascular effects, hypertonic saline and the antidiabetic metformin.

5.1. Hypertonic Saline

No significant changes in mean arteriolar and venular diameters and blood flow as well as on mean arterial and venous pressures could be detected in hamsters in which no blood was withdrawn as a result of infusion of 7.5% NaCl [106]. Similarly, Velasco and co-workers [107] reported that an identical injection of hyperosmotic NaCl solution into normotensive normovolaemic dogs was practically without effects. It must be noted, however, that this is not an entirely valid control. Normovolaemic animals have roughly twice the plasma volume of the shocked one, and this means that the injection or infusion of the hypertonic NaCl will dilute in a larger pool (hence at lower concentration) in the normovolaemic animal.

In hamster subjected to haemorrhage, smaller arterioles dilated while larger ones constricted during hypotension [106]. Similar observations have been reported for the cat tenuissimus muscle [108], cat sartorius muscle [109] and rat cremaster muscle [110] as well as for skin preparations of the unaenesthetized bat [111] and hamster [112] and rat intestine [113]. Conflicting results have also been reported [114,115].

It seems that the variation between arterioles in their response to haemorrhage could be partly attributable to differences in their initial diameter [116]. However, part of the resistance increase in the microcirculation during haemorrhagic shock might also be attributed to luminal narrowing and endothelial cell swelling observed in capillaries [117].

The main differences between the infusions after haemorrhage are a significant increase in mean arterial pressure and arteriolar blood flow, venoconstriction and a tendency for the smaller arterioles to remain more dilated and the larger ones more constricted after the hypertonic infusion [106]. Attenuation of leucocyte activation and of endothelial adhesion molecules have also been reported, possibly explaining reductions in microvascular permeability [118].

5.2. Metformin

Since several reviews have been published on microvascular effects of metformin [51, 52,119] this section will only stress out the main characteristics of this fascinating drug in this area. Metformin belongs to the chemical class of biguanides, which were known very early to exert potent fibrinolytic effects. However more investigations on vascular aspects awaited the mid 80's when it was found that metformin activated directly precapillary vasomotion in non diabetic animals [51]. Interestingly metformin exerts no significant direct effect on large arterial vessels. In addition to stimulating basal slow wave vasomotion, it restored failing vasomotion in several situations of insulin resistance or ischemia [51]. Of particular interest for the topic of this book is the observation that topically applied insulin blunted vasomotion in the hamster cheek pouch and that metformin administration was able to restore it [120]. Illustrating the beneficial consequences of activated vasomotion, metformin increased functional capillary density in insulin-resistant, fructose-fed and in diabetic animals [51]. Furthermore, metformin was shown to strongly inhibit microvascular permeability in various cardiovascular or metabolic pathological situations. In hemorrhagic shock, metformin restored vasomotion, capillary perfusion and inhibited almost completely leukocyte adhesion without significantly increasing in blood pressure [119]. Inhibition of leukocyte adhesion in ischemic situations is also known for AICAR, an activator of AMPK [121], an effect which is shared by metformin [122,123], thereby providing a possible mechanistic explanation for this important effect. A most fascinating finding was the almost 100% survival of a group of hamsters subjected to hemorrhagic shock receiving acute intravenous metformin [119], a finding which lends support to the efficacy of microvascular flow maintenance despite severe circulatory failure. Recent investigations strongly support that metformin may stimulate/restore vasomotion by activating chloride channels. As shown in Fig. (**2**) (E.Bouskela, unpublished results) metformin increases arteriolar spontaneous, low frequency vasomotion, which is blunted by the chloride channel blockers bumetanide and niflumic acid. In particular niflumic acid completely abolishes the metformin effect, while bumetanide is a weaker inhibitor.

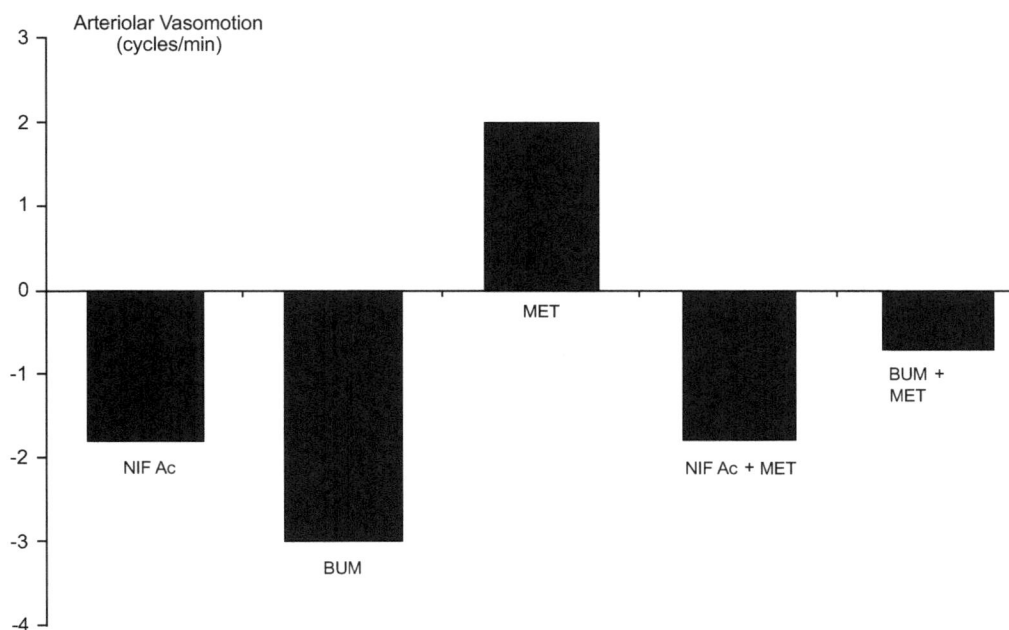

Figure 2: Variations in spontaneous arteriolar vasomotion of hamster cheek pouch arterioles by chloride channel blockers (Bumetanide=BUM and Niflumic Acid=NIFAc) or metformin (MET) and their combination.

Finally we should also consider the positive actions of metformin on intravascular components prone to interfere with capillary perfusion: metformin is known to improve fibrinolysis by reducing PAI-1 levels [119,124], to reduce the expression of adhesion molecules [125] and to improve red cell rheological properties [51]. The combination of all these positive effects clearly explains its beneficial effects on functional capillary density and related features. These properties make metformin a unique drug for targeting microcirculation and a clinical benefit has indeed been observed in the long-term, large scale UKPDS trial [126], where diabetic patients placed under different antidiabetic therapies were followed for close to 20 years. Although glycemic control was equivalent for all treatments, only metformin led to a significant improvement in all case mortality and cardiovascular complications; statistical analysis revealed that the beneficial effect was mainly due to its effects on microvascular disturbances [127].

6. MACROVASCULAR AND MICROVASCULAR RELATIONSHIPS

The marked differences mentioned above between macro- and microcirculation reflects their largely independent physiological roles and pathophysiological specificities. This is also reflected in the respective relevance of the techniques and data interpretation applied for their evaluation. Although these two parts of the vascular bed form a continuum, their show nevertheless both interdependent and independent characteristics. According to the test and technique employed, vasomotor reactions reflect poorly, little or largely feature occurring in the microvascular part [Kraemer, this book]. Thus, flow-mediated dilatation, a classical clinical test now widely used to study vascular reactivity, has little or no correlation with microcirculation in healthy [128,129], hypertensive [130], diabetic [131] or insulin resistant subjects [132]. This consideration is of course of major importance when data are to be interpreted.

On the other hand, the role of microcirculation in cardiovascular physiology is unfortunately largely underestimated. In particular one should be aware that post-ischemic recovery is determined for the greatest part by the quality of acute microflow recovery and of mid-term remodelling, such as in acute myocardial infarction or in chronic heart failure. Thus while cardiovascular accidents occur mainly in large vessels, microcirculation determines the extent of healing [134,135]. Moreover, microcirculation is also important in the initiation of cardiovascular diseases due to its immense endothelial surface which makes it an endocrine organ, where it also represents a main source of inflammatory factors ultimately involved in cardiovascular and metabolic disorders [132,136-139].

7. CONCLUSION

Clearly microcirculation is widely different from macrocirculation. Its role is to permanently adapt local perfusion in most tiny tissue areas to local metabolic demands, the fractal organization and a vast series of local regulatory mechanisms make the microvascular bed a whole and extremely heterogeneous physiological entity. Specific processes in microvascular reactivity, structural characteristics of microvessel architecture and locally adapted mechanisms allow this complicated machinery to work. Nevertheless a lot is still to be learned, because its *in vivo* examination is limited by the low number of accessible tissues, the technology and the number of potential artefacts. The development of new technologies and the increasing awareness of the role played by the microcirculation as an integral cause of diseases have yielded unsuspected new insights into our knowledge of pathophysiology. Although we are at the beginning of this story, one of the most fascinating concepts is the very early occurrence of microvascular disturbances in situations of insulin resistance (or even in situations "at risk of"), raising the question of its possible role in the genesis and/or aggravation of metabolic defects which lead today to the burden of cardiovascular diseases and diabetes over the world.

8. REFERENCES

[1]   Pohl U, De Wit C, Gloe T. Large arterioles in the control of blood flow: role of endothelium-dependent dilation. Acta Physiol Scand 2000 Apr; 168(4): 505-10.
[2]   Souza FM, Padilha AS, Stefanon I, Vassallo DV. Differences in functional and structural properties of segments of the rat tail artery. Braz J Med Biol Res 2008 May; 41(5): 416-23.
[3]   Thijssen DH, Dawson EA, Black MA, Hopman MT, Cable NT, Green DJ. Heterogeneity in conduit artery function in humans: impact of arterial size. Am J Physiol Heart Circ Physiol 2008 Nov; 295(5): H1927-34.
[4]   McAllister RM. Endothelium-dependent vasodilation in different rat hindlimb skeletal muscles. J Appl Physiol 2003 May; 94(5): 1777-84.
[5]   dela Paz NG, D'Amore PA. Arterial versus venous endothelial cells. Cell Tissue Res 2009 Jan; 335(1): 5-16.
[6]   Jackson CJ, Nguyen M. Human microvascular endothelial cells differ from macrovascular endothelial cells in their expression of matrix metalloproteinases. Int J Biochem Cell Biol 1997 Oct; 29(10): 1167-77.
[7]   Sandow SL, Haddock RE, Hill CE, Chadha PS, Kerr PM, Welsh DG, *et al.* What'S where and why at a vascular myoendothelial microdomain signalling complex. Clin Exp Pharmacol Physiol 2009 Jan; 36(1): 67-76.
[8]   Davis MJ. Myogenic response gradient in an arteriolar network. Am J Physiol 1993 Jun; 264(6 Pt 2): H2168-79.
[9]   Tooke JE. Capillary hypertension and microvascular complications. Transplant Proc 1994 Apr; 26(2): 373-4.
[10]   Pries AR, Secomb TW. Origins of heterogeneity in tissue perfusion and metabolism. Cardiovasc Res 2009 Feb 1; 81(2): 328-35.
[11]   Berg BR, Cohen KD, Sarelius IH. Direct coupling between blood flow and metabolism at the capillary level in striated muscle. Am J Physiol 1997 Jun; 272(6 Pt 2): H2693-700.
[12]   Collins DM, McCullough WT, Ellsworth ML. Conducted vascular responses: communication across the capillary bed. Microvasc Res 1998 Jul; 56(1): 43-53.
[13]   Ellis CG, Wrigley SM, Groom AC. Heterogeneity of red blood cell perfusion in capillary networks supplied by a single arteriole in resting skeletal muscle. Circ Res 1994 Aug; 75(2): 357-68.
[14]   Lo A, Fuglevand AJ, Secomb TW. Oxygen delivery to skeletal muscle fibers: effects of microvascular unit structure and control mechanisms. Am J Physiol Heart Circ Physiol 2003 Sep; 285(3): H955-63.
[15]   Kayar SR, Banchero N. Sequential perfusion of skeletal muscle capillaries. Microvasc Res 1985 Nov; 30(3): 298-305.
[16]   Slaaf DW, Oude Egbrink MG. Capillaries and flow redistribution play an important role in muscle blood flow reserve capacity. J Mal Vasc 2002 Apr; 27(2): 63-7.

[17] Lindbom L, Arfors KE. Mechanisms and site of control for variation in the number of perfused capillaries in skeletal muscle. Int J Microirc Clin Exp1985; 4(1): 19-30.

[18] Clark MG, Rattigan S, Barrett EJ. Nutritive blood flow as an essential element supporting muscle anabolism. Curr Opin Clin Nutr Metab Care 2006 May; 9(3): 185-9.

[19] Vetterlein F, Schmidt G. Effects of vasodilating agents on the microcirculation in marginal parts of the skeletal muscle. Arch Int Pharmacodyn Ther1975 Jan; 213(1): 4-16.

[20] Eringa EC, Bakker W, Smulders YM, Serne EH, Yudkin JS, Stehouwer CD. Regulation of vascular function and insulin sensitivity by adipose tissue: focus on perivascular adipose tissue. Microcirculation 2007 Jun-Jul; 14(4-5): 389-402.

[21] Yudkin JS, Eringa E, Stehouwer CD. "Vasocrine" signalling from perivascular fat: a mechanism linking insulin resistance to vascular disease. Lancet 2005 May 21-27; 365(9473): 1817-20.

[22] Intaglietta M. Arteriolar vasomotion: implications for tissue ischemia. Blood Vessels 1991; 28 Suppl 1: 1-7.

[23] Bouskela E. Vasomotion frequency and amplitude related to intraluminal pressure and temperature in the wing of the intact, unanesthetized bat. Microvasc Res1989 May; 37(3): 339-51.

[24] Bartlett IS, Crane GJ, Neild TO, Segal SS. Electrophysiological basis of arteriolar vasomotion in vivo. J Vasc Res 2000 Nov-Dec; 37(6): 568-75.

[25] Lamboley M, Schuster A, Beny JL, Meister JJ. Recruitment of smooth muscle cells and arterial vasomotion. Am J Physiol Heart Circ Physiol 2003 Aug; 285(2): H562-9.

[26] Duza T, Sarelius IH. Localized transient increases in endothelial cell Ca2+ in arterioles in situ: implications for coordination of vascular function. Am J Physiol Heart Circ Physiol 2004 Jun; 286(6): H2322-31.

[27] Boedtkjer DM, Matchkov VV, Boedtkjer E, Nilsson H, Aalkjaer C. Vasomotion has chloride-dependency in rat mesenteric small arteries. Pflugers Arch 2008 Nov; 457(2): 389-404.

[28] Jacobsen JC, Aalkjaer C, Nilsson H, Matchkov VV, Freiberg J, Holstein-Rathlou NH. A model of smooth muscle cell synchronization in the arterial wall. Am J Physiol Heart Circ Physiol 2007 Jul; 293(1): H229-37.

[29] Jacobsen JC, Aalkjaer C, Nilsson H, Matchkov VV, Freiberg J, Holstein-Rathlou NH. Activation of a cGMP-sensitive calcium-dependent chloride channel may cause transition from calcium waves to whole cell oscillations in smooth muscle cells. Am J Physiol Heart Circ Physiol 2007 Jul; 293(1): H215-28.

[30] Aalkaer C, Nilsson H. Vasomotion: cellular background for the oscillator and for the synchronization of smooth muscle cells. Br J Pharmacol 2005 Mar; 144(5): 605-16.

[31] Nilsson H, Aalkjaer C. Vasomotion: mechanisms and physiological importance. Mol Interv 2003 Mar; 3(2): 79-89, 51.

[32] Ursino M, Colantuoni A, Bertuglia S. Vasomotion and blood flow regulation in hamster skeletal muscle microcirculation: A theoretical and experimental study. Microvasc Res 1998 Nov; 56(3): 233-52.

[33] Renaudin C, Michoud E, Rapin JR, Lagarde M, Wiernsperger N. Hyperglycaemia modifies the reaction of microvessels to insulin in rat skeletal muscle. Diabetologia 1998 Jan; 41(1): 26-33.

[34] Takenaka T, Kanno Y, Kitamura Y, Hayashi K, Suzuki H, Saruta T. Role of chloride channels in afferent arteriolar constriction. Kidney Int 1996 Sep; 50(3): 864-72.

[35] Pekanmaki K, Kolari PJ, Kiistala U. Laser Doppler vasomotion among patients with post-thrombotic venous insufficiency: effect of intermittent pneumatic compression. Vasa 1991; 20(4): 394-7.

[36] Rucker M, Strobel O, Vollmar B, Spitzer WJ, Menger MD. Protective skeletal muscle arteriolar vasomotion during critical perfusion conditions of osteomyocutaneous flaps is not mediated by nitric oxide and endothelins. Langenbecks Arch Surg 2003 Oct; 388(5): 339-43.

[37] Clark MG. Impaired microvascular perfusion: a consequence of vascular dysfunction and a potential cause of insulin resistance in muscle. Am J Physiol Endocrinol Metab 2008 Oct; 295(4): E732-50.

[38] Rossi M, Maurizio S, Carpi A. Skin blood flowmotion response to insulin iontophoresis in normal subjects. Microvasc Res 2005 Jul; 70(1-2): 17-22.

[39] de Jongh RT, Serne EH, RG IJ, Jorstad HT, Stehouwer CD. Impaired local microvascular vasodilatory effects of insulin and reduced skin microvascular vasomotion in obese women. Microvasc Res 2008 Mar; 75(2): 256-62.

[40] Stewart JM, Taneja I, Goligorsky MS, Medow MS. Noninvasive measure of microvascular nitric oxide function in humans using very low-frequency cutaneous laser Doppler flow spectra. Microcirculation 2007 Apr-May; 14(3): 169-80.

[41] de Jongh RT, Clark AD, RG IJ, Serne EH, de Vries G, Stehouwer CD. Physiological hyperinsulinaemia increases intramuscular microvascular reactive hyperaemia and vasomotion in healthy volunteers. Diabetologia 2004 Jun; 47(6): 978-86.

[42] Schmiedel O, Schroeter ML, Harvey JN. Microalbuminuria in Type 2 diabetes indicates impaired microvascular vasomotion and perfusion. Am J Physiol Heart Circ Physiol 2007 Dec; 293(6): H3424-31.

[43] Jaffer U, Aslam M, Standfield N. Impaired hyperaemic and rhythmic vasomotor response in type 1 diabetes mellitus patients: a predictor of early peripheral vascular disease. Eur J Vasc Endovasc Surg 2008 May; 35(5): 603-6.

[44] Rossi M, Carpi A, Galetta F, Franzoni F, Santoro G. Skin vasomotion investigation: a useful tool for clinical evaluation of microvascular endothelial function? Biomed Pharmacother 2008 Oct; 62(8): 541-5.

[45] Pradhan RK, Chakravarthy VS. A computational model that links non-periodic vasomotion to enhanced oxygenation in skeletal muscle. Math Biosci 2007 Oct; 209(2): 486-99.

[46]   Rucker M, Strobel O, Vollmar B, Roesken F, Menger MD. Vasomotion in critically perfused muscle protects adjacent tissues from capillary perfusion failure. Am J Physiol Heart Circ Physiol 2000 Aug; 279(2): H550-8.

[47]   Seifert H, Jager K, Bollinger A. Analysis of flow motion by the laser Doppler technique in patients with peripheral arterial occlusive disease. Int J Microcirc Clin Exp1988 Aug; 7(3): 223-36.

[48]   Christensen NJ. Spontaneous variations in resting blood flow, postischaemic peak flow and vibratory perception in the feet of diabetics. Diabetologia1969 Jun; 5(3): 171-8.

[49]   Meyer MF, Rose CJ, Hulsmann JO, Schatz H, Pfohl M. Impairment of cutaneous arteriolar 0.1 Hz vasomotion in diabetes. Exp Clin Endocrinol Diabetes 2003 Apr; 111(2): 104-10.

[50]   Renaudin C, Michoud E, Lagarde M, Wiernsperger N. Impaired microvascular responses to acute hyperglycemia in type I diabetic rats. J Diabetes Complications 1999 Jan-Feb; 13(1): 39-44.

[51]   Wiernsperger N. 50years later: is metformin a vascular drug with antidiabetic properties ? Br J Diabetes Vasc Dis 2007; 7: 204-10.

[52]   Wiernsperger NF, Bouskela E. Microcirculation in insulin resistance and diabetes: more than just a complication. Diabetes Metab 2003 Sep; 29(4 Pt 2): 6S77-87.

[53]   Schubert R, Mulvany MJ. The myogenic response: established facts and attractive hypotheses. Clin Sci (Lond) 1999 Apr; 96(4): 313-26.

[54]   Meininger GA, Mack CA, Fehr KL, Bohlen HG. Myogenic vasoregulation overrides local metabolic control in resting rat skeletal muscle. Circ Res1987 Jun; 60(6): 861-70.

[55]   Vissing SF, Secher NH, Victor RG. Mechanisms of cutaneous vasoconstriction during upright posture. Acta Physiol Scand 1997 Feb; 159(2): 131-8.

[56]   Vayssairat M, Tribout L, Gouny P, Gaitz JP, Baudot N, Cheynel C, *et al.* Importance of cutaneous postural reflex vasoconstriction in patients with atherosclerotic occlusive disease of the lower extremities. Int Angiol 1998 Mar; 17(1): 53-7.

[57]   Khiabani HZ, Anvar MD, Kroese AJ, Stranden E. The role of the veno-arteriolar reflex (VAR) in the pathogenesis of peripheral oedema in patients with chronic critical limb ischaemia (CLI). Ann Chir Gynaecol 2000; 89(2): 93-8.

[58]   Husmann M, Willenberg T, Keo HH, Spring S, Kalodiki E, Delis KT. Integrity of venoarteriolar reflex determines level of microvascular skin flow enhancement with intermittent pneumatic compression. J Vasc Surg 2008 Dec; 48(6): 1509-13.

[59]   Cacciatori V, Dellera A, Bellavere F, Bongiovanni LG, Teatini F, Gemma ML, *et al.* Comparative assessment of peripheral sympathetic function by postural vasoconstriction arteriolar reflex and sympathetic skin response in NIDDM patients. Am J Med 1997 Apr; 102(4): 365-70.

[60]   Golster H, Hyllienmark L, Ledin T, Ludvigsson J, Sjoberg F. Impaired microvascular function related to poor metabolic control in young patients with diabetes. Clin Physiol Funct Imaging 2005 Mar; 25(2): 100-5.

[61]   Belcaro G, Nicolaides AN. The venoarteriolar response in diabetics. Angiology 1991 Oct; 42(10): 827-35.

[62]   Rai A, Riemann M, Gustafsson F, Holstein-Rathlou NH, Torp-Pedersen C. Streptozotocin-induced diabetes decreases conducted vasoconstrictor response in mouse cremaster arterioles. Horm Metab Res 2008 Sep; 40(9): 651-4.

[63]   Shore AC, Price KJ, Sandeman DD, Tripp JH, Tooke JE. Posturally induced vasoconstriction in diabetes mellitus. Arch Dis Child 1994 Jan; 70(1): 22-6

[64]   Wiernsperger NF. In defense of microvascular constriction in diabetes. Clin Hemorheol Microcirc 2001; 25(2): 55-62.

[65]   Sarelius IH, Kuebel JM, Wang J, Huxley VH. Macromolecule permeability of in situ and excised rodent skeletal muscle arterioles and venules. Am J Physiol Heart Circ Physiol 2006 Jan; 290(1): H474-80.

[66]   Fu BM, Chen B, Chen W. An electrodiffusion model for effects of surface glycocalyx layer on microvessel permeability. Am J Physiol Heart Circ Physiol 2003 Apr; 284(4): H1240-50.

[67]   Noble MI, Drake-Holland AJ, Vink H. Hypothesis: arterial glycocalyx dysfunction is the first step in the atherothrombotic process. QJM 2008 Jul; 101(7): 513-8.

[68]   Perrin RM, Harper SJ, Bates DO. A role for the endothelial glycocalyx in regulating microvascular permeability in diabetes mellitus. Cell Biochem Biophys 2007; 49(2): 65-72.

[69]   Dell'Omo G, Penno G, Pucci L, Mariani M, Del Prato S, Pedrinelli R. Abnormal capillary permeability and endothelial dysfunction in hypertension with comorbid Metabolic Syndrome. Atherosclerosis 2004 Feb; 172(2): 383-9.

[70]   Minshall RD, Malik AB. Transport across the endothelium: regulation of endothelial permeability. Handb Exp Pharmacol 2006(176 Pt 1): 107-44.

[71]   Yuan SY, Breslin JW, Perrin R, Gaudreault N, Guo M, Kargozaran H, *et al.* Microvascular permeability in diabetes and insulin resistance. Microcirculation 2007 Jun-Jul; 14(4-5): 363-73.

[72]   Michel CC, Curry FE. Microvascular permeability. Physiol Rev 1999 Jul; 79(3): 703-61.

[73]   Moan A, Nordby G, Os I, Birkeland KI, Kjeldsen SE. Relationship between hemorrheologic factors and insulin sensitivity in healthy young men. Metabolism 1994 Apr; 43(4): 423-7.

[74]   Brun JF, Aloulou I, Varlet-Marie E. Hemorheological aspects of the metabolic syndrome: markers of insulin resistance, obesity or hyperinsulinemia? Clin Hemorheol Microcirc 2004; 30(3-4): 203-9.

[75]   Sola E, Vaya A, Simo M, Hernandez-Mijares A, Morillas C, Espana F, *et al.* Fibrinogen, plasma viscosity and blood viscosity in obesity. Relationship with insulin resistance. Clin Hemorheol Microcirc 2007; 37(4): 309-18.

[76] McHedlishvili G, Varazashvili M, Gobejishvili L. Local RBC aggregation disturbing blood fluidity and causing stasis in microvessels. Clin Hemorheol Microcirc 2002; 26(2): 99-106.

[77] Minetti M, Agati L, Malorni W. The microenvironment can shift erythrocytes from a friendly to a harmful behavior: pathogenetic implications for vascular diseases. Cardiovasc Res 2007 Jul 1; 75(1): 21-8.

[78] Sprague RS, Stephenson AH, Ellsworth ML. Red not dead: signaling in and from erythrocytes. Trends Endocrinol Metab 2007 Nov; 18(9): 350-5.

[79] Anichkov DA, Maksina AG, Shostak NA. Relationships between erythrocyte membrane properties and components of metabolic syndrome in women. Med Sci Monit 2005 Apr; 11(4): CR203-10.

[80] Justo D, Marilus R, Mardi T, Tolchinsky T, Goldin Y, Rozenblat M, et al. The appearance of aggregated erythrocytes in the peripheral blood of individuals with insulin resistance. Diabetes Metab Res Rev 2003 Sep-Oct; 19(5): 386-91.

[81] Kaul DK, Koshkaryev A, Artmann G, Barshtein G, Yedgar S. Additive effect of red blood cell rigidity and adherence to endothelial cells in inducing vascular resistance. Am J Physiol Heart Circ Physiol 2008 Oct; 295(4): H1788-93.

[82] Yalcin O, Uyuklu M, Armstrong JK, Meiselman HJ, Baskurt OK. Graded alterations of RBC aggregation influence in vivo blood flow resistance. Am J Physiol Heart Circ Physiol 2004 Dec; 287(6): H2644-50.

[83] Aloulou I, Varlet-Marie E, Mercier J, Brun JF. Hemorheological disturbances correlate with the lipid profile but not with the NCEP-ATPIII score of the metabolic syndrome. Clin Hemorheol Microcirc 2006; 35(1-2): 207-12.

[84] Aloulou I, Varlet-Marie E, Mercier J, Brun JF. The hemorheological aspects of the metabolic syndrome are a combination of separate effects of insulin resistance, hyperinsulinemia and adiposity. Clin Hemorheol Microcirc 2006; 35(1-2): 113-9.

[85] Sola E, Vaya A, Corella D, Santaolaria ML, Espana F, Estelles A, et al. Erythrocyte hyperaggregation in obesity: determining factors and weight loss influence. Obesity (Silver Spring) 2007 Aug; 15(8): 2128-34.

[86] Rucker M, Schafer T, Scheuer C, Harder Y, Vollmar B, Menger MD. Local heat shock priming promotes recanalization of thromboembolized microvasculature by upregulation of plasminogen activators. Arterioscler Thromb Vasc Biol 2006 Jul; 26(7): 1632-9.

[87] Brodsky SV, Malinowski K, Golightly M, Jesty J, Goligorsky MS. Plasminogen activator inhibitor-1 promotes formation of endothelial microparticles with procoagulant potential. Circulation 2002 Oct 29; 106(18): 2372-8.

[88] Kraja AT, Province MA, Arnett D, Wagenknecht L, Tang W, Hopkins PN, et al. Do inflammation and procoagulation biomarkers contribute to the metabolic syndrome cluster? Nutr Metab (Lond) 2007; 4: 28.

[89] Lindahl B, Asplund K, Eliasson M, Evrin PE. Insulin resistance syndrome and fibrinolytic activity: the northern Sweden MONICA study. Int J Epidemiol 1996 Apr; 25(2): 291-9.

[90] Scelles V, Raccah D, Alessi MC, Vialle JM, Juhan-Vague I, Vague P. Plasminogen activator inhibitor 1 and insulin levels in various insulin resistance states. Diabete Metab 1992 Jan-Feb; 18(1): 38-42.

[91] Westrick RJ, Eitzman DT. Plasminogen activator inhibitor-1 in vascular thrombosis. Curr Drug Targets 2007 Sep; 8(9): 966-1002.

[92] Gurlek A, Bayraktar M, Kirazli S. Increased plasminogen activator inhibitor-1 activity in offspring of type 2 diabetic patients: lack of association with plasma insulin levels. Diabetes Care 2000 Jan; 23(1): 88-92.

[93] Bastard JP, Pieroni L, Hainque B. Relationship between plasma plasminogen activator inhibitor 1 and insulin resistance. Diabetes Metab Res Rev 2000 May-Jun; 16(3): 192-201.

[94] Juhan-Vague I, Alessi MC. PAI-1, obesity, insulin resistance and risk of cardiovascular events. Thromb Haemost 1997 Jul; 78(1): 656-60.

[95] Fitzgerald SM, Bashari H, Cox JA, Parkington HC, Evans RG. Contributions of endothelium-derived relaxing factors to control of hindlimb blood flow in the mouse in vivo. Am J Physiol Heart Circ Physiol 2007 Aug; 293(2): H1072-82.

[96] Katakam PV, Hoenig M, Ujhelyi MR, Miller AW. Cytochrome P450 activity and endothelial dysfunction in insulin resistance. J Vasc Res 2000 Sep-Oct; 37(5): 426-34.

[97] Triggle CR, Ding H, Anderson TJ, Pannirselvam M. The endothelium in health and disease: a discussion of the contribution of non-nitric oxide endothelium-derived vasoactive mediators to vascular homeostasis in normal vessels and in type II diabetes. Mol Cell Biochem 2004 Aug; 263(1-2): 21-7.

[98] Kohler R, Hoyer J. The endothelium-derived hyperpolarizing factor: insights from genetic animal models. Kidney Int 2007 Jul; 72(2): 145-50.

[99] Shimokawa H, Yasutake H, Fujii K, Owada MK, Nakaike R, Fukumoto Y, et al. The importance of the hyperpolarizing mechanism increases as the vessel size decreases in endothelium-dependent relaxations in rat mesenteric circulation. J Cardiovasc Pharmacol 1996 Nov; 28(5): 703-11.

[100] Coleman HA, Tare M, Parkington HC. Endothelial potassium channels, endothelium-dependent hyperpolarization and the regulation of vascular tone in health and disease. Clin Exp Pharmacol Physiol 2004 Sep; 31(9): 641-9.

[101] Park Y, Capobianco S, Gao X, Falck JR, Dellsperger KC, Zhang C. Role of EDHF in type 2 diabetes-induced endothelial dysfunction. Am J Physiol Heart Circ Physiol 2008 Nov; 295(5): H1982-8.

[102] Folgering JH, Sharif-Naeini R, Dedman A, Patel A, Delmas P, Honore E. Molecular basis of the mammalian pressure-sensitive ion channels: focus on vascular mechanotransduction. Prog Biophys Mol Biol 2008 Jun-Jul; 97(2-3): 180-95.

[103] Gautam M, Gojova A, Barakat AI. Flow-activated ion channels in vascular endothelium. Cell Biochem Biophys 2006; 46(3): 277-84.

[104] Jentsch TJ, Stein V, Weinreich F, Zdebik AA. Molecular structure and physiological function of chloride channels. Physiol Rev 2002 Apr; 82(2): 503-68.

[105] McGahon MK, Needham MA, Scholfield CN, McGeown JG, Curtis TM. Ca2+-activated Cl- current in retinal arteriolar smooth muscle. Invest Ophthalmol Vis Sci 2009 Jan; 50(1): 364-71.

[106] Bouskela E, Grampp W, Mellander S. Effects of hypertonic NaCl solution on microvascular haemodynamics in normo- and hypovolaemia. Acta Physiol Scand 1990 Sep; 140(1): 85-94.

[107] Velasco IT, Pontieri V, Rocha e Silva M, Jr., Lopes OU. Hyperosmotic NaCl and severe hemorrhagic shock. Am J Physiol1980 Nov; 239(5): H664-73.

[108] Eriksson E, Lisander B. Low flow states in the microvessels of skeletal muscle in cat. Acta Physiol Scand1972 Oct; 86(2): 202-10.

[109] Torres Filho IP, Boegehold MA, Bouskela E, House SD, Johnson PC. Microcirculatory responses in cat sartorius muscle to hemorrhagic hypotension. Am J Physiol1989 Nov; 257(5 Pt 2): H1647-55.

[110] Hutchins PM, Goldstone J, Wells R. Effects of hemorrhagic shock on the microvasculature of skeletal muscle. Microvasc Res1973 Mar; 5(2): 131-40.

[111] Harris PD, Greenwald EK, Nicoll PA. Neural mechanisms in small vessel response to hemorrhage in the unanesthetized bat. Am J Physiol1970 Feb; 218(2): 560-5.

[112] Colantuoni A, Bertuglia S, Intaglietta M. Microvessel diameter changes during hemorrhagic shock in unanesthetized hamsters. Microvasc Res1985 Sep; 30(2): 133-42.

[113] Zakaria el R, Tsakadze NL, Garrison RN. Hypertonic saline resuscitation improves intestinal microcirculation in a rat model of hemorrhagic shock. Surgery 2006 Oct; 140(4): 579-87; discussion 87-8.

[114] Gray SD. Microscopic observation of skeletal muscle vascular responses to vasopressors during severe hemorrhagic hypotension. J Trauma1972 Feb; 12(2): 147-60.

[115] Zhao KS, Junker D, Delano FA, Zweifach BW. Microvascular adjustments during irreversible hemorrhagic shock in rat skeletal muscle. Microvasc Res1985 Sep; 30(2): 143-53.

[116] Boegehold MA, Johnson PC. Response of arteriolar network of skeletal muscle to sympathetic nerve stimulation. Am J Physiol1988 May; 254(5 Pt 2): H919-28.

[117] Mazzoni MC, Borgstrom P, Intaglietta M, Arfors KE. Lumenal narrowing and endothelial cell swelling in skeletal muscle capillaries during hemorrhagic shock. Circ Shock1989 Sep; 29(1): 27-39.

[118] Victorino GP, Newton CR, Curran B. Effect of hypertonic saline on microvascular permeability in the activated endothelium. J Surg Res 2003 Jun 1; 112(1): 79-83.

[119] Wiernsperger NF. Metformin: intrinsic vasculoprotective properties. Diabetes Technol Ther 2000 Summer; 2(2): 259-72.

[120] Bouskela E, Cyrino FZ, Wiernsperger N. Effects of insulin and the combination of insulin plus metformin (glucophage) on microvascular reactivity in control and diabetic hamsters. Angiology 1997 Jun; 48(6): 503-14.

[121] Gaskin FS, Kamada K, Yusof M, Durante W, Gross G, Korthuis RJ. AICAR preconditioning prevents postischemic leukocyte rolling and adhesion: role of K(ATP) channels and heme oxygenase. Microcirculation 2009 Feb; 16(2): 167-76.

[122] Fujii N, Ho RC, Manabe Y, Jessen N, Toyoda T, Holland WL, et al. Ablation of AMP-activated protein kinase alpha2 activity exacerbates insulin resistance induced by high-fat feeding of mice. Diabetes 2008 Nov; 57(11): 2958-66.

[123] Hardie DG. Role of AMP-activated protein kinase in the metabolic syndrome and in heart disease. FEBS Lett 2008 Jan 9; 582(1): 81-9.

[124] Grant PJ. Beneficial effects of metformin on haemostasis and vascular function in man. Diabetes Metab 2003 Sep; 29(4 Pt 2): 6S44-52.

[125] Mamputu JC, Wiernsperger NF, Renier G. Antiatherogenic properties of metformin: the experimental evidence. Diabetes Metab 2003 Sep; 29(4 Pt 2): 6S71-6.

[126] Scheen AJ, Paquot N, Lefebvre PJ. [United Kingdom Prospective Diabetes Study (UKPDS): 10 years later]. Rev Med Liege 2008 Oct; 63(10): 624-9.

[127] Holman RR, Paul SK, Bethel MA, Matthews DR, Neil HA. 10-year follow-up of intensive glucose control in type 2 diabetes. N Engl J Med 2008 Oct 9; 359(15): 1577-89.

[128] Dhindsa M, Sommerlad SM, DeVan AE, Barnes JN, Sugawara J, Ley O, et al. Interrelationships among noninvasive measures of postischemic macro- and microvascular reactivity. J Appl Physiol 2008 Aug; 105(2): 427-32.

[129] Gori T, Di Stolfo G, Sicuro S, Dragoni S, Lisi M, Parker JD, et al. Correlation analysis between different parameters of conduit artery and microvascular vasodilation. Clin Hemorheol Microcirc 2006; 35(4): 509-15.

[130] Kullo IJ, Malik AR, Santos S, Ehrsam JE, Turner ST. Association of cardiovascular risk factors with microvascular and conduit artery function in hypertensive subjects. Am J Hypertens 2007 Jul; 20(7): 735-42.

[131] Meyer MF, Lieps D, Schatz H, Pfohl M. Impaired flow-mediated vasodilation in type 2 diabetes: lack of relation to microvascular dysfunction. Microvasc Res 2008 May; 76(1): 61-5.

[132] Title LM, Lonn E, Charbonneau F, Fung M, Mather KJ, Verma S, et al. Relationship between brachial artery flow-mediated dilatation, hyperemic shear stress, and the metabolic syndrome. Vasc Med 2008 Nov; 13(4): 263-70.

[133] Ren G, Michael LH, Entman ML, Frangogiannis NG. Morphological characteristics of the microvasculature in healing myocardial infarcts. J Histochem Cytochem 2002 Jan; 50(1): 71-9.

[134] Sambuceti G, L'Abbate A, Marzilli M. Why should we study the coronary microcirculation? Am J Physiol Heart Circ Physiol 2000 Dec; 279(6): H2581-4.

[135] Urbancic-Rovan V, Bernjak A, Stefanovska A, Azman-Juvan K, Kocijancic A. Macro- and microcirculation in the lower extremities--possible relationship. Diabetes Res Clin Pract 2006 Aug; 73(2): 166-73.

[136] Lockhart CJ, Hamilton PK, Quinn CE, McVeigh GE. End-organ dysfunction and cardiovascular outcomes: the role of the microcirculation. Clin Sci (Lond) 2009 Feb; 116(3): 175-90.

[137] Krentz AJ, Clough G, Byrne CD. Interactions between microvascular and macrovascular disease in diabetes: pathophysiology and therapeutic implications. Diabetes Obes Metab 2007 Nov; 9(6): 781-91.

[138] Stokes KY, Granger DN. The microcirculation: a motor for the systemic inflammatory response and large vessel disease induced by hypercholesterolaemia? J Physiol 2005 Feb 1; 562(Pt 3): 647-53.

[139] Abularrage CJ, Sidawy AN, Aidinian G, Singh N, Weiswasser JM, Arora S. Evaluation of the microcirculation in vascular disease. J Vasc Surg 2005 Sep; 42(3): 574-81.

CHAPTER 2

Techniques to Measure Microcirculatory Parameters in Insulin Resistant States in Humans

Luiz Guilherme Kraemer-Aguiar and Eliete Bouskela

Department of Clinical Medicine and Physiology - Biomedical Center BioVasc – Clinical and Experimental Research Laboratory on Vascular Biology State University of Rio de Janeiro, Rio de Janeiro, Brazil

Address correspondence: Luiz G. Kraemer-Aguiar, Endocrinology - Department of Internal Medicine, Biomedical Center, State University of Rio de Janeiro, Brazil. Tel. 55-21-2587-7771;Fax 55-21-2587-7760; E-mail: gkraemer@ig.com.br

Abstract: Obesity and insulin resistance show increasing incidence in all ages, especially but not only, in western countries. The world epidemic on obesity imposes a higher prevalence of subjects with insulin resistance. This latter condition is associated with impairments on macro and microvascular function of different degrees. The exact interrelationship and meaning of this association and subsequent result on glucose homeostasis, vascular damage and end-organ impairments deserve further investigations. Techniques used to study the microcirculation could help researchers to clarify these questions. This chapter will focus on techniques employed in humans to investigate the microcirculation, endothelial reactivity, their significance and importance for the understanding of microcirculatory function with special focus on those employed and experienced by the authors.

Keywords: Microcirculation, techniques, insulin resistance.

1. INTRODUCTION

In the microcirculation the most purposeful function of the circulation occurs, transport of nutrients to tissues and removal of cellular excreta in response to variations in demand. In fact, microvessels are the true site of blood/tissue nutrition and exchange and, accordingly, represent the largest part of vessels subjected to multiple, fine tuning regulation. Small arterioles control blood flow to each tissue area and local conditions in tissues themselves control diameters of arterioles in turn. A second important function is to avoid large fluctuations in hydrostatic pressure at capillary level that otherwise would impair blood-tissue exchange. At microcirculation, the substantial proportion of hydrostatic pressure drop occurs, making it an important site in determining overall peripheral resistance [1]. The microcirculation encompasses vessels <150μm in mean internal diameter including arterioles, capillaries and venules. Nowadays it is possible to define the microcirculation using a new focus, as any vessel that respond to increasing pressure by a reduction in lumen diameter, the so-called myogenic response, including not only those in the microcirculatory bed considered as such but also some of the smallest arteries in tissues [1,2].

In the pathogenesis of cardiovascular diseases, one of the earliest vascular changes is an impairment of endothelial vascular signaling leading to endothelial dysfunction, a systemic disease [3,4] process consisting of attenuated endothelial-dependent vasodilation (EDV), augmented vasoconstriction and structural microvessel remodeling. Microvascular dysfunction (MD) should be viewed as the loss of local metabolic and myogenic autoregulatory mechanisms that ensure adequate functions [5,6].

Overweight and obesity are becoming epidemic, particularly because of increasing nourishment and decreasing physical exercise [7,8]. This excessive accumulation of adiposity is the soil for most cardiovascular diseases, insulin resistance and type 2 diabetes mellitus. Classically microvascular damage is related to hyperglycaemia, but there are also cumulative evidences of a relationship between impaired glucose tolerance and renal and retinal microvascular injuries [9]. The latter has been also associated with blood pressure, lipid concentration and body mass index [10], supporting the concept that not only hyperglycaemia but also previous metabolic disturbances could impair precociously the human microcirculation. Obesity-associated microvascular dysfunction may contribute to diseases caused by microangiopathy, such as nephropathy [11] and heart failure [12] and it has been postulated

Nicolas Wiernsperger (Ed.)

that MD participate in the development of insulin resistance by limiting glucose and insulin delivery to muscle cells [1,13-16]. Experimentally, it has been demonstrated that graded occlusion of perfused rat muscle vasculature markedly impaired insulin delivery, insulin-mediated Akt phosphorilation and glucose uptake, suggesting a pre-receptor defect on insulin signalling pathway [17]. Techniques for testing microcirculatory behavior and function should be viewed as a new diagnostic tool in clinical and research settings. Investigation of human microcirculation has been generally performed only on easily accessible microcirculatory beds. This short review will focus on techniques employed, especially in *in vivo* human studies, related to insulin resistance states.

Muscle and coronary circulation would be most relevant from a pathophysiological standpoint but they require complicated techniques for assessment - forearm perfusion technique and coronary vessels reactivity, respectively. These methods are usually employed to explore muscle and coronary microvascular function in hypertensive and insulin resistant patients [18]. Additionally and unfortunately, both need invasive procedures. Regarding the contribution of endothelial dysfunction to the pathophysiology of cardiovascular diseases, the development of less invasive methods is a great challenge for both clinical risk assessment and monitoring the responses to treatment. There is a need for non- to minimally-invasive techniques to investigate effects of chronic diseases on vascular and endothelial functions.

Taking this point of view, one of the main sites for microcirculatory investigation is the skin, the largest organ in the body, weighing on average 4 kg and covering an approximate area of 2 m^2, it is now considered by many authors as a model of generalized microvascular function [19]. Skin acts as a barrier to protect the body from the external environment and as a thermoregulatory organ. Small blood vessels supplying the skin are highly organized into two horizontal plexuses, the upper one lying 1 to 5 mm below the epidermis and form dermal papillary loops, the major site for gas and nutrient exchange within the skin. The lower plexus is located on the dermal-hypodermal junction. These vessels supply the upper plexus and their branches supply dermal appendages, such as hair follicles and sweat glands. In acral or nonhairy skin, the two plexuses are additionally connected by arteriovenous anastomoses, important in the thermoregulatory shunting of blood between upper and lower plexuses. As much as 60 percent of cutaneous blood can be shunted through these anastomoses away from the capillary loops and to venous plexus reducing connective heat loss, and as a result blood flow in skin is extremely variable [19,20]. The control of this labile vascular bed is complex and involves neural, humoral, and local influences. Another challenge to use cutaneous microcirculation as a model might be its complex vascular network, which in human skin includes both nutritional and non-nutritional components [19]. Nonnutritional cutaneous blood flow includes responses to several thermal and nonthermal stimuli.

2. LASER DOPPLER FLOWMETRY

Techniques involving the study of skin microvascular blood flow should be viewed as those able to visualize microvessels, called intravital microscopy such as videocapillaroscopy or ortogonal polarization spectral imaging; and those able to quantify the microflow, such as laser-Doppler flowmetry (LDF). By some estimates, nutritional blood flow may represent only 5-10% of the laser-Doppler signal, being the reminder nonnutritional [21]. This latter method was designed to provide continuos noninvasive measurement of microvascular perfusion. In LDF, low-power laser light impinges on the tissue surface individual photons that migrate through the tissue in a random fashion, the exact statistical pattern of which is determined by tissue optical properties [22]. Interaction with one or more moving objects (blood cells) shifts scattered photons in frequency by an amount determined by the scattering angle, the wavelenght of the laser light and the velocity of the scatterer. The back-scattered and Doppler-broadened light carries information about both the speed of blood cells traversing the scattering volume, reflected by the broadening frequency of the backscattered signal and their concentration, derived from the fraction of total photons that is frequency-shifted. The perfusion value is usually expressed in volts (V), in arbitrary units (AU) or in perfusion units (PU).

Currrently available LDF systems cannot express measurements in absolute units because of the enormous inter- and intra-individual variation in microvascular architecture, physiology and optical properties [22-24]. Independent of this limitation, methodologies used to explore cutaneous microcirculation evoke an integrative physiology that is not unique to the cutaneous microvascular bed [19]. Thus, when used in the correct manner, and accounting for possible endothelial, neural and smooth muscle pathways involved [25], the skin circulation offers great potential as a valuable, easily accessible site for monitoring the development and progression of MD [26], and for characterizing overall cardiovasular risk [27,28].

Relative changes in skin blood flow over large areas of skin can be measured using laser-Doppler imagery to examine the spatial distribution of microvessel reactivity [29]. Alternatively, laser-Doppler flowmetry can be used to measure dynamic changes in laser-Doppler flux over a small area of skin to vasoreactive stimuli. Cutaneous vasodilation or vasoconstriction can be elicited through post-occlusive reactive hyperemia (PORH) [30], whole body heating [31], whole body cooling, local heating [32], local cooling [33], and the application of specific vasoactive pharmacological agents by iontophoresis [14,15,34] or intradermal microdialysis. Related to thermal and PORH responses in skin, it was observed that the late plateau of thermal hyperemia is partly nitric oxide (NO)-dependent [35], but controversy still exists over the implication of NO in the PORH response [19,27]. Although flow-mediated dilation (FMD) of the brachial artery, an index of macrovascular reactivity at PORH, is currently used as a marker of the NO-dependent vasodilation of conductance arteries; cutaneuous responses seems to be mediated by different mechanisms. Recently, it was demonstrated that endothelium-derived hyperpolarizing factors (EDHF) are implicated in the PORH responses in skin [36]. These methodologies combined provide a unique non-invasive opportunity to investigate microvessels physiology, with specific interest in EDHF and NO.

3. VASOACTIVE SUBSTANCES AND EVALUATION OF ENDOTHELIUM FUNCTION ON THE SKIN

Historically, pharmacologically active agents used to study vascular function have been introduced either into the systemic circulation, or locally via intradermal injection or topical application. These methods used to test microvascular reactivity in response to vasocactive agents suffer from limitations related to systemic reactions in consequence of systemic administration, to the invasive characteristic of methods applied and also to knowledge that even small volumes injected will cause major changes in local tissue pressure that may stimulate confounding reflexes, and finally related to topical application, wich it is known that the stratum corneum is only permeable to relative small lipophilic molecules.

In recent years, cutaneous iontophoresis has been developed; it delivers charged pharmacological agents in a vehicle solution to a localized area of skin using opposing electrical current. This is a non-invasive method associated with the delivery of large amount of the drug in large areas of the skin. Coupled with laser-Doppler flowmetry, iontophoresis has been used to study the role of endothelium in the modulation of blood flow in the skin. Examples of drugs used are responses to acetylcholine and sodium nitroprusside, respectively, endothelial-dependent and independent vasodilation. It should be pointed out that in skin the endothelial-mediated phenomenon elicited by acetylcholine appears not to be dependent on NO [37,38]. Intradermal microdyalisis is a minimally invasive technique that allows bidirectional exchange of small molecular weight substances through a porous cellulose membrane with continuous drug (or combination of drugs) delivery to a small localized area of skin while measuring the effects of that drug via laser-Doppler flowmetry. These microdialized small molecular weight substances can also be sampled and analysed from the microdialysis effluent. Intradermal microdialysis has not the potential confounding effect of electrical current-induced hyperemia as may occur with iontophoresis, although the potential confound of needle insertion trauma does exist with the first one.

4. VASOMOTION

Circulatory system should be considered as a single entity, which in about 1 minute let the circulation of 5 liters of human blood through its vascular network, including those of the skin. Additionally there are two major pumps impacting on the dynamics of the cardiovascular system: the heart, generating arterial pressure differences and the lungs, generating the pressure difference necessary for the venous return. Each of them imprints oscillatory motion on flow and vessels. This propagating oscillatory pattern is further modulated by regulatory mechanisms (related to myogenic, neurogenic and endothelial behavior) oscillating at widely different frequencies to alter vessel conductance and adjust flow velocity [37,39]. In addition to techniques described, digital power frequency analysis domains of laser-Doppler flowmeter signal can be performed to partition vascular endothelial, myogenic, local sympathetic activity, hemodynamic and respiratory influences on cutaneous microvascular reactivity [39].

5. TRANSCUTANEOUS OXYGEN TENSION (TCPO₂)

Transcutaneous oxygen tension ($TCpO_2$) is an integral part of the noninvasive assessment of microcirculatory blood flow [40] related mainly to peripheral vascular disease. $TCpO_2$ quantifies oxygen molecules transferred to the skin microcirculation after heating it with a transducer to more than 40°C. Limitations are related to tha fact that $TCpO_2$ is time consuming and does not assess all ischemic regions of the skin unless the probe is specifically placed on the studied tissue.

One of the major limitations of laser-Doppler flowmetry is that it is not possible to measure absolute perfusion values (i.e. cutaneous blood flow in ml/min relative to volume or weight of tissue). Although some researchers have tried to convert milivolts to conventional blood units using theoretical calculations, this is not widely accepted. Measurements in most studies are expressed as arbitrary perfusion units (PU) or milivolts (1 PU = 10mV) and are often referred to as flux rather than flow. Although, reproducibility of laser-Doppler was considered poor, it is possible related to the site of investigation. When the recording site is standardized, the day-to-day reproducibility of PORH, thermal hyperemia and acetylcholine iontoforesis compares well with the FMD of the brachial artery, with each having a coeficient of variation <10% [23,41].

6. INTRAVITAL MICROSCOPY

Intravital microscopy can be applied in animals using various tissue preparations, and in humans, where it has been primarily used within the nailfold. It allows visualization of a living system in real time and provides 2-D projection of a 3-D capillary network. Intravital microscopy of human capillaries, or capillaroscopy, used in the nailfold allows the visualization of the complete capillary loop because at this site it parallels the skin Fig. (1). The orientation of capillaries changes to become perpendicular or oblique to the surface by moving proximally along the digit. It can also be used in the skinfold, lip or bulbar conjunctiva [42,43]. Microvessels in the papillary dermis, observed by capillaroscopy, range from 10 to 35 μm whereas those in the mid to deep dermis are 40 to 50 μm with an occasional arteriole as large as 100 μm being observed [44]. Capillaries play a vital role in nutrient and waste product exchange and their functional density determines the total surface area available for exchange, the maximum distance between a cell and blood and thus diffusion time, and contribute to total resistance at the capillary bed [45]. Alterations in capillary blood flow and pressure may influence transcapillary exchange processes, the magnitude of this effect being influenced by lipid-solubility and size of concerned molecules and tissue metabolic requirements. They also play a key role in tissue fluid homeostasis.

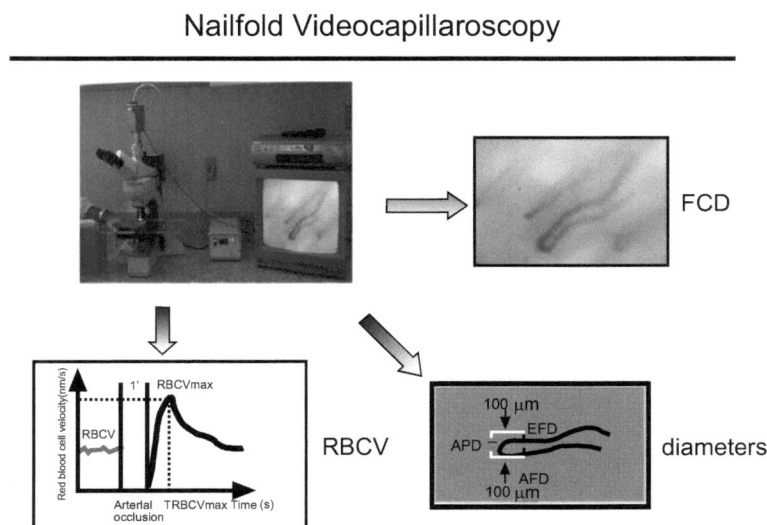

Nailfold Videocapillaroscopy

Figure 1: Nailfold videocapillaroscopy technique with assessment on the 4th finger. Imaging of capillaries with determination of functional capillary density (FCD). Schematic representation of measurements of red blood cell velocity (RBCV) at baseline and after 1 min arterial occlusion and the time taken to reach it. Schematic representation of capillary diameter measurements on different locations which ultimately represent the measuremtent of the red blood cell column.

This technique may be used to assess capillary morphology, capillary functional density, capillary blood cell velocity (dynamic capillaroscopy), and width of the capillary red cell column ("capillary diameter") or to facilitate direct capillary cannulation. In combination with fluorescent dyes (e.g sodium fluorescein or indocyanide green – fluorescence video microscopy), capillaroscopy was used to examine heterogeneity of capillary flow distribution, to visualize structures not detectable by native capillaroscopy such as aneurysms, and to follow transcapillary diffusion of tracer as a marker of capillary permeability to small solutes [46], but safety and ethical problems hinder its use for research in humans. The capillary wall cannot be visualized and fluorescent dye studies using indocyanide green have demonstrated that the width of the red blood cell column occupies nearly 70% of the total capillary diameter [47].

Dynamic videocapillaroscopy visualizes nutritive microvessels and quantify microvessel flow. Initially frame-to-frame analysis was used to assess the movement of plasma gaps along a given capillary [48]. Subsequently this measurement of capillary flow was improved and simplified in a video-photometric cross correlation technique [49]. This latter allowed continuous assessment of capillary red blood cell velocity over longer period of time, although considered technically difficult to proceed. Variables related to functional measurement of capillary flow are red blood cell velocity (RBCV) at resting state and also at PORH and, finally, the time taken to reach RBCV at PORH. Testing variables at PORH may minimize differences between capillaries, standardize the temporal changes in flow between vessels and thus reduce variability between individuals [50,51], allowing human studies related to microvascular responses to drugs Fig. (**2**). Additionally at capillaroscopy, it is possible to quantify the number of capillary loops with flowing red blood cells in a pre-specified area resulting in the so-called functional capillary density (FCD). Cannulation of human capillaries and direct measurement of capillary pressure is also possible to be assessed [45].

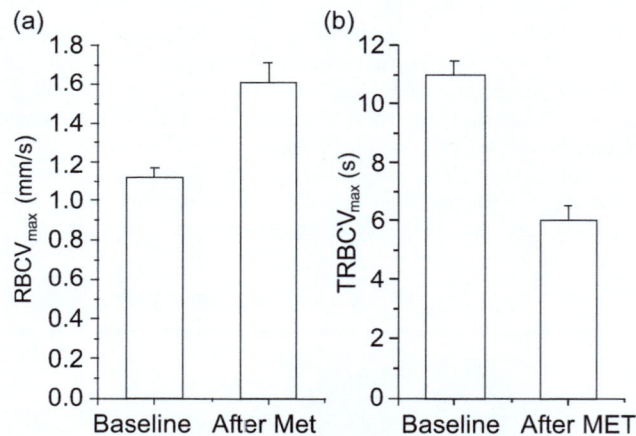

Figure 2: Microvascular responses after the use of an insulin-sensitising agent (metformin - MET) demonstrating improvement on peak red blood cell velocity (a - RBCVmax), and on time taken to reach it after 1 min arterial occlusion (b - TRBCVmax) in normoglycaemic subjects with the metabolic syndrome ($P<0.001$). Redrawn from Kraemer de Aguiar *et al.* [50].

Ageing is accompanied by a loss of dermal volume, a reduction in capillary density, shortened capillary loops, and rarefaction of larger microvessels [52]. Although initially this technique was extensively used to study of rheumatic diseases, nowadays FCD at PORH, also called capillary recruitment, is an important index related to insulin-resistant states and hypertension [14,51], obesity [53] and diabetes mellitus [45]. At PORH, RBCV and the time taken to reach it were both related to metabolic syndrome diagnosis and body mass index even without any degree of glucose intolerance Figs. (**3**) and (**4**) [51]. Capillaroscopic parameters represent entirely nutritional flow morphology and dynamics and possibly reproduce well the physiology and pathophysiology of insulin resistant states, even knowing that cutaneous tissue is not a primary insulin target tissue such as muscle. However, even at skin capillary, recruitment was induced by physiological hyperinsulinemia [15].

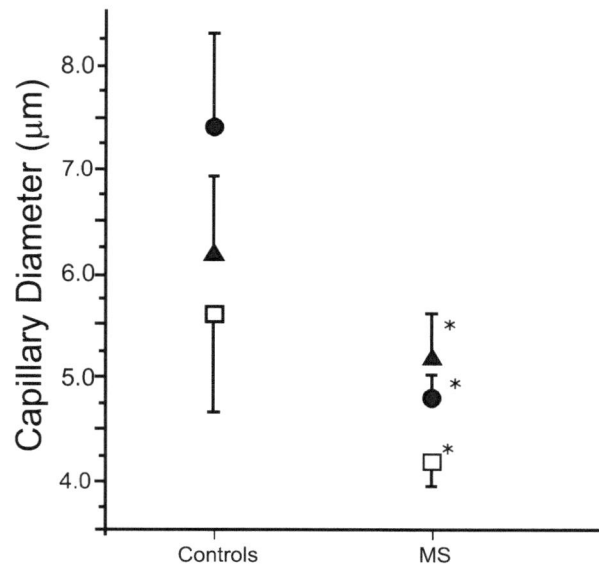

Figure 3: Capillary diameters on afferent (□), apical (●) and efferent (▲) capillary loops in subjects with metabolic syndrome at normoglycemic milieu (MS) *P<0.01. Redrawn from Kraemer de Aguiar *et al.* [51].

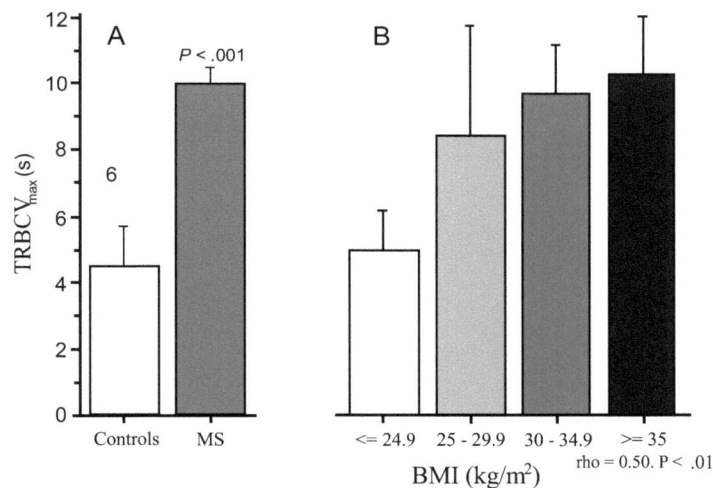

Figure 4: A, Time taken to reach peak red blood cell velocity (TRBCVmax) during post-occlusive reactive hyperemia (PORH) in subjects with metabolic syndrome at normoglycemic milieu. **B**, Stepwise progression of impaired TRBCVmax associated with body mass index (BMI). Redrawn from Kraemer de Aguiar *et al.* [51].

The skin pigment, melanin, absorbs light strongly and the use of capillaroscopy in highly pigmented skin is difficult and limits its use. A common factor to all examinations using capillaroscopy is the requirement for excellent images, in particular high black/white contrast with no movement artifacts. To achieve this, it is necessary to immobilize the digit but this must be achieved without affecting blood flow. Questions about capillarosocopy variability and also if this method is able to reproduce microvascular dysfunction in other tissues still remain. Although questionable [54], some data demonstrated its relationship in patients with cardiovascular risk [28] and coronary microvascular dysfunction [55,56].

7. SPECTRAL IMAGING TECHNIQUE

For many years, capillary microscopy has been the only method for assessment of the human microcirculation at microscopic level *in vivo*. The spectral imaging technique obtained using the developed method of orthogonal polarization of light, also called orthogonal polarization spectral (OPS) imaging allows for the *in vivo* noninvasively transcutaneous evaluation of the microcirculation [57], with real time observations Figs. (**5**) and (**6**) [58]. OPS´s successor technique, the so-called sidestream dark-field (SDF) imaging is relatively new and use similar principles [59]. Microcirculation studies assessed by these techniques in insulin resistant states are lacking, on the opposite because nailfold microcirculation is extremely sensitive to external temperature and vasoconstrictive agents limiting videocapillaroscopy use, there are some studies in critically ill patients [60].

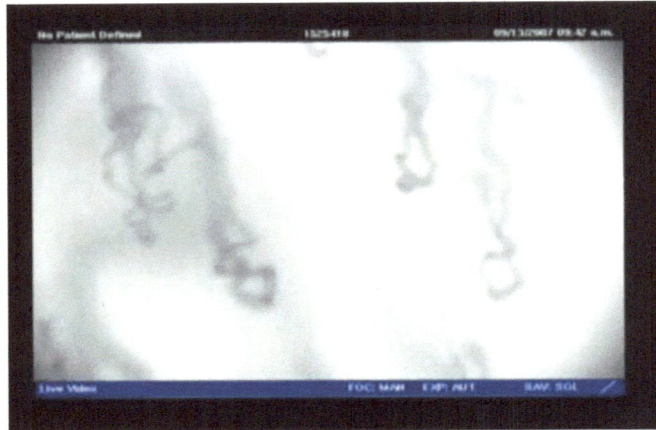

Figure 5: Evaluation of skin microcirculation by orthogonal polarization spectral (OPS) technique with detection of the rate of displacement of erythrocytes in arterioles and venules, functional capillary density (number of flowing capillaries per unit area), diameter of the dermal papilla, and capillary diameter. Redrawn from Lupi *et al.* [58].

CYTOSCAN - OPS

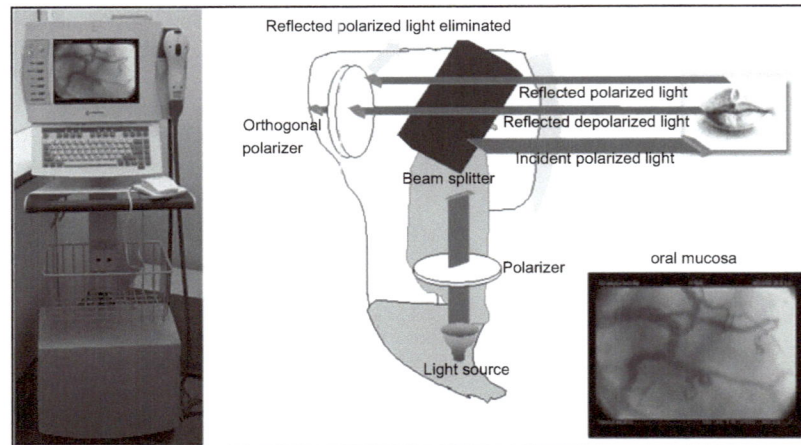

Figure 6: Portable device that allows inspection of individual capillaries of the cutaneous microcirculation and flow through these vessels in real time. Cytoscan© by Cytometrics© and schematic representation of how the image is obtained.

Two innovations, however, have been introduced recently: epiillumination and the assessment of images obtained from objects illuminated with rays of light that originate from the same direction as the observer [57,61]. The utilization of polarized light is applied to the skin surface, a large part of the radiation is simply reflected and retains its original polarization [61]. A small amount of this light penetrates to deeper layers and undergoes multiple dispersion events before being depolarized and reissued to the surface. The reissued light is the fraction of original light which, as a result of reflection or dispersion, returns from the illuminated object. The degree of penetration of polarized light depends on the density of studied tissue and the power of the polarized radiation [57,61]. Depolarized light reissued from a deeper origin needs to be evaluated separately from the light reflected by more superficial layers of tissue under study because this light retains photon polarization, whereas the former one undergoes real depolarization. A second polarizer, placed in a precise orthogonal position allows the rejection of all photons not depolarized, i.e. the ones originated from more superficial layers of the tissue [61,62] and analyzes only the depolarized light that comes from deeper layers of the skin. The image formed when immersion objectives are correctly placed is that of the microcirculation in contrast with an illuminated background [62], allowing the *in vivo* assessment, in real time, of the microcirculation situated up to 3 mm in depth in the skin. When the light is absorbed by hemoglobin, an image of the illuminated hemoglobin-carrying structures in negative contrast is created. SDF imaging is based on light-emiting diodes arranged in a ring formation at the tip of the light guide emitting green light (540±50nm), which illuminates directly tissue microcirculation [59]. This "virtual backlighting" technology allows the visualization and measurement of real-time images of the microcirculation without the use of fluorescent dyes or transillumination [57]. OPS and SDF, although the latter technique seems to improve resolution and clarity of images compared to the former one, have been implemented in a hand-held videomicroscope convenient for both clinical and experimental conditions. The variation in skin thickness allows some areas, such as the face, thorax, dorsum, and limbs to be examined easily by the OPS technique: the skin in these regions is not very thick and presents abundant vascularization. Mucosal surfaces are ideal areas for the method because they lack a corneal or granular layer and are richly vascularized [63-65]. Skin microcirculation is mainly found within the papillary dermis, approximately 3–4 mm below the surface, and therefore within reach of the OPS technique [63-65]. As well as in videocapillaroscopy [66], the visualization of the dermal microcirculation is influenced, however, by the amount of melanin present at the dermal–epidermal junction.

In summary, despite limitations, the OPS technique is a very promising tool for researchers in both experimental and clinical studies. The OPS method was validated in comparison with videomicroscopy in both experimental and clinical settings and resulted in good agreement of analysed variables [67-72]. As observed with videocapillaroscopy [50], the OPS technique could also enable the monitoring of the microcirculatory response to therapy [73], and thus may become a valuable clinical tool once a standardized and automated analysis routine is established in skin microcirculation.

8. EVALUATION OF ENDOTHELIUM FUNCTION ON SKELETAL MUSCLE

The endothelium plays a key role on vascular homeostasis by the release of a variety of autocrine and paracrine substances [74]. In addition to vasodilation, a healthy endothelium is antiatherogenic due to effects like inhibition of platelet aggregation and adhesion, smooth muscle cell proliferation and leukocyte adhesion. Endothelial dysfunction is a systemic process, considered as the initiating event in atherosclerosis and important in ischemic manifestation of the disease process as well. During the last two decades, much attention has been given to the evaluation of NO contribution to vasodilatory process in humans. Originally, endothelium-dependent vasodilation (EDV) was assessed during coronary angiography by measuring the response to acetylcholine infused into a coronary artery [75-77]. Quantitative assessment of myocardial blood flow and of its metabolic activity may be performed by positron emission tomography scanning [78,79]. However, as these methods are both expensive and restricted to subjects undergoing coronary angiography, other methods have been developed to measure EDV in the peripheral circulation.

Limb blood flow can be directly assessed by electrically calibrated pletysmography [80]. The invasive peripheral technique to test limb blood flow uses a similar concept described for coronary arteries Fig. (7). Using this technique at forearm site, acetylcholine, or some other muscarinic receptor agonist [81], is infused into the brachial artery and the increase in forearm blood flow (FBF), expressed in ml/min/100 ml of tissue, is taken as an index of EDV. Blunted EDV has been found in patients with coronary heart disease, hypertension, hypercholesterolemia or diabetes [82-87]. Endothelium-independent vasodilation (EIDV) is evaluated by sodium nitropruside infusion. This technique, in contrast with most studies on coronary circulation, evaluates vasodilation mainly in resistance vessels, which will partly represent endothelial reactivity at the microcirculatory level, i.e. small arteries with myogenic response [1,2] and arterioles. FMD, an index to evaluate vasodilation on a conduit artery also during post-occlusion reactive hyperemia (PORH), has gained popularity in recent years, attenuated in patients with hypertension, hypercholesterolemia or diabetes [88-91] reflecting mainly the macrovascular reactivity. Both measurements, FBF and FMD are of value for testing endothelial dysfunction and can also be considered a prognostic predictor for cardiovascular events [4,92,93]. Although it was established that endothelial responses to pharmacologic and ischemic stimuli, respectively FBF and FMD, differ between resistance and conduit arteries in the same patient they do not demonstrated good correlation between them [94,95]. Therefore, the exact meaning of the endothelial response is dependent on which technique has been employed on the peripheral circulation.

Venous Occlusion Plethysmography

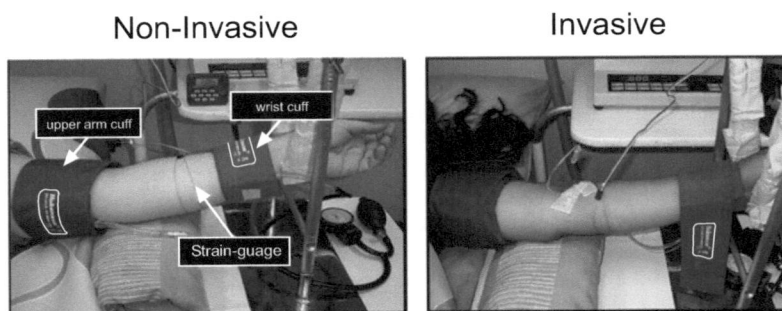

Figure 7: Venous occlusion pletismography tested by non- and invasive techniques. The latter (right-sided) shows the catheter inserted into the brachial artery for continuous infusion of vasoactive drugs.

There is no ideal technique to measure muscle blood flow in humans. Flow to contracting muscles can be much higher than once thought and careful considerations about what fraction of limb blood flow is going to limb's nonmuscle elements are required to estimate changes in muscle blood flow. FBF is much more important in respect to muscle microcirculation, the main site of insulin action, and there are some studies relating it with glucose homesostasis and insulin resitance [96,96-98].

Skeletal muscle is the largest organ in the body and muscle contractions increase energy use and activate numerous metabolic pathways in an effort to meet the muscles' increased demand for energy. Owing to muscle ability to increase its metabolism more than 100 fold, rise in blood flow to active muscles can be vast and is generally proportional to metabolism rise. In this context, whole body and local muscle 'fuel homeostasis' are linked by the cardiovascular system [99], which transports substrate to the active muscle and removes byproducts of contraction.

9. VENOUS OCCLUSION PLETHYSMOGRAPHY (VOP)

The use of VOP to measure blood flow in humans was first described 100 years ago [100] and with the advent of mercury-in-silastic strain gauges this technique greatly increased its applicability. The general principle of VOP is that a pneumatic cuff is inflated (40–50mmHg) around the upper arm or thigh to occlude blood flow in veins but not preventing arterial inflow. A second cuff is placed at wrist or ankle level and inflated to suprasystolic pressure to exclude hand or foot blood flow, respectively. VOP provides a measure of blood flow to that part of forearm comprised by two cuffs. Mercury-in-silastic strain gauges placed around the widest part of the limb (forearm or leg) where flow should be measured are commonly used to detect changes on limb circumference and calculate the corresponding percentage increase in volume. Blood flow is measured as linear increases in forearm volume over time and is thought to be proportional to the rate of arterial inflow [101]. When measurements are conducted in a quiet, temperature-controlled room (22-26°C), with the subject resting in a comfortable supine position, measurement of FBF by strain gauge VOP compares favourably with values obtained by other established techniques [102].

VOP has been extensively used to determine human vascular reactivitivy *in vivo* and it also allows detailed studies in vascular pharmacology, usually through infusion of receptor agonists, and physiology, mainly by infusion of receptor antagonists. Indeed, forearm VOP with local brachial artery infusion has become one of the "gold-standards" for assessment of vascular function in health and disease, and an accurate, reproducible and convenient method to assess the effect of new vasoactive drugs and hormones in humans *in vivo* [103]. Indeed, patients with established risk factors for cardiovascular disease (i.e. hypertension, hyperlipidemia and aging) demonstrate blunted dose–response curves to acetylcholine, indicative of endothelial dysfunction [104-106].

The use of VOP has provided several fundamental observations and advanced our understanding of limb blood flow responses to exercise in humans. This technique has provided critical information regarding dynamics and timing of muscle blood flow at the onset of exercise, mechanisms responsible for changes on muscle blood flow during exercise and the balance between vasoconstricting and vasodilating substances contributing to muscle blood flow regulation at rest and during exercise [107]. Interventions such as aerobic exercise [105,108,109], weight loss [110], administration of antioxidant vitamins [109,111] or vasculo-protective drugs [112,113] have been shown to improve endothelial function in different high-risk populations Fig. (**8**).

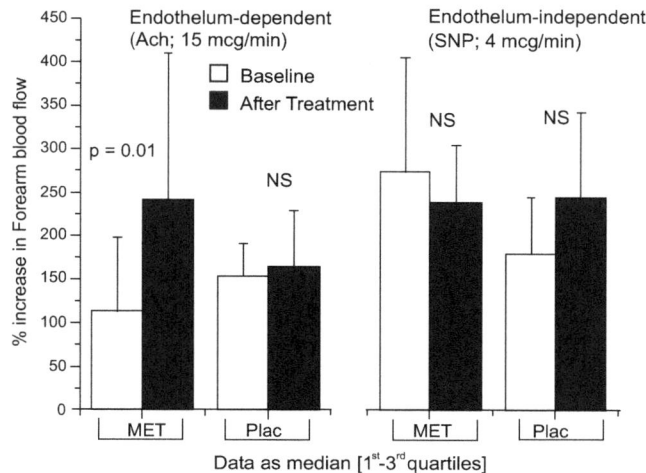

Figure 8: Forearm blood flow responses in endothelium-dependent vasodilation after acetylcholine infusion, before (baseline) and after treatment with an insulin-sensitising agent (metformin) on metabolic syndrome subjects. Met, metformin; Plac, placebo. Redrawn from de Aguiar *et al.* [112].

Following limb ischaemia there is a rapid increase in FBF, which slowly returns to baseline values and is termed reactive hyperemia Fig. (**9**). The maximum flow and area under the curve for this increase in blood flow are directly related to the duration of ischaemia until approximately 13 min [100]. This principle allows the evaluation of FBF time-response curve during reactive hyperemia by assessing it using VOP [114]. Indeed, the maximal post-ischaemic FBF is not influenced by sympathetic tone [115] or vasodilator administration [100] and seems to represent the minimum forearm vascular resistance, which is a function of the average wall:lumen ratio of resistance vessels [116]. Therefore, it provides indirect information concerning the structure of resistance vessels on tested limb. Increased minimum vascular resistance has been demonstrated in hypertension [116,117], borderline hypertension [115], white-coat hypertension [118] and obesity [114]. Finally, VOP can also assess deep forearm veins compliance [119] and microvascular permeability [120].

Venous Occlusion Plethysmography

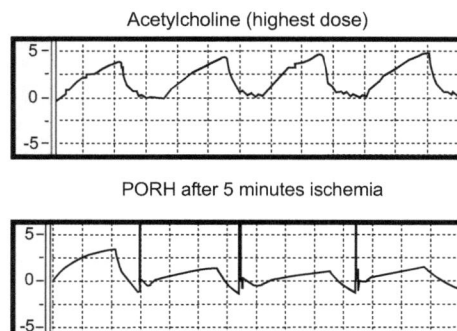

Figure 9: Venous occlusion pletismography curves observed after infusion of a vasoactive drug (acetylcholine) by invasive technique (upper) and after ischemia during post-occlusive reactive hyperemia (PORH) by non-invasive (lower) technique. Continuous infusion of a drug into the brachial artery allows curves with almost the same pattern during recordings. On the opposite, curves obtained in the PORH period decay during the analysis.

Several groups have assessed the reproducibility of VOP, demonstrating good within-subject reproducibility for unilateral blood flow measurements with aproximately 10% for the coefficient of variation [121]. Although different values of this coefficient appear in other studies [122-124] reaching values of up to 39% when testing for unilateral flows at rest. However, some of these authors when testing absolute values of FBF after pharmacological stimuli, inspite of the percentage change on the FBF ratio, observed lower values for the variation coefficient [123,124].

10. RADIOLABELED MICROSPHERES

Radiolabeled microspheres have been used extensively in animal studies to measure local and regional blood flow [125] but are not used in human research. However, a similar technique that uses ultrasonography has recently been used for the assessment of skeletal muscle microcirculation and may have widespread applications. The so-called technique, contrast-enhanced ultrasonography (CEU), originally developed to measure myocardial perfusion [126] has been adapted for the quantification of skeletal muscle perfusion [127]. The gas-filled microbubbles, infused systemically to provide contrast for ultrasound detection, are both simultaneously imaged and destroyed by an ultrasound probe positioned over the muscle bed of interest [128,129]. The intensity of the signal emitted from microbubbles destruction is proportional to their concentration and is recorded as acoustic intensity. A series of images are collected over a given period of time in a specified region of interest and a replenishment curve is generated that describes the refilling rate and the volume of microvasculature filled by microbubbles [128]. The ability of CEU to detect perfusion deficits over a populational range with known microvascular disorders is yet to be determined. Experimentally it was demonstrated a vascular recruitment in skeletal muscle during exercise and hyperinsulinemia assessed by CEU [130], which was also observed in human muscle [131]. Muscle contraction, which causes vasodilation, is a strong stimulator of capillary recruitment and occurs at low intensities during muscle activity [131]. Bradykinin and epinephrine are muscle vasodilators but although they increase muscle total blood flow they do not cause capillary recruitment and therefore do not change microvascular blood volume by CEU assessment [132,133]. On the opposite, metacholine was able to induce an increment on total flow and capillary recruitment with this technique [132]. Insulin is another strong stimulator of capillary recruitment and CEU was used to measure changes on microvascular volume sequentially, each 20 s. After the commencement of a 3 mU.min^{-1}.kg^{-1} insulin clamp, it was observed that insulin-mediated capillary recruitment occurred before insulin signaling or glucose uptake was stimulated in the muscle [134]. Additionally, studies of the relationship between insulin dose and capillary recruitment also indicated that recruitment could occur in the absence of changes in total blood flow and glucose metabolism [135]. CEU has the advantage of being highly sensitive, even to blood flow within capillaries, noninvasive and can be used during voluntary exercise. Finally, CEU has great potential for clinical implementation because of its portability, low cost and requirement for equipment already in place in most vascular laboratories. Limitations to the technique include: perfusion has to be measured at a single representative muscle region and therefore, may not give representative results for the whole muscle group, and CEU data acquisition lasts for 90–120 s, therefore, realtime measurement of perfusion is not possible [127].

Muscle blood flow should be viewed as a key link between systemic and regional metabolism [136,137] and there are other techniques employed for measuring or assessing it. Indicator dilution methods for measuring blood flow include thermodilution and dye dilution that are useful to perform measurements at steady state, including at rest and during maximal and submaximal exercise. A number of different techniques have been utilized to measure local tissue blood flow, most dependent on measuring appearance or disappearance of various tracers, including radioactive isotope clearance (e.g. 133Xe) [138] and ethanol from microdialysis fibers. However, the radioactive isotope clearance technique is limited by its ability to be used for repetitive measurements owing to its inaccuracy in injecting the tracer in the same spot and also by variable perfusion at rest [139]. Although newer imaging techniques such as magnetic resonance imaging (MRI) [140], near-infrared spectroscopy (NIRS) [141], and positron emission tomography (PET) [142], require sophisticated and expensive equipment, they are all being adapted to measurements of blood flow and offer the promise of measurements of local blood flow in regions that have not been able to be easily measured before and at very high resolution.

Microvascular abnormalities that lead to impaired tissue perfusion appear to represent a generalized condition affecting multiple tissues and organs. This assertion seemed to be true also in states of insulin resistance. Therefore, impaired tissue perfusion may be involved in target-organ damage and complications involving several vascular beds. For practical purposes, intravital microscopy and LDF measurements seem to be feasible in clinical and research practice, and both techniques, express mainly microcirculatory physiology and pathophysilogy, and also pharmacologic responses on the microcirculation better than others techniques discussed. Since a reasonable proportion of microvessels are not perfused under resting conditions, but can be recruited during hyperemia, a useful overall index of microvascular status of the cutanneous microvascular bed may be obtained by estimating the available flow reserve, the so-called capillary recruitment, either in terms of number of microvessels that can be recruited or maximal increase in blood flow, respectively by intravital microscopy and LDF measurements. This index seems sensitive to disorders associated with insulin resistance and metabolic disarrengemnts in humans. Techniques employed to investigate the microcirculation specifically on target-organ are actually invasive in the majority of cases and also have high cost-effective ratio, puting the skin on central focus on studies of microcirculation in humans. New techniques that assess microvascular blood flow in skeletal muscle appear to be promising, mainly in studies of insulin resistance states, but still deserve further validation.

11. CONCLUSION

Several techniques are available to assess human microcirculation and endothelial reactivity. Most commonly used ones to assess the microcirculation in humans rely on measurements of microvacular blood flow and/or visualization at cutanneous site, also used to investigate endothelial reactivity. At the skin it is possible to visualize capillaries and to quantify microvascular blood flow. Insulin resistant states are related to impaired responses of the vascular tissue already described in different organs. Muscle is the main target tissue to study the interrelationship between insulin action, glucose homeostasis and vascular physiology and pathophysiology related to obesity, insulin resistance and type 2 diabetes mellitus. Blood flow and considerations about its changes on muscle require careful analysis about assumptions on how different interventions influence flow to other (especially skin) tissues. In humans, skeletal muscle blood flow and microvascular blood volume can be assessed by noninvasive techniques. Finally, the study of the microcirculation in states of insulin resitance provides a unique opportunity for the study of pathophysiology and its implication as cause/effect of insulin resistance and vascular damage, and also on pharmacology. Recognizing the advantages and limitations of each technique is essential to translational researchers studying effects of nutrition and metabolism on the microcirculation.

12. ACKNOLEDGEMENTS

The authors wish to thank Professor Daniel A. Bottino for excellent technical assistance.

13. REFERENCES

[1]   Levy BI, Ambrosio G, Pries AR, Struijker-Boudier HA: Microcirculation in hypertension: a new target for treatment? Circulation 104:735-740, 2001.

[2]   Feihl F, Liaudet L, Waeber B, Levy BI: Hypertension: a disease of the microcirculation? Hypertension 48:1012-1017, 2006.

[3]   Sax FL, Cannon RO, III, Hanson C, Epstein SE: Impaired forearm vasodilator reserve in patients with microvascular angina. Evidence of a generalized disorder of vascular function? N Engl J Med 317:1366-1370, 1987.

[4]   Fichtlscherer S, Breuer S, Zeiher AM: Prognostic value of systemic endothelial dysfunction in patients with acute coronary syndromes: further evidence for the existence of the "vulnerable" patient. Circulation 110:1926-1932, 2004.

[5]   Johnson PC: Active and passive determinants of capillary density: a historical perspective. Int J Microcirc Clin Exp 15:218-222, 1995.

[6]   Verdant C, De BD: How monitoring of the microcirculation may help us at the bedside. Curr Opin Crit Care 11:240-244, 2005.

[7]   Haslam DW, James WP: Obesity. Lancet 366:1197-1209, 2005.

[8]   Mokdad AH, Bowman BA, Ford ES, Vinicor F, Marks JS, Koplan JP: The continuing epidemics of obesity and diabetes in the United States. JAMA 286:1195-1200, 2001.

[9]   Singleton JR, Smith AG, Russell JW, Feldman EL: Microvascular complications of impaired glucose tolerance. Diabetes 52:2867-2873, 2003.

[10]   van Leiden HA, Dekker JM, Moll AC, Nijpels G, Heine RJ, Bouter LM, Stehouwer CD, Polak BC: Blood pressure, lipids, and obesity are associated with retinopathy: the hoorn study. Diabetes Care 25:1320-1325, 2002.

[11]   de Jongh PE, Verhave J.C., Pinto-Siestma S.J., Hillege H.L.: Obesity and target organ damage: the kidney. Int J Obes Relat Metab Disord 26:S21-S24, 2002.

[12]   Kenchaiah S, Gaziano JM, Vasan RS: Impact of obesity on the risk of heart failure and survival after the onset of heart failure. Med Clin North Am 88:1273-1294, 2004.

[13]   Clark MG, Wallis MG, Barrett EJ, Vincent MA, Richards SM, Clerk LH, Rattigan S: Blood flow and muscle metabolism: a focus on insulin action. Am J Physiol Endocrinol Metab 284:E241-E258, 2003.

[14]   de Jongh RT, Serne EH, Ijzerman RG, de VG, Stehouwer CD: Impaired microvascular function in obesity: implications for obesity-associated microangiopathy, hypertension, and insulin resistance. Circulation 109:2529-2535, 2004.

[15]   Serne EH, Ijzerman RG, Gans RO, Nijveldt R, de VG, Evertz R, Donker AJ, Stehouwer CD: Direct evidence for insulin-induced capillary recruitment in skin of healthy subjects during physiological hyperinsulinemia. Diabetes 51:1515-1522, 2002.

[16]   Serne EH, Stehouwer CD, ter Maaten JC, ter Wee PM, Rauwerda JA, Donker AJ, Gans RO: Microvascular function relates to insulin sensitivity and blood pressure in normal subjects. Circulation 99:896-902, 1999.

[17]   Vollus GC, Bradley EA, Roberts MK, Newman JM, Richards SM, Rattigan S, Barrett EJ, Clark MG: Graded occlusion of perfused rat muscle vasculature decreases insulin action. Clin Sci (Lond) 112:457-466, 2007.

[18]   Barac A, Campia U, Panza JA: Methods for evaluating endothelial function in humans. Hypertension 49:748-760, 2007.

[19]   Holowatz LA, Thompson-Torgerson CS, Kenney WL: The human cutaneous circulation as a model of generalized microvascular function. J Appl Physiol 105:370-372, 2008.

[20]   Johnson PC: Active and passive determinants of capillary density: a historical perspective. Int J Microcirc Clin Exp 15:218-222, 1995.

[21]   Wright CI, Kroner CI, Draijer R: Non-invasive methods and stimuli for evaluating the skin's microcirculation. J Pharmacol Toxicol Methods 54:1-25, 2006.

[22]   Leahy MJ, de Mul FF, Nilsson GE, Maniewski R: Principles and practice of the laser-Doppler perfusion technique. Technol Health Care 7:143-162, 1999.

[23]   Kubli S, Waeber B, le-Ave A, Feihl F: Reproducibility of laser Doppler imaging of skin blood flow as a tool to assess endothelial function. J Cardiovasc Pharmacol 36:640-648, 2000.

[24]   Newton DJ, Khan F, Belch JJ: Assessment of microvascular endothelial function in human skin. Clin Sci (Lond) 101:567-572, 2001.

[25]   Cracowski JL, Minson CT, Salvat-Melis M, Halliwill JR: Methodological issues in the assessment of skin microvascular endothelial function in humans. Trends Pharmacol Sci 27:503-508, 2006.

[26]   Khan F, Elhadd TA, Greene SA, Belch JJ: Impaired skin microvascular function in children, adolescents, and young adults with type 1 diabetes. Diabetes Care 23:215-220, 2000.

[27]   Kruger A, Stewart J, Sahityani R, O'Riordan E, Thompson C, Adler S, Garrick R, Vallance P, Goligorsky MS: Laser Doppler flowmetry detection of endothelial dysfunction in end-stage renal disease patients: correlation with cardiovascular risk. Kidney Int 70:157-164, 2006.

[28]   Ijzerman RG, de Jongh RT, Beijk MA, van Weissenbruch MM, Delemarre-van de Waal HA, Serne EH, Stehouwer CD: Individuals at increased coronary heart disease risk are characterized by an impaired microvascular function in skin. Eur J Clin Invest 33:536-542, 2003.

[29]   Pierzga JM, Frymoyer A, Kenney WL: Delayed distribution of active vasodilation and altered vascular conductance in aged skin. J Appl Physiol 94:1045-1053, 2003.

[30]   Wong BJ, Wilkins BW, Holowatz LA, Minson CT: Nitric oxide synthase inhibition does not alter the reactive hyperemic response in the cutaneous circulation. J Appl Physiol 95:504-510, 2003.

[31]   Holowatz LA, Thompson CS, Kenney WL: L-Arginine supplementation or arginase inhibition augments reflex cutaneous vasodilatation in aged human skin. J Physiol 574:573-581, 2006.

[32]   Minson CT, Holowatz LA, Wong BJ, Kenney WL, Wilkins BW: Decreased nitric oxide- and axon reflex-mediated cutaneous vasodilation with age during local heating. J Appl Physiol 93:1644-1649, 2002.

[33]   Thompson-Torgerson CS, Holowatz LA, Flavahan NA, Kenney WL: Cold-induced cutaneous vasoconstriction is mediated by Rho kinase in vivo in human skin. Am J Physiol Heart Circ Physiol 292:H1700-H1705, 2007.

[34]   Abahji TN, Nill L, Ide N, Keller C, Hoffmann U, Weiss N: Acute hyperhomocysteinemia induces microvascular and macrovascular endothelial dysfunction. Arch Med Res 38:411-416, 2007.

[35]   Minson CT, Berry LT, Joyner MJ: Nitric oxide and neurally mediated regulation of skin blood flow during local heating. J Appl Physiol 91:1619-1626, 2001.

[36]   Lorenzo S, Minson CT: Human cutaneous reactive hyperaemia: role of BKCa channels and sensory nerves. J Physiol 585:295-303, 2007.

[37]   Kvandal P, Stefanovska A, Veber M, Kvernmo HD, Kirkeboen KA: Regulation of human cutaneous circulation evaluated by laser Doppler flowmetry, iontophoresis, and spectral analysis: importance of nitric oxide and prostaglandines. Microvasc Res 65:160-171, 2003.

[38]   Celermajer DS: Statins, skin, and the search for a test of endothelial function. J Am Coll Cardiol 42:78-80, 2003.

[39]   Stefanovska A, Bracic M, Kvernmo HD: Wavelet analysis of oscillations in the peripheral blood circulation measured by laser Doppler technique. IEEE Trans Biomed Eng 46:1230-1239, 1999.

[40]   Abularrage CJ, Sidawy AN, Aidinian G, Singh N, Weiswasser JM, Arora S: Evaluation of the microcirculation in vascular disease. J Vasc Surg 42:574-581, 2005.

[41]   Boignard A, Salvat-Melis M, Carpentier PH, Minson CT, Grange L, Duc C, Sarrot-Reynauld F, Cracowski JL: Local hyperemia to heating is impaired in secondary Raynaud's phenomenon. Arthritis Res Ther 7:R1103-R1112, 2005.
[42]   Fagrell B, Intaglietta M: Microcirculation: its significance in clinical and molecular medicine. J Intern Med 241:349-362, 1997.
[43]   Fagrell B: Microcirculatory methods for the clinical assessment of hypertension, hypotension, and ischemia. Ann Biomed Eng 14:163-173, 1986.
[44]   Braverman IM: The cutaneous microcirculation: ultrastructure and microanatomical organization. Microcirculation 4:329-340, 1997.
[45]   Shore AC: Capillaroscopy and the measurement of capillary pressure. Br J Clin Pharmacol 50:501-513, 2000.
[46]   Bollinger A, Saesseli B, Hoffmann U, Franzeck UK: Intravital detection of skin capillary aneurysms by videomicroscopy with indocyanine green in patients with progressive systemic sclerosis and related disorders. Circulation 83:546-551, 1991.
[47]   Moneta G, Brulisauer M, Jager K, Bollinger A: Infrared fluorescence videomicroscopy of skin capillaries with indocyanine green. Int J Microcirc Clin Exp 6:25-34, 1987.
[48]   Bollinger A, Butti P, Barras JP, Trachsler H, Siegenthaler W: Red blood cell velocity in nailfold capillaries of man measured by a television microscopy technique. Microvasc Res 7:61-72, 1974.
[49]   Fagrell B, Fronek A, Intaglietta M: A microscope-television system for studying flow velocity in human skin capillaries. Am J Physiol 233:H318-H321, 1977.
[50]   Kraemer de Aguiar LG, Laflor CM, Bahia L, Villela NR, Wiernsperger N, Bottino DA, Bouskela E: Metformin improves skin capillary reactivity in normoglycaemic subjects with the metabolic syndrome. Diabet Med 24:272-279, 2007.
[51]   Kraemer-Aguiar LG, Laflor CM, Bouskela E: Skin microcirculatory dysfunction is already present in normoglycemic subjects with metabolic syndrome. Metabolism 57:1740-1746, 2008.
[52]   Montagna W, Carlisle K: Structural changes in aging human skin. J Invest Dermatol 73:47-53, 1979.
[53]   de Jongh RT, Ijzerman RG, Serne EH, Voordouw JJ, Yudkin JS, de Waal HA, Stehouwer CD, van Weissenbruch MM: Visceral and truncal subcutaneous adipose tissue are associated with impaired capillary recruitment in healthy individuals. J Clin Endocrinol Metab 91:5100-5106, 2006.
[54]   Shamim-Uzzaman QA, Pfenninger D, Kehrer C, Chakrabarti A, Kacirotti N, Rubenfire M, Brook R, Rajagopalan S: Altered cutaneous microvascular responses to reactive hyperaemia in coronary artery disease: a comparative study with conduit vessel responses. Clin Sci (Lond) 103:267-273, 2002.
[55]   Antonios TF, Kaski JC, Hasan KM, Brown SJ, Singer DR: Rarefaction of skin capillaries in patients with anginal chest pain and normal coronary arteriograms. Eur Heart J 22:1144-1148, 2001.
[56]   Pasqui AL, Puccetti L, Di RM, Bruni F, Camarri A, Palazzuoli A, Biagi F, Servi M, Bischeri D, Auteri A, Pastorelli M: Structural and functional abnormality of systemic microvessels in cardiac syndrome X. Nutr Metab Cardiovasc Dis 15:56-64, 2005.
[57]   Schiessler C, Schaudig S, Harris AG, Christ F: [Orthogonal polarization spectral imaging--a new clinical method for monitoring of microcirculation]. Anaesthesist 51:576-579, 2002.
[58]   Lupi O, Semenovitch I, Treu C, Bouskela E: Orthogonal polarization technique in the assessment of human skin microcirculation. Int J Dermatol 47:425-431, 2008.
[59]   Turek Z, Cerny V, Parizkova R: Noninvasive in vivo assessment of the skeletal muscle and small intestine serous surface microcirculation in rat: sidestream dark-field (SDF) imaging. Physiol Res 57:365-371, 2008.
[60]   De BD, Dubois MJ: Assessment of the microcirculatory flow in patients in the intensive care unit. Curr Opin Crit Care 7:200-203, 2001.
[61]   Cerny V, Turek Z, Parizkova R: Orthogonal polarization spectral imaging. Physiol Res 56:141-147, 2007.
[62]   Groner W, Winkelman JW, Harris AG, Ince C, Bouma GJ, Messmer K, et al: Orthogonal polarization spectral imaging: A new method for study of the microcirculation. Nature Medicine 5:1209-1213, 1999.
[63]   Milner SM, Bhat S, Gulati S, Gherardini G, Smith CE, Bick RJ: Observations on the microcirculation of the human burn wound using orthogonal polarization spectral imaging. Burns 31:316-319, 2005.
[64]   Erdmann D, Sweis R, Wong MS, Eyler CE, Olbrich KC, Levin LS, Germann G, Klitzman B: [Current perspectives of orthogonal polarization spectral imaging in plastic surgery]. Chirurg 73:827-832, 2002.
[65]   Chierego M, Verdant C, De BD: Microcirculatory alterations in critically ill patients. Minerva Anestesiol 72:199-205, 2006.
[66]   Lipowsky HH, Sheikh NU, Katz DM: Intravital microscopy of capillary hemodynamics in sickle cell disease. J Clin Invest 80:117-127, 1987.
[67]   De BD: OPS techniques. Minerva Anestesiol 69:388-391, 2003.
[68]   Pahernik S, Harris AG, Schmitt-Sody M, Krasnici S, Goetz AE, Dellian M, Messmer K: Orthogonal polarisation spectral imaging as a new tool for the assessment of antivascular tumour treatment in vivo: a validation study. Br J Cancer 86:1622-1627, 2002.
[69]   Harris AG, Sinitsina I, Messmer K: The Cytoscan Model E-II, a new reflectance microscope for intravital microscopy: comparison with the standard fluorescence method. J Vasc Res 37:469-476, 2000.
[70]   Harris AG, Sinitsina I, Messmer K: Validation of OPS imaging for microvascular measurements during isovolumic hemodilution and low hematocrits. Am J Physiol Heart Circ Physiol 282:H1502-H1509, 2002.
[71]   Mathura KR, Vollebregt KC, Boer K, De Graaff JC, Ubbink DT, Ince C: Comparison of OPS imaging and conventional capillary microscopy to study the human microcirculation. J Appl Physiol 91:74-78, 2001.

[72]   Langer S, Harris AG, Biberthaler P, von DE, Messmer K: Orthogonal polarization spectral imaging as a tool for the assessment of hepatic microcirculation: a validation study. Transplantation 71:1249-1256, 2001.

[73]   Lascasas-Porto CL, Milhomens AL, Virgin-Magalhaes CE, Fernandes FF, Sicuro FL, Bouskela E: Use of microcirculatory parameters to evaluate clinical treatments of chronic venous disorder (CVD). Microvasc Res 76:66-72, 2008.

[74]   Moncada S, Higgs A: The L-arginine-nitric oxide pathway. N Engl J Med 329:2002-2012, 1993.

[75]   Ludmer PL, Selwyn AP, Shook TL, Wayne RR, Mudge GH, Alexander RW, Ganz P: Paradoxical vasoconstriction induced by acetylcholine in atherosclerotic coronary arteries. N Engl J Med 315:1046-1051, 1986.

[76]   Werns SW, Walton JA, Hsia HH, Nabel EG, Sanz ML, Pitt B: Evidence of endothelial dysfunction in angiographically normal coronary arteries of patients with coronary artery disease. Circulation 79:287-291, 1989.

[77]   Zeiher AM, Drexler H, Wollschlager H, Just H: Endothelial dysfunction of the coronary microvasculature is associated with coronary blood flow regulation in patients with early atherosclerosis. Circulation 84:1984-1992, 1991.

[78]   Gould KL, Martucci JP, Goldberg DI, Hess MJ, Edens RP, Latifi R, Dudrick SJ: Short-term cholesterol lowering decreases size and severity of perfusion abnormalities by positron emission tomography after dipyridamole in patients with coronary artery disease. A potential noninvasive marker of healing coronary endothelium. Circulation 89:1530-1538, 1994.

[79]   Aengevaeren WR, Uijen GJ, Jukema JW, Bruschke AV, van der WT: Functional evaluation of lipid-lowering therapy by pravastatin in the Regression Growth Evaluation Statin Study (REGRESS). Circulation 96:429-435, 1997.

[80]   Hokanson DE, Sumner DS, Strandness DE, Jr.: An electrically calibrated plethysmograph for direct measurement of limb blood flow. IEEE Trans Biomed Eng 22:25-29, 1975.

[81]   Anderson TJ: Assessment and treatment of endothelial dysfunction in humans. J Am Coll Cardiol 34:631-638, 1999.

[82]   Linder L, Kiowski W, Buhler FR, Luscher TF: Indirect evidence for release of endothelium-derived relaxing factor in human forearm circulation in vivo. Blunted response in essential hypertension. Circulation 81:1762-1767, 1990.

[83]   Panza JA, Quyyuml AA, Brush Jr JE, Epstein SE: Abnormal endothelium-dependent vascular relaxation in patients with essential hypertension. New England Journal of Medicine 323:22-27, 1990.

[84]   Creager MA, Cooke JP, Mendelsohn ME, Gallagher SJ, Coleman SM, Loscalzo J, Dzau VJ: Impaired vasodilation of forearm resistance vessels in hypercholesterolemic humans. J Clin Invest 86:228-234, 1990.

[85]   Johnstone MT, Creager SJ, Scales KM, Cusco JA, Lee BK, Creager MA: Impaired endothelium-dependent vasodilation in patients with insulin-dependent diabetes mellitus. Circulation 88:2510-2516, 1993.

[86]   Chowienczyk PJ, Watts GF, Cockcroft JR, Ritter JM: Impaired endothelium-dependent vasodilation of forearm resistance vessels in hypercholesterolaemia. Lancet 340:1430-1432, 1992.

[87]   Williams SB, Cusco JA, Roddy MA, Johnstone MT, Creager MA: Impaired nitric oxide-mediated vasodilation in patients with non-insulin-dependent diabetes mellitus. J Am Coll Cardiol 27:567-574, 1996.

[88]   Anderson TJ, Uehata A, Gerard MD, Meredith IT, Knab S, Delagrange D, et al: Close relation of endothelial function in the human coronary and peripheral circulations. Journal of the American College of Cardiology 26:1235-1241, 1995.

[89]   Celermajer DS, Sorensen KE, Bull C, Robinson J, Deanfield JE: Endothelium-dependent dilation in the systemic arteries of asymptomatic subjects relates to coronary risk factors and their interaction. J Am Coll Cardiol 24:1468-1474, 1994.

[90]   Clarkson P, Celermajer DS, Donald AE, Sampson M, Sorensen KE, Adams M, Yue DK, Betteridge DJ, Deanfield JE: Impaired vascular reactivity in insulin-dependent diabetes mellitus is related to disease duration and low density lipoprotein cholesterol levels. J Am Coll Cardiol 28:573-579, 1996.

[91]   Lambert J, Aarsen M, Donker AJ, Stehouwer CD: Endothelium-dependent and -independent vasodilation of large arteries in normoalbuminuric insulin-dependent diabetes mellitus. Arterioscler Thromb Vasc Biol 16:705-711, 1996.

[92]   Schachinger V, Britten MB, Zeiher AM: Prognostic impact of coronary vasodilator dysfunction on adverse long-term outcome of coronary heart disease. Circulation 101:1899-1906, 2000.

[93]   Suwaidi JA, Hamasaki S, Higano ST, Nishimura RA, Holmes DR, Jr., Lerman A: Long-term follow-up of patients with mild coronary artery disease and endothelial dysfunction. Circulation 101:948-954, 2000.

[94]   Lind L, Hall J, Johansson K: Evaluation of four different methods to measure endothelium-dependent vasodilation in the human peripheral circulation. Clin Sci (Lond) 102:561-567, 2002.

[95]   Lind L, Hall J, Larsson A, Annuk M, Fellstrom B, Lithell H: Evaluation of endothelium-dependent vasodilation in the human peripheral circulation. Clin Physiol 20:440-448, 2000.

[96]   Laakso M, Edelman SV, Brechtel G, Baron AD: Decreased effect of insulin to stimulate skeletal muscle blood flow in obese man. A novel mechanism for insulin resistance. J Clin Invest 85:1844-1852, 1990.

[97]   Baron AD, Laakso M, Brechtel G, Edelman SV: Reduced capacity and affinity of skeletal muscle for insulin-mediated glucose uptake in noninsulin-dependent diabetic subjects. Effects of insulin therapy. J Clin Invest 87:1186-1194, 1991.

[98]   Baron AD, Steinberg HO, Chaker H, Leaming R, Johnson A, Brechtel G: Insulin-mediated skeletal muscle vasodilation contributes to both insulin sensitivity and responsiveness in lean humans. J Clin Invest 96:786-792, 1995.

[99] Cleland SJ, Petrie JR, Ueda S, Elliott HL, Connell JM: Insulin-mediated vasodilation and glucose uptake are functionally linked in humans. Hypertension 33:554-558, 1999.

[100] Wilkinson IB, Webb DJ: Venous occlusion plethysmography in cardiovascular research: methodology and clinical applications. Br J Clin Pharmacol 52:631-646, 2001.

[101] Joannides R, Bellien J, Thuillez C: Clinical methods for the evaluation of endothelial function-- a focus on resistance arteries. Fundam Clin Pharmacol 20:311-320, 2006.

[102] Dahn I, Hallbook T: Simultaneous blood flow measurements by water and strain gauge plethysmography. Scand J Clin Lab Invest 25:419-428, 1970.

[103] Webb DJ: The pharmacology of human blood vessels in vivo. J Vasc Res 32:2-15, 1995.

[104] Gilligan DM, Guetta V, Panza JA, Garcia CE, Quyyumi AA, Cannon RO, III: Selective loss of microvascular endothelial function in human hypercholesterolemia. Circulation 90:35-41, 1994.

[105] Higashi Y, Sasaki S, Kurisu S, Yoshimizu A, Sasaki N, Matsuura H, Kajiyama G, Oshima T: Regular aerobic exercise augments endothelium-dependent vascular relaxation in normotensive as well as hypertensive subjects: role of endothelium-derived nitric oxide. Circulation 100:1194-1202, 1999.

[106] Taddei S, Virdis A, Ghiadoni L, Mattei P, Sudano I, Bernini G, Pinto S, Salvetti A: Menopause is associated with endothelial dysfunction in women. Hypertension 28:576-582, 1996.

[107] Joyner MJ, Dietz NM, Shepherd JT: From Belfast to Mayo and beyond: the use and future of plethysmography to study blood flow in human limbs. J Appl Physiol 91:2431-2441, 2001.

[108] DeSouza CA, Shapiro LF, Clevenger CM, Dinenno FA, Monahan KD, Tanaka H, Seals DR: Regular aerobic exercise prevents and restores age-related declines in endothelium-dependent vasodilation in healthy men. Circulation 102:1351-1357, 2000.

[109] Taddei S, Galetta F, Virdis A, Ghiadoni L, Salvetti G, Franzoni F, Giusti C, Salvetti A: Physical activity prevents age-related impairment in nitric oxide availability in elderly athletes. Circulation 101:2896-2901, 2000.

[110] Sasaki S, Higashi Y, Nakagawa K, Kimura M, Noma K, Sasaki S, Hara K, Matsuura H, Goto C, Oshima T, Chayama K: A low-calorie diet improves endothelium-dependent vasodilation in obese patients with essential hypertension. Am J Hypertens 15:302-309, 2002.

[111] Taddei S, Virdis A, Ghiadoni L, Magagna A, Salvetti A: Vitamin C improves endothelium-dependent vasodilation by restoring nitric oxide activity in essential hypertension. Circulation 97:2222-2229, 1998.

[112] de Aguiar LG, Bahia LR, Villela N, Laflor C, Sicuro F, Wiernsperger N, Bottino D, Bouskela E: Metformin improves endothelial vascular reactivity in first-degree relatives of type 2 diabetic patients with metabolic syndrome and normal glucose tolerance. Diabetes Care 29:1083-1089, 2006.

[113] Bahia L, Aguiar LG, Villela N, Bottino D, Godoy-Matos AE, Geloneze B, Tambascia M, Bouskela E: Adiponectin is associated with improvement of endothelial function after rosiglitazone treatment in non-diabetic individuals with metabolic syndrome. Atherosclerosis 195:138-146, 2007.

[114] Pasimeni G, Ribaudo MC, Capoccia D, Rossi F, Bertone C, Leonetti F, Santiemma V: Non-invasive evaluation of endothelial dysfunction in uncomplicated obesity: relationship with insulin resistance. Microvasc Res 71:115-120, 2006.

[115] Takeshita A, Mark AL: Decreased vasodilator capacity of forearm resistance vessels in borderline hypertension. Hypertension 2:610-616, 1980.

[116] Conway J: A vascular abnormality in hypertension. A study of blood flow in the forearm. Circulation 27:520-529, 1963.

[117] Folkow B: Physiological aspects of primary hypertension. Physiol Rev 62:347-504, 1982.

[118] Julius S, Mejia A, Jones K, Krause L, Schork N, van d, V, Johnson E, Petrin J, Sekkarie MA, Kjeldsen SE, .: "White coat" versus "sustained" borderline hypertension in Tecumseh, Michigan. Hypertension 16:617-623, 1990.

[119] Brown E, Greenfield DM, Goei JS, Plassaras G: Filling and emptying of the low-pressure blood vessels of the human forearm. J Appl Physiol 21:573-582, 1966.

[120] Gamble J, Gartside IB, Christ F: A reassessment of mercury in silastic strain gauge plethysmography for microvascular permeability assessment in man. J Physiol 464:407-422, 1993.

[121] Roberts DH, Tsao Y, Breckenridge AM: The reproducibility of limb blood flow measurements in human volunteers at rest and after exercise by using mercury-in-Silastic strain gauge plethysmography under standardized conditions. Clin Sci (Lond) 70:635-638, 1986.

[122] Cooke JP, Dzau VJ: Nitric oxide synthase: role in the genesis of vascular disease. Annu Rev Med 48:489-509, 1997.

[123] Petrie JR, Ueda S, Morris AD, Murray LS, Elliott HL, Connell JM: How reproducible is bilateral forearm plethysmography? Br J Clin Pharmacol 45:131-139, 1998.

[124] Walker HA, Jackson G, Ritter JM, Chowienczyk PJ: Assessment of forearm vasodilator responses to acetylcholine and albuterol by strain gauge plethysmography: reproducibility and influence of strain gauge placement. Br J Clin Pharmacol 51:225-229, 2001.

[125] Chou CC, Hsieh CP, Yu YM, Kvietys P, Yu LC, Pittman R, Dabney JM: Localization of mesenteric hyperemia during digestion in dogs. Am J Physiol 230:583-589, 1976.

[126] Wei K, Jayaweera AR, Firoozan S, Linka A, Skyba DM, Kaul S: Quantification of myocardial blood flow with ultrasound-induced destruction of microbubbles administered as a constant venous infusion. Circulation 97:473-483, 1998.

[127]   Krix M, Weber MA, Krakowski-Roosen H, Huttner HB, Delorme S, Kauczor HU, Hildebrandt W: Assessment of skeletal muscle perfusion using contrast-enhanced ultrasonography. J Ultrasound Med 24:431-441, 2005.

[128]   Clark MG, Rattigan S, Barrett EJ, Vincent MA: Point: There is capillary recruitment in active skeletal muscle during exercise. J Appl Physiol 104:889-891, 2008.

[129]   Wei K, Skyba DM, Firschke C, Jayaweera AR, Lindner JR, Kaul S: Interactions between microbubbles and ultrasound: in vitro and in vivo observations. J Am Coll Cardiol 29:1081-1088, 1997.

[130]   Dawson D, Vincent MA, Barrett EJ, Kaul S, Clark A, Leong-Poi H, Lindner JR: Vascular recruitment in skeletal muscle during exercise and hyperinsulinemia assessed by contrast ultrasound. Am J Physiol Endocrinol Metab 282:E714-E720, 2002.

[131]   Vincent MA, Clerk LH, Lindner JR, Price WJ, Jahn LA, Leong-Poi H, Barrett EJ: Mixed meal and light exercise each recruit muscle capillaries in healthy humans. Am J Physiol Endocrinol Metab 290:E1191-E1197, 2006.

[132]   Mahajan H, Richards SM, Rattigan S, Clark MG: Local methacholine but not bradykinin potentiates insulin-mediated glucose uptake in muscle in vivo by augmenting capillary recruitment. Diabetologia 47:2226-2234, 2004.

[133]   Rattigan S, Clark MG, Barrett EJ: Hemodynamic actions of insulin in rat skeletal muscle: evidence for capillary recruitment. Diabetes 46:1381-1388, 1997.

[134]   Vincent MA, Clerk LH, Lindner JR, Klibanov AL, Clark MG, Rattigan S, Barrett EJ: Microvascular recruitment is an early insulin effect that regulates skeletal muscle glucose uptake in vivo. Diabetes 53:1418-1423, 2004.

[135]   Zhang L, Vincent MA, Richards SM, Clerk LH, Rattigan S, Clark MG, Barrett EJ: Insulin sensitivity of muscle capillary recruitment in vivo. Diabetes 53:447-453, 2004.

[136]   Mahajan H, Kolka CM, Newman JM, Rattigan S, Richards SM, Clark MG: Vascular and metabolic effects of methacholine in relation to insulin action in muscle. Diabetologia 49:713-723, 2006.

[137]   Rattigan S, Zhang L, Mahajan H, Kolka CM, Richards SM, Clark MG: Factors influencing the hemodynamic and metabolic effects of insulin in muscle. Curr Diabetes Rev 2:61-70, 2006.

[138]   Coppack SW, Persson M, Miles JM: Phenylalanine kinetics in human adipose tissue. J Clin Invest 98:692-697, 1996.

[139]   Kjellmer I, Lindbjerg I, Prerovsky I, Tonnesen H: The relation between blood flow in an isolated muscle measured with the Xe133 clearance and a direct recording technique. Acta Physiol Scand 69:69-78, 1967.

[140]   Lalande S, Gusso S, Hofman PL, Baldi JC: Reduced leg blood flow during submaximal exercise in type 2 diabetes. Med Sci Sports Exerc 40:612-617, 2008.

[141]   Hachiya T, Blaber AP, Saito M: Near-infrared spectroscopy provides an index of blood flow and vasoconstriction in calf skeletal muscle during lower body negative pressure. Acta Physiol (Oxf) 193:117-127, 2008.

[142]   Heinonen I, Nesterov SV, Kemppainen J, Nuutila P, Knuuti J, Laitio R, Kjaer M, Boushel R, Kalliokoski KK: Role of adenosine in regulating the heterogeneity of skeletal muscle blood flow during exercise in humans. J Appl Physiol 103:2042-2048, 2007.

CHAPTER 3

Microvascular Dysfunction in Insulin Resistance

Jefferson C. Frisbee and Robert W. Brock

Department of Physiology and Pharmacology, Center for Cardiovascular and Respiratory Sciences, West Virginia University Health Sciences Center, Morgantown, WV

Address Correspondence: Dr. Jefferson C. Frisbee. Department of Physiology and Pharmacology, Center for Cardiovascular and Respiratory Sciences, 1 Medical Center Drive; HSN 3152, West Virginia University Health Sciences Center, Morgantown, WV 26506; Phone: (304)293-6527; Fax:(304)293-5513; Email: jfrisbee@hsc.wvu.edu

Abstract: The increasing incidence and prevalence of insulin resistance and its associated co-morbidities represents a growing concern to public health policy across developed economies world wide. While the economic and psycho-social implications of insulin resistance and the ultimate development of type II diabetes mellitus are profound, much of this is associated with the increased probability of afflicted individuals for the development of peripheral vascular disease; with the hallmark characteristics of impaired matching of skeletal muscle perfusion with elevated metabolic demand. Two models of insulin resistance are highlighted in this chapter: the fructose-fed rodent model (which develops insulin resistance in the absence of obesity) and the obese Zucker rat (which develops insulin resistance subsequent to a chronic hyperphagia). While this chapter provides an overview of some of the skeletal muscle perfusion impairments associated with insulin resistance and its satellite co-morbidities, it also provides a discussion of key contributing elements to this relative ischemic condition. Specifically, this chapter will discuss the contributions of altered vascular reactivity from the perspective of both dilator and constrictor responses, the impact of insulin resistance on potassium channel function, structural alterations to microvascular networks (microvascular rarefaction), and the impact of insulin resistance on patterns of capillary recruitment. What rapidly becomes apparent is that the profound impact of pathological states such as insulin resistance on skeletal muscle perfusion represents a spatially and temporally distributed outcome with many contributors resulting in an integrated negative outcome.

Keywords: Vascular reactivity, vasculopathy, impaired glycemic control, skeletal muscle perfusion.

1. INTRODUCTION

Insulin resistance is defined as an evolving impairment to the body's ability to respond to insulin secreted from the pancreas in response to hyperglycemic stimuli, and can be characterized by normoglycemic hyperinsulinemia or fasting hyperinsulinemia [1, 2]. This is reflective of a condition wherein the ability of insulin secreted by the pancreas to reduce plasma glucose levels through either suppression of hepatic glucose production or increased skeletal muscle or adipose tissue glucose utilization is compromised. The origins of insulin resistance are divergent across afflicted individuals, existing within both polygenic and environmental cues [3]. Genetic mutations, while rare, can impair function at the insulin receptor, although more commonly, mutations at sites distal to insulin binding (tyrosine kinase activity, GLUT-4 transporter activity, glycogen synthase activity) are also potential sites for dysfunction [3]. Additional sites for impairment include genes encoding insulin receptor substrate 1 [4], glycogen synthase [5] and the regulatory subunits of protein tyrosine phosphatase-1β [6] have all been associated with insulin resistance, although their importance remains unclear. Alternately, chronic consumption of an excess of dietary caloric intake, creating a condition of positive energy balance, coupled with a sedentary lifestyle increases the risk for the development of increased adiposity, a key risk factor for the development of insulin resistance [2].

Given the considerable importance of insulin resistance, and the potential for the development of type II diabetes mellitus on public health and health outcomes, numerous animal models of insulin resistance have been developed for interrogating vascular function within this setting, including both mouse [7], and rat models [8]. With specific regard to the alterations in vascular reactivity, two rat models of insulin resistance have recently undergone intensive study; the obese Zucker rat (*fa/fa*) and the high fructose-diet fed rat. The obese Zucker rat (OZR) is characterized by a dysfunctional leptin receptor gene, and as such exhibits profound leptin resistance. Due to this genetic alteration, OZR demonstrate an impaired satiety reflex, and experience profound chronic hyperphagia [9] with the ensuing development of obesity, insulin resistance, dyslipidemia and moderate hypertension versus its control strain, the lean Zucker rat. The OZR represents an excellent candidate model for the study of the effects of insulin resistance, as evolution of this condition parallels that most commonly found in the afflicted human population (i.e., chronic elevations in food intake). In contrast, the fructose-fed rat (FFR) model of insulin resistance employs otherwise normal animals chronically ingesting a diet consisting of ~66% fructose [10]. After several weeks, these animals develop severe insulin resistance, yet lack the confounding influences of obesity and fasting hyperglycemia. Hypertriglyceridemia and a moderate, clinically relevant, hypertension are present to a comparable extent in both the OZR and the fructose-fed rat (FFR) models of insulin resistance.

2. INSULIN RESISTANCE AND SKELETAL MUSCLE PERFUSION

The regulation of skeletal muscle perfusion is ultimately tied to its local metabolic demands, as elevated metabolic rate mandates an increased convective and diffusive delivery of substrate (and removal of metabolic end-product). This response is termed active or functional hyperemia and is associated with a reduction in vascular tone, resulting in an increased perfusion. Multiple contributing parameters are associated with the regulation of skeletal muscle perfusion, including the production of metabolic end-products from skeletal muscle metabolism which cause dilator responses, intralumenal pressure-induced (myogenic) responses, propagated/conducted responses, adrenergic tone and the production and release of endothelium-derived factors (i.e., nitric oxide, prostaglandins, and hyperpolarizing factors which can impact potassium channel function). In addition to these 'active' processes, an array of structural elements of vascular biology can also impact skeletal muscle perfusion, including the mechanical characteristics of the vascular wall and the capillary density within skeletal muscle.

As insulin resistance represents a systemic pathology of metabolic origin, it can lead to a profound increase in the risk for developing peripheral vascular disease, with its defining characteristic of impaired perfusion:metabolic demand matching. This negative outcome has been demonstrated previously in multiple clinical populations with impaired glycemic control [11-14]. Additionally, in OZR, impaired functional hyperemia in skeletal muscle has been indentified by multiple investigators using numerous tissue preparations [15, 16]. However, individual mechanisms regulating vascular tone integrate to produce this negative perfusion outcome are currently unclear and will be discussed below.

3. INSULIN RESISTANCE AND VASCULAR REACTIVITY

Almost without exception, the existing literature clearly indicates that the evolution of insulin resistance in both OZR and FFR models results in a dramatic impairment to the dilator reactivity of small arteries and arterioles throughout the body. Using OZR, endothelial dependent dilation of skeletal muscle [17, 18], cerebral [19], renal [20] and mesenteric [21] arteries and arterioles are strongly impaired versus responses in control rats Fig. (**1**). As representative examples, the ability of renal arterioles to dilate in response to challenge with acetylcholine in OZR was significantly impaired versus responses determined in control strains [20]. Further, the ability of norepinephrine-preconstricted mesenteric arteries to dilate in response to challenge with acetylcholine or sodium nitroprusside was reduced in OZR versus controls [21]. More recently, Frisbee and colleagues demonstrated that the ability of skeletal muscle arterioles to dilate in response to reduced oxygen tension or elevated wall shear rate is strongly impaired in OZR versus lean Zucker rats.

Microvessels from FFR demonstrate a similar pattern of impaired dilator reactivity to endothelium-dependent stimuli as demonstrated in OZR. Initial studies by Miller and colleagues have clearly demonstrated that the dilator responses of isolated coronary [22] and mesenteric arteries [23] in response to acetylcholine were impaired in FFR as compared to responses determined in vessels from rats fed a normal diet. Specifically, the authors demonstrated that acetylcholine-induced dilation of mesenteric arteries was impaired in vessels from FFR [23], while a supplemental study by this same group found that a similar pattern of impaired vasodilator responses was also present in coronary arteries of FFR, as vasodilation in response to application of acetylcholine was impaired in these vessels as well [22]. However, while Miller *et al.* suggested that this impaired reactivity was not associated with arachidonic acid metabolism via cyclooxygenase, it might be due to a decrease in an endothelial-derived hyperpolarizing factor, as a pharmacological blockade of Ca^{2+}-activated K^+ channels with a combination of charybdotoxin and apamin, while severely attenuating acetylcholine-induced dilation of coronary arteries of control rats, had a negligible effect in insulin resistant animals. Further, Katakam *et al.* determined that this pattern of impaired vasomotor responses in mesenteric arteries of FFR was most likely due to the progression of insulin resistance, *per se*, as the impaired dilator responses of these vessels in response to application of acetylcholine significantly preceded the evolution of any elevation in mean arterial pressure [10], similar to responses demonstratd in the cerebral circulation of FFR by Erdos *et al.* [24].

4. INSULIN RESISTANCE AND POTASSIUM CHANNEL FUNCTION

A recent study, using primarily the FFR model of insulin resistance, has specifically addressed alterations to the behavior of K^+ channels in vascular smooth muscle which could contribute to impaired dilator reactivity Fig. (**1**). In insulin-resistant FFR, mesenteric arterial dilation in response to application of 11, 12-epoxyeicosatrienoic acids (11,12 EETs) and 14,15-EETs [dependent primarily on an increased open probability of K_{Ca} in vascular smooth muscle] was reduced compared to responses in arteries from control rats [25]. Further, arterial dilation in response to EET application was attenuated in vessels from control animals following blockade of K_{Ca} channels, although treatment of vessels from FFR with these agents had no effect on responses to EETs. Additional investigation of K^+ channel function in mesenteric arterial myocytes from FFR indicated that, in the cell-attached configuration, the ability of EETs to increase K_{Ca} channel activity was reduced in cells from FFR versus control animals. In contrast, in the inside-out patch clamp configuration, K_{Ca} channel activity was elevated following application of EETs to a comparable extent between insulin resistant rats and control animals. The results from this study clearly suggested that the impaired dilator reactivity to EET application in vessels from insulin-resistant rats may be due to an alteration in the signal transduction pathways regulating the open state probability of K_{Ca} channels rather than a specific alteration in their function *per se*.

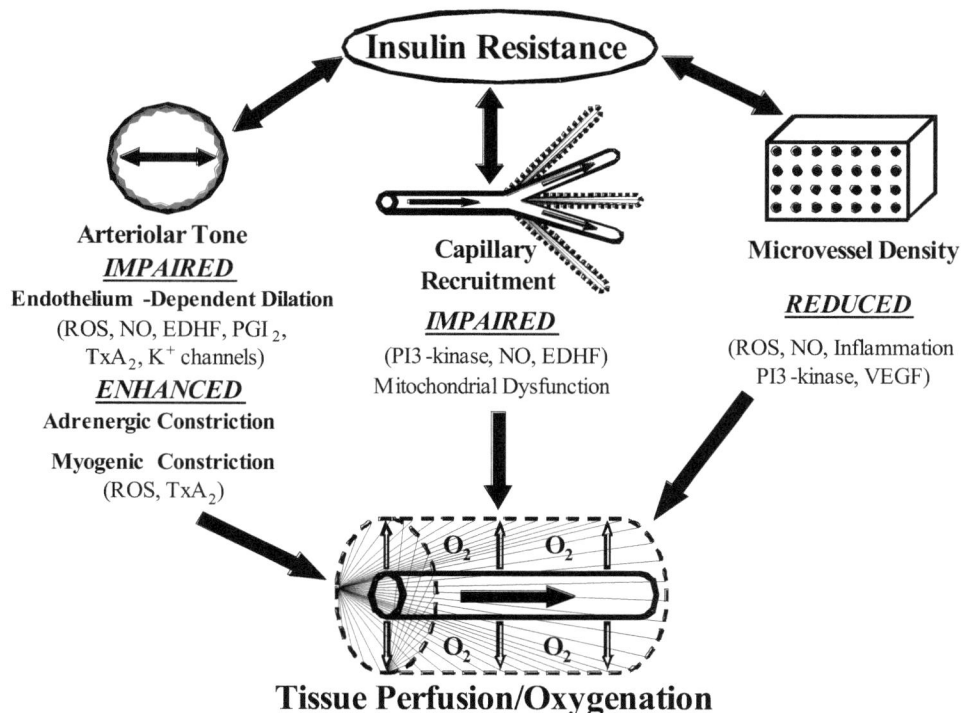

Figure 1: Schematic depiction of the integrated effects of insulin resistance on arteriolar tone regulation, capillary recruitment and microvessel density, and their impact on outcomes for tissue perfusion and oxygenation (O_2). Abbreviations: ROS=reactive oxygen species, NO=nitric oxide, EDHF=endothelium-derived hyperpolarizing factor, VEGF=vascular endothelial growth factor, PGI$_2$=prostacyclin, TxA$_2$=thromboxane A$_2$, K^+ channels=potassium channels (K_{Ca}, K_{ATP}).

In a follow-up study, it was demonstrated that current density via K_{Ca} channels was reduced in mesenteric arteries from insulin-resistant FFR versus control animals [26]. Further, the authors demonstrated that pharmacological inhibition of K_{Ca} channels from FFR caused a greater reduction in the K^+ current in arterial myocytes from control animals than from insulin resistant ones, while pharmacological activation of K_{Ca} channels was more effective at increasing outward current in control versus insulin-resistant rats. These results strongly suggested that a decreased K^+ current in vessels from insulin-resistant rats was not due to alterations in either channel expression or the inherent physical properties of the individual channels themselves, but rather that a distinct external mechanism might contribute to impaired K_{Ca} channel function.

Additional study [23, 24] has supported these observations, demonstrating that a qualitatively similar impairment in the function of both K_{ATP} and K_{Ca} channel activity was also occurring in the middle cerebral and mesenteric arteries of FFR and may contribute to the compromised dilator reactivity of those vessels as well. Somewhat contrasting results were identified in the OZR model of insulin resistance, as dilator responses of skeletal muscle arterioles was not impaired in response to application of K_{ATP} channel activators [17], although the effects of iberiotoxin on vascular tone [27] were similar to that determined in the arteries of FFR, discussed above.

One of the most consistent observations regarding vascular function in insulin resistance is an impaired endothelium-dependent vasodilation across tissues and organs, suggesting the likelihood of common mechanisms underlying this compromised outcome. As examples, within skeletal muscles of OZR, dilator responses to elevated wall shear [28], acetylcholine [28, 29] or arachidonic acid [16, 28] have consistently been demonstrated to be reduced below that in lean rats. The impairments to endothelium-dependent dilation have also been verified using isolated skeletal muscle arterioles, as Johnson *et al.* [30] demonstrated an impaired acetylcholine- and shear-induced dilation in arterioles from OZR, results that are consistent with previous studies demonstrating an impaired endothelium-dependent dilation of isolated arterioles in response to acetylcholine, reduced oxygen tension, and arachidonic acid. While isolated reports of an impaired vasodilation in response to endothelium-independent stimuli exist, the overwhelming majority of the literature suggests that dilator reactivity following direct activation of the smooth muscle is near normal across vascular beds within OZR.

As many of the studies cited above have employed shear-induced and acetylcholine-induced dilation, both highly dependent on the appropriate production and bioavailability of NO from the endothelium, several studies have targeted these processes for elucidating mechanisms of the impaired response in OZR. Fulton *et al.* [31] demonstrated that eNOS expression patterns, phosphorylation and binding to HSP-90 are not altered in OZR relative to controls, and concluded that mechanisms underlying the reduced vascular reactivity to endothelium- and NO-dependent stimuli must lie elsewhere, citing possible cofactor or substrate bioavailability limitations or elevated scavenging actions of superoxide anion.

An elevated vascular oxidant stress in insulin resistance has been well documented, and several investigators have pursued this, treating animals with an array of oxidative radical scavengers in an attempt to restore NO bioavailability and vascular reactivity. In general, treatment of OZR with antioxidants has improved vasodilator responses to NO-dependent stimuli in microvessels [15, 28], suggesting that endothelium-dependent dilation can be improved by acute treatment with oxidative radical scavengers which, by extension, implicates scavenging of NO as a key contributor to compromised dilator responses in OZR. Interestingly, recent study by Geakelman *et al.* [32] provided insight into this area as they determined that chronic treatment of Zucker diabetic fatty rats (which develop type II diabetes mellitus more rapidly than do OZR), with a peroxynitrite scavenger improved acetylcholine-induced dilation of renal microvessels, bringing into question the concept of which process is more important, the reduction in NO bioavailability or the generation of peroxynitrite. This may be a key consideration as it has been identified that peroxynitrite can antagonize calcium-activated potassium (K_{Ca}) channels in smooth muscle cells, thereby preventing membrane hyperpolarization in the face of elevated calcium [33]. A number of other mechanisms have been investigated in OZR which could contribute to a reduction in NO bioavailability and compromised arterial/arteriolar dilator reactivity, including increased expression and activity of protein kinase □II which act to constrain stimulus-induced NO formation [34], and the role of heme oxygenase derived carbon monoxide production as a contributor to inhibiting NOS [30].

The demonstration that peroxynitrite, produced via the interaction of superoxide anion with nitric oxide, had the potential to impact the regulation of vascular tone by inhibiting the open state probability of vascular K_{Ca} channels, has significant implications for the vascular reactivity within the setting of insulin resistance. In an initial study, it was demonstrated that this process may be central to the increased myogenic activation of skeletal muscle resistance arterioles of OZR in response to elevated intralumenal pressure [27]. Additionally, it was determined in this study that direct application of peroxynitrite to arterioles of OZR caused a pronounced pressure-dependent vasoconstriction, which was completely blocked by prior incubation of vessels with iberiotoxin.

More recently, Erdos and colleagues examined the role of elevated oxidant tone in contributing to the altered vascular reactivity determined in small resistance arteries of the cerebral circulation within both the FFR [35] and OZR [19] models of insulin resistance. Using isolated middle cerebral arteries, Erdos *et al.* [35] demonstrated that dilator responses to both K_{Ca} channel-dependent and K_{ATP} channel-dependent agonists were impaired in FFR versus responses in vessels from control animals. However, incubation of vessels with anti-oxidants restored the dilator reactivity of vessels from FFR. Interestingly, vasodilator responses mediated through the inward-rectifier K^+ channels (K_{IR}, elevated extracellular K^+), were unaltered between vessels of the two animal groups, and pharmacological blockade of both K_{IR} (barium) and K_v channels (4-aminopyridine) resulted in a comparable constriction of middle cerebral arteries between the two groups.

5. VASOCONSTRICTOR REACTIVITY

Although having received considerably less attention, there is evidence that pathways associated with vasoconstriction may also be markedly altered in OZR and that that these may exhibit a much stronger influence on the evolving ischemia in skeletal muscle of these animals than do pathways of vasodilation. While isolated reports of increased vascular tone exists due to an increased myogenic activation [27], an elevated expression and activity of serotonin [36], and endothelin receptors [37] in skeletal muscle have been reported, it is unclear how these results would impact skeletal muscle perfusion, as the necessary analyses have not been performed.

With the development of obesity, an increased adrenergic activity is frequently observed [38], which can have a profound impact on the perfusion of tissues that are sensitive to adrenergic modulation. Carlson *et al.* [39] demonstrated that, with development of the metabolic syndrome in OZR, sympathetic nervous system activity was elevated as compared to levels in control animals. Building from this, it was determined that norepinephrine-induced constriction of skeletal muscle resistance arterioles was increased in OZR relative to that in lean animals, and that intravenous infusion of the $\Box_1$-adrenoreceptor antagonist prazosin caused a pronounced dilation of *in vivo* arterioles, significantly greater than in controls [40]. Moreover, phenylephrine-induced elevation in vascular resistance in the hindlimb of OZR was greater than that in lean Zucker rats [41]. Attempts at elucidating the mechanism underlying this increased adrenergic reactivity of skeletal muscle resistance arterioles in OZR have only recently been undertaken, although Naik *et al.* [42] has provided evidence suggesting that RhoA-kinase may play a significant role in increasing the sensitivity of the contractile machinery of the vascular smooth muscle cell of OZR in response to elevations in intracellular calcium levels.

Recent studies have begun to elucidate the significance of this increased adrenergic reactivity of the skeletal muscle microvessel of OZR for muscle perfusion. In *in situ* gastrocnemius muscle of OZR, the increased adrenergic vasoconstriction contributes to reduced skeletal muscle perfusion at rest, and in response to mild and moderate elevations in metabolic demand, as intravenous infusion of adrenergic antagonists restored perfusion in OZR to levels that were near those in control animals [43].

6. INSULIN RESISTANCE AND CAPILLARY RECRUITMENT

While previous study demonstrated that challenge with insulin increased muscle perfusion, correlated with glucose uptake [44], it has also been determined that this outcome is impaired in insulin resistant, obese subjects [44, 45]; Fig. (1). This difference highlights questions of whether insulin-mediated perfusion outcomes are associated with impairment in insulin resistant states, and the extent to which this contributes to impaired insulin-stimulated muscle glucose uptake. The issues began to become clarified when it was postulated that the importance of insulin's hemodynamic actions was associated with an increased capillary surface area for substrate (e.g., glucose) exchange [46]. Using recently developed techniques [14,15,18], including metabolism of 1-methylxanthine (1-MX) and contrast enhanced ultrasound (CEU), it has been demonstrated that skeletal muscle microcirculation is not fully perfused under resting conditions, and that both insulin and increased metabolic demand result in an increased microvascular volume or capillary recruitment [47].

Infusion of insulin results in capillary recruitment in both human subjects and rodent models [48, 49], and ongoing studies have demonstrated that this recruitment precedes any detectable alterations to bulk skeletal muscle perfusion [50]. This is a critical observation, as it suggests a temporal disconnect between changes to blood flow and glucose metabolism within perfused muscle [47], a concept that received further support when CEU demonstrated that insulin-mediated capillary recruitment not only preceded changes to bulk blood flow, but also downstream insulin signaling/glucose uptake [51]. Furthermore, it shows that insulin-induced capillary recruitment can occur independent of changes in total blood flow and glucose metabolism [52]. While the temporal nature of insulin-mediated capillary recruitment suggests independence from parenchymal myocytes [51], additional studies suggest the importance of PI3-kinase [9], endothelial nitric oxide production and bioavailability [54], as well as other endothelium derived hyperpolarizing factors [55].

A significant question that remains unanswered is whether the acute loss of insulin-mediated capillary recruitment contributes substantially to the development of insulin resistance within the skeletal muscle myocyte, essentially a "cause versus effect" issue. One hypothesis states that with impairment of insulin delivery to the muscle due to poor recruitment, plasma glucose levels will experience a retarded clearance, resulting in hyperglycemia that will then further impair insulin signaling in the skeletal muscle. Additionally, it has been suggested that mitochrondrial dysfunction associated with impaired glycemic control may also be associated with poor insulin-mediated capillary recruitment [56].

7. MICROVASCULAR RAREFACTION AND INSULIN RESISTANCE

While observations of obesity and insulin resistance as a pathological condition predisposing individuals to either a reduced tissue/organ microvessel density or an impaired response to an angiogenic stimulus have been made repeatedly in the existing literature [32, 57-59], it has also been frequently demonstrated that a reduced microvessel density (rarefaction) within the vascular networks can contribute to impairments in mass transport and exchange through two mechanisms. First, and most importantly, a loss of microvessel density will increase diffusion distances between adjacent microvessels [60], while secondly, it will also lead to an elevation in vascular resistance across tissues or organs owing to a reduction in the number of parallel pathways [61]. However, the mechanistic pathways leading to this microvessel loss have been less clearly elucidated.

In OZR, a progressive reduction in skeletal muscle microvessel density has been previously been demonstrated. However, while OZR also manifest a moderate hypertension, and hypertension has long been considered to be a strong stimulus for microvessel loss, it can be difficult to discern the extent to which either of these conditions (insulin resistance or elevated blood pressure, or both) contributes to the microvessel loss. As a further complication, the impact of these combined pathological states on microvascular outcomes can be difficult to discern owing to the close interrelationships between hypertension, insulin resistance, obesity and vascular dysfunction [62, 63]. In addition it is extremely complicated to determine the extent to which the progressive vascular dysfunction causes the increased insulin resistance and elevations in arterial pressure, or whether the systemic pathologies lead to the poor vascular outcomes. Previous study has addressed this issue in OZR, suggesting that microvessel loss does not reflect an adaptive response to hypertension, as the rarefaction significantly precedes the development of any discernible elevation in mean arterial pressure [64]. Similar results have also been identified by Toblli *et al.* [65, 66], wherein chronic treatment of OZR with the angiotensin converting enzyme inhibitor perindopril improved myocardial microvessel density over that determined in untreated control rats, and that these improvements were associated with increased expression of both vascular endothelial growth factor (VEGF) and endothelial nitric oxide synthase (eNOS), but were poorly associated with alterations to blood pressure Fig. (**1**).

Based on data discussed above, the role of eNOS and vascular NO bioavailability has recently received some attention in the literature. The importance of vascular NO bioavailability in terms of the regulation of microvascular density under obese, insulin resistant conditions was further emphasized when it was demonstrated that chronic treatment of the Zucker diabetic fatty rat with a peroxynitrite scavenger, blunted the nephropathy that develops in these animals and improves both the renal capillary density and the angiogenic competence of renal explants [32]. This concept was advanced further in recent studies, where chronic treatment of OZR with anti-oxidants only improved skeletal muscle microvessel density if this was associated with an increased vascular NO bioavailability [67]. More recent work from King's laboratory has suggested that the reduction in myocardial microvascular density in OZR was associated with an inhibition of the PI3K/Akt pathway activation and a consequent decrease in VEGF expression and a reduction in microvessel density, further implicating NO as a central mechanistic pathway underlying microvessel density regulation under these conditions [68].

One of the most powerful and clinically relevant for patients with insulin resistance, stimuli for increasing vascular NO bioavailability is chronic exercise [69, 70]. However, specific mechanisms responsible for the increased vascular NO bioavailability remain controversial, and may include eNOS gene transcription, protein translation, and oxidant defense mechanisms. The effects of chronic exercise training, of sufficient intensity, on increasing capillary density in control human and animal subjects has been well documented [58, 70-74], and this has been associated with a chronic increase in vascular NO bioavailability [75-77], and alterations to the profile of angiogenic/angiostatic growth factors [75, 78-80]. However, the study of chronic exercise training on peripheral microvascular density has not been thoroughly investigated in obese, insulin resistant subjects.

Although isolated reports exist to the contrary [81], the observation that exercise training can improve microvessel density have been well established in both the OZR model of obesity and insulin resistance [74, 82, 83], as well as in human subjects [58, 84]. Consistent among these observations is the demonstration that the severity of insulin resistance was also reduced as a result of exercise training and that this was tightly associated with an improvement in microvessel density. Despite a growing number of studies investigating the effects of exercise and microvessel density in obesity and insulin resistance, these have produced a fairly limited amount of information with regard to the mechanisms underlying these potentially ameliorative effects on skeletal muscle vascularity. Of some interest, however, was evidence that the improvement to microvacular density in the skeletal muscle of obese, insulin resistant Zucker rats as a result of chronic exercise may be well predicted by a reduction in chronic sub-acute inflammation [82]. Specifically, individual markers of inflammation that have previously been identified as being negatively correlated with both nitric oxide bioavailability and microvessel density, while putative pro-angiogenic markers were positively associated with both of these outcomes. Clearly, given the profound evidence for chronic inflammation as a contributor to vascular dysfunction in the obese and insulin resistant state [63], these interrelationships between NO bioavailability, oxidant stress and inflammation, and how they impact microvascular density through the effects on the angiogenic/angiostatic growth factor profiles will require considerable future investigation.

8. REFERENCES

[1]   American Diabetes Association. All About Insulin Resistance, Toolkit No. 5. American Diabetes Association Type II Diabetes Information: 2004.
[2]   American Heart Association. Insulin Resistance. American Heart Association Diseases and Conditions: 2004.
[3]   Perez-Martin A, Raynaud E, and Mercier J. Insulin resistance and associated metabolic abnormalities in muscle: effects of exercise. Obes.Rev. 2: 47-59, 2001.
[4]   Clausen JO, Hansen T, Bjorbaek C, Echwald SM, Urhammer SA, Rasmussen S, Andersen CB, Hansen L, Almind K, Winther K, and . Insulin resistance: interactions between obesity and a common variant of insulin receptor substrate-1. Lancet 346: 397-402, 1995.
[5]   Zouali H, Velho G, and Froguel P. Polymorphism of the glycogen synthase gene and non-insulin-dependent diabetes mellitus. N.Engl.J.Med. 328: 1568, 1993.
[6]   Olivier M, Hsiung CA, Chuang LM, Ho LT, Ting CT, Bustos VI, Lee TM, De Witte A, Chen YD, Olshen R, Rodriguez B, Wen CC, and Cox DR. Single nucleotide polymorphisms in protein tyrosine phosphatase 1{beta} (PTPN1) are associated with essential hypertension and obesity. Hum.Mol.Genet. 13: 1885-1892, 2004.
[7]   Nandi A, Kitamura Y, Kahn CR, and Accili D. Mouse models of insulin resistance. Physiol Rev. 84: 623-647, 2004.
[8]   Brindley DN, Russell JC. Animal models of insulin resistance and cardiovascular disease: some therapeutic approaches using JCR: LA-cp rat. Diabetes Obes.Metab 4: 1-10, 2002.
[9]   Mathe D. Dyslipidemia and diabetes: animal models. Diabete Metab 21: 106-111, 1995.
[10]   Katakam PV, Ujhelyi MR, Hoenig ME, and Miller AW. Endothelial dysfunction precedes hypertension in diet-induced insulin resistance. Am.J.Physiol 275: R788-R792, 1998.
[11]   Ribeiro MM, Silva AG, Santos NS, Guazzelle I, Matos LNJ, Trombetta IC, Halpern A, Negrao CE, Villares SMF. (2005). Diet and exercise training restore blood pressure and vasodilatory responses during physiological maneuvers in obese children. Circulation 111: 19151923.
[12]   Negrao CE, Trombetta IC, Batalha LT, Ribeiro MM, Rondon MUPB, Tinucci T, Forjaz CLM, Barretto ACP, Halpern A, Villares SMF. (2001). Muscle metaboreflex control is diminished in normotensive obese women. Am J Physiol Heart Circ Physiol 281: H469-H475.
[13]   Menon RK, Grace AA, Burgoyne W, Fonseca VA, James IM, Dandona P. (1992). Muscle blood flow in diabetes mellitus. Evidence of abnormality after exercise. Diabetes Care 15: 693-695.

[14]   Young JL, Pendergast DR, Steinbach J. (1991). Oxygen transport and peripheral microcirculation in long-term diabetes. Proc Soc Exp Biol Med 196: 61-68.

[15]   Frisbee JC. (2003). Impaired skeletal muscle perfusion in obese Zucker rats. Am J Physiol Regul Integr Comp Physiol 285: R1124-R1134.

[16]   Xiang L, Naik JS, Hodnett BL, Hester RL. (2006). Altered arachidonic acid metabolism impairs functional vasodilation in metabolic syndrome. Am J Physiol Regul Integr Comp Physiol 290: R134-R138.

[17]   Frisbee JC. Impaired dilation of skeletal muscle microvessels to reduced oxygen tension in diabetic obese Zucker rats. Am.J.Physiol Heart Circ.Physiol 281: H1568-H1574, 2001.

[18]   Laight DW, Desai KM, Anggard EE, and Carrier MJ. Endothelial dysfunction accompanies a pro-oxidant, pro-diabetic challenge in the insulin resistant, obese Zucker rat in vivo. Eur.J.Pharmacol. 402: 95-99, 2000.

[19]   Erdos B, Snipes JA, Miller AW, and Busija DW. Cerebrovascular dysfunction in Zucker obese rats is mediated by oxidative stress and protein kinase C. Diabetes 53: 1352-1359, 2004.

[20]   Hayashi K, Kanda T, Homma K, Tokuyama H, Okubo K, Takamatsu I, Tatematsu S, Kumagai H, and Saruta T. Altered renal microvascular response in Zucker obese rats. Metabolism 51: 1553-1561, 2002.

[21]   Wu X, Makynen H, Kahonen M, Arvola P, and Porsti I. Mesenteric arterial function in vitro in three models of experimental hypertension. J.Hypertens. 14: 365-372, 1996.

[22]   Miller AW, Katakam PV, and Ujhelyi MR. Impaired endothelium-mediated relaxation in coronary arteries from insulin-resistant rats. J.Vasc.Res. 36: 385-392, 1999.

[23]   Katakam PV, Ujhelyi MR, and Miller AW. EDHF-mediated relaxation is impaired in fructose-fed rats. J.Cardiovasc.Pharmacol. 34: 461-467, 1999.

[24]   Erdos B, Miller AW, and Busija DW. Impaired endothelium-mediated relaxation in isolated cerebral arteries from insulin-resistant rats. Am.J.Physiol Heart Circ.Physiol 282: H2060-H2065, 2002.

[25]   Miller AW, Dimitropoulou C, Han G, White RE, Busija DW, and Carrier GO. Epoxyeicosatrienoic acid-induced relaxation is impaired in insulin resistance. Am.J.Physiol Heart Circ.Physiol 281: H1524-H1531, 2001.

[26]   Dimitropoulou C, Han G, Miller AW, Molero M, Fuchs LC, White RE, and Carrier GO. Potassium (BK_{Ca}) currents are reduced in microvascular smooth muscle cells from insulin-resistant rats. Am.J.Physiol Heart Circ.Physiol 282: H908-H917, 2002.

[27]   Frisbee JC, Maier KG, and Stepp DW. Oxidant stress-induced increase in myogenic activation of skeletal muscle resistance arteries in obese Zucker rats. Am.J.Physiol Heart Circ.Physiol 283: H2160-H2168, 2002.

[28]   Frisbee JC, Stepp DW. Impaired NO-dependent dilation of skeletal muscle arterioles in hypertensive diabetic obese Zucker rats. Am J Physiol Heart Circ Physiol. 281: H1304-H1311, 2001.

[29]   Xiang L, Naik J, Hester RL. Exercise-induced increase in skeletal muscle vasodilatory responses in obese Zucker rats. Am J Physiol Regul Integr Comp Physiol. 288: R987-R991, 2005.

[30]   Johnson FK, Johnson RA, Durante W, Jackson KE, Stevenson BK, Peyton KJ. Metabolic syndrome increases endogenous carbon monoxide production to promote hypertension and endothelial dysfunction in obese Zucker rats. Am J Physiol Regul Integr Comp Physiol. 290: R601-R608, 2006.

[31]   Fulton D, Harris MB, Kemp BE, Venema RC, Marrero MB, Stepp DW. Insulin resistance does not diminish eNOS expression, phosphorylation, or binding to HSP-90. Am J Physiol Heart Circ Physiol. 287: H2384-H2393, 2004.

[32]   Geakelman O, Brodsky SV, Zhang F, Chander PN, Friedli C, Nasjletti A, Goligorsky MS. Endothelial dysfunction as a modifier of angiogenic response in Zucker diabetic fat rat: amelioration with Ebselen. Kidney Int. 66: 2337-2347, 2004.

[33]   Brzezinska AK, Gebremedhin D, Chilian WM, Kalyanaraman B, Elliott SJ. Peroxynitrite reversibly inhibits Ca(2+)-activated K(+) channels in rat cerebral artery smooth muscle cells. Am J Physiol Heart Circ Physiol. 278: H1883-H1890, 2000.

[34]   Bohlen HG. Protein kinase betaII in Zucker obese rats compromises oxygen and flow-mediated regulation of nitric oxide formation. Am J Physiol Heart Circ Physiol. 286: H492-H497, 2004.

[35]   Erdos B, Simandle SA, Snipes JA, Miller AW, and Busija DW. Potassium channel dysfunction in cerebral arteries of insulin-resistant rats is mediated by reactive oxygen species. Stroke 35: 964-969, 2004.

[36]   Janiak P, Lainee P, Grataloup Y, Luyt CE, Bidouard JP, Michel JB, O'Connor SE, Herbert JM. Serotonin receptor blockade improves distal perfusion after lower limb ischemia in the fatty Zucker rat. Cardiovasc Res. 56: 293-302, 2002.

[37]   Wu SQ, Hopfner RL, McNeill JR, Wilson TW, Gopalakrishnan V. Altered paracrine effect of endothelin in blood vessels of the hyperinsulinemic, insulin resistant obese Zucker rat. Cardiovasc Res. 45: 994-1000, 2000.

[38]   van Baak MA. The peripheral sympathetic nervous system in human obesity. Obes Rev. 2: 3-14, 2001.

[39]   Carlson SH, Shelton J, White CR, Wyss JM. Elevated sympathetic activity contributes to hypertension and salt sensitivity in diabetic obese Zucker rats. Hypertension. 35: 403-408, 2000.

[40]   Stepp DW, Frisbee JC. Augmented adrenergic vasoconstriction in hypertensive diabetic obese Zucker rats. Am J Physiol Heart Circ Physiol. 282: H816-H820, 2002.

[41]   Schreihofer AM, Hair CD, Stepp DW. Reduced plasma volume and mesenteric vascular reactivity in obese Zucker rats. Am J Physiol Regul Integr Comp Physiol. 288: R253-R261, 2005.

[42]   Naik JS, Xiang L, Hester RL. Enhanced role for RhoA-associated kinase in adrenergic-mediated vasoconstriction in gracilis arteries from obese Zucker rats. Am J Physiol Regul Integr Comp Physiol. 290: R154-R161, 2006.

[43] Frisbee JC. Enhanced arteriolar alpha-adrenergic constriction impairs dilator responses and skeletal muscle perfusion in obese Zucker rats. J Appl Physiol. 97: 764-772, 2004.

[44] Laakso, M., Edelman, S., Brechtel, G., Baron, A. (1990). Decreased effect of insulin to stimulate skeletal muscle blood flow in obese man. J Clin Invest 85: 1844-1852.

[45] Baron, A., Laakso, M., Brechtel, G., Edelman, S. (1991). Reduced capacity and affinity of skeletal muscle for insulin- mediated glucose uptake in noninsulin-dependent diabetic subjects. J Clin Invest 87: 1186-1194.

[46] Baron, A. (1994). Hemodynamic actions of insulin. Am J Physiol 267: E187-E202.

[47] Clark, M., Wallis, M., Barrett, E., Vincent, M., Richards, S., Clerk, L., Rattigan, S. (2003). Blood flow and muscle metabolism: a focus on insulin action. Am J Physiol Endocrinol Metab 284: E241-E258.

[48] Coggins, M., Lindner, J., Rattigan, S., Jahn, L., Fasy, E., Kaul, S., Barrett, E. (2001). Physiologic hyperinsulinemia enhances human skeletal muscle perfusion by capillary recruitment. Diabetes 50: 2682-2690.

[49] Rattigan, S., Clark, M., Barrett, E. (1999). Acute vasoconstriction-induced insulin resistance in rat muscle in vivo. Diabetes 48: 564-569.

[50] Vincent, M., Dawson, D., Clark, A., Lindner, J., Rattigan, S., Clark, M., Barrett, E. (2002). Skeletal muscle microvascular recruitment by physiological hyperinsulinemia precedes increases in total blood flow. Diabetes 51: 42-48.

[51] Vincent, M., Clerk, L., Lindner, J., Klibanov, A., Clark, M., Rattigan, S., Barrett, E. (2004). Microvascular recruitment is an early insulin effect that regulates skeletal muscle glucose uptake in vivo. Diabetes 53: 1418-1423.

[52] Zhang, L., Vincent, M., Richards, S., Clerk, L., Rattigan, S., Clark, M., Barrett, E. (2004). Insulin sensitivity of muscle capillary recruitment in vivo. Diabetes 53: 447-453.

[53] Bradley, E., Clark, M., Rattigan, S. (2006). Acute effects of wortmannin on insulin's hemodynamic and metabolic actions in vivo. Am J Physiol Endocrinol Metab In press.

[54] Vincent, M., Barrett, E., Lindner, J., Clark, M., Rattigan, S. (2003). Inhibiting NOS blocks microvascular recruitment and blunts muscle glucose uptake in response to insulin. Am J Physiol Endocrinol Metab 285: E123-E129.

[55] Rattigan, S., Zhang, L., Mahajan, H., Kolka, C., Richards, S., Clark, M. (2006). Factors influencing the hemodynamic and metabolic effects of insulin in muscle. Curr Diab Rev 2: 61-70.

[56] LeBrasseur, N., Ruderman, N. (2005). Why might thiazolidinediones increase exercise capacity in patients with type 2 diabetes? Diabetes Care 28: 2975-2977.

[57] Frisbee JC. Remodeling of the skeletal muscle microcirculation increases resistance to perfusion in obese Zucker rats. Am J Physiol Heart Circ Physiol. 2003; 285: H104-11.

[58] Gavin TP, Stallings HW 3rd, Zwetsloot KA, Westerkamp LM, Ryan NA, Moore RA, Pofahl WE, Hickner RC. Lower capillary density but no difference in VEGF expression in obese vs. lean young skeletal muscle in humans. J Appl Physiol. 2005; 98: 315-21.

[59] Green DJ, Maiorana A, O'Driscoll G, Taylor R. Effect of exercise training on endothelium-derived nitric oxide function in humans. J Physiol. 2004; 561: 1-25.

[60] Stainsby WN, Snyder B, Welch HG. A pictographic essay on blood and tissue oxygen transport. Med Sci Sports Exerc. 1988; 20: 213-21.

[61] Greene AS, Tonellato PJ, Zhang Z, Lombard JH, Cowley AW Jr. Effect of microvascular rarefaction on tissue oxygen delivery in hypertension. Am J Physiol. 1992; 262: H1486-93.

[62] Sharma AM, Chetty VT. Obesity, hypertension and insulin resistance. Acta Diabetol. 2005; 42 Suppl 1: S3-8.

[63] Dandona P, Aljada A, Chaudhuri A, Mohanty P, Garg R. Metabolic syndrome: a comprehensive perspective based on interactions between obesity, diabetes, and inflammation. Circulation. 2005; 111: 1448-54.

[64] Frisbee JC. Hypertension-independent microvascular rarefaction in the obese Zucker rat model of the metabolic syndrome. Microcirculation. 2005; 12: 383-92.

[65] Toblli JE, Cao G, DeRosa G, Di Gennaro F, Forcada P. Angiotensin-converting enzyme inhibition and angiogenesis in myocardium of obese Zucker rats. Am J Hypertens. 2004; 17: 172-80.

[66] Toblli JE, DeRosa G, Rivas C, Cao G, Piorno P, Pagano P, Forcada P. Cardiovascular protective role of a low-dose antihypertensive combination in obese Zucker rats. J Hypertens. 2003; 21: 611-20.

[67] Frisbee JC. Reduced nitric oxide bioavailability contributes to skeletal muscle microvessel rarefaction in the metabolic syndrome. Am J Physiol Regul Integr Comp Physiol. 2005; 289: R307-R316.

[68] He Z, Opland DM, Way KJ, Ueki K, Bodyak N, Kang PM, Izumo S, Kulkarni RN, Wang B, Liao R, Kahn CR, King GL. Regulation of vascular endothelial growth factor expression and vascularization in the myocardium by insulin receptor and PI3K/Akt pathways in insulin resistance and ischemia. Arterioscler Thromb Vasc Biol. 2006; 26: 787-93.

[69] Green DJ, Maiorana A, O'Driscoll G, Taylor R. Effect of exercise training on endothelium-derived nitric oxide function in humans. J Physiol. 2004; 561: 1-25.

[70] Maiorana A, O'Driscoll G, Taylor R, Green D. Exercise and the nitric oxide vasodilator system. Sports Med. 2003; 33: 1013-35.

[71] Ivy JL. Role of exercise training in the prevention and treatment of insulin resistance and non-insulin-dependent diabetes mellitus. Sports Med. 1997; 24: 321-36.

[72] Krotkiewski M, Bylund-Fallenius AC, Holm J, Bjorntorp P, Grimby G, Mandroukas K. Relationship between muscle morphology and metabolism in obese women: the effects of long-term physical training. Eur J Clin Invest. 1983; 13: 5-12.

[73]   Krotkiewski M. Physical training in the prophylaxis and treatment of obesity, hypertension and diabetes. Scand J Rehabil Med Suppl. 1983; 9: 55-70.

[74]   Lash JM, Sherman WM, Hamlin RL. Capillary basement membrane thickness and capillary density in sedentary and trained obese Zucker rats. Diabetes. 1989; 38: 854-60.

[75]   Benoit H, Jordan M, Wagner H, Wagner PD. Effect of NO, vasodilator prostaglandins, and adenosine on skeletal muscle angiogenic growth factor gene expression. J Appl Physiol. 1999; 86: 1513-8.

[76]   Buckwalter JB, Curtis VC, Valic Z, Ruble SB, Clifford PS. Endogenous vascular remodeling in ischemic skeletal muscle: a role for nitric oxide. J Appl Physiol. 2003; 94: 935-40.

[77]   Laufs U, Werner N, Link A, Endres M, Wassmann S, Jurgens K, Miche E, Bohm M, Nickenig G. Physical training increases endothelial progenitor cells, inhibits neointima formation, and enhances angiogenesis. Circulation. 2004; 109: 220-6.

[78]   Lloyd PG, Prior BM, Yang HT, Terjung RL. Angiogenic growth factor expression in rat skeletal muscle in response to exercise training. Am J Physiol Heart Circ Physiol. 2003; 284: H1668-78.

[79]   Lloyd PG, Prior BM, Li H, Yang HT, Terjung RL. VEGF receptor antagonism blocks arteriogenesis, but only partially inhibits angiogenesis, in skeletal muscle of exercise-trained rats. Am J Physiol Heart Circ Physiol. 2005; 288: H759-68.

[80]   Suzuki J. L-arginine supplementation causes additional effects on exercise-induced angiogenesis and VEGF expression in the heart and hind-leg muscles of middle-aged rats. J Physiol Sci. 2006; 56: 39-44.

[81]   Lithell H, Krotkiewski M, Kiens B, Wroblewski Z, Holm G, Stromblad G, Grimby G, Bjorntorp P. Non-response of muscle capillary density and lipoprotein-lipase activity to regular training in diabetic patients. Diabetes Res. 1985; 2: 17-21.

[82]   Frisbee JC, Samora JB, Peterson J, Bryner R. Exercise training blunts microvascular rarefaction in the metabolic syndrome. Am J Physiol Heart Circ Physiol. 2006; 291: H2483-92.

[83]   Torgan CE, Brozinick JT Jr, Kastello GM, Ivy JL. Muscle morphological and biochemical adaptations to training in obese Zucker rats. J Appl Physiol. 1989; 67: 1807-13.

[84]   Kern PA, Simsolo RB, Fournier M. Effect of weight loss on muscle fiber type, fiber size, capillarity, and succinate dehydrogenase activity in humans. J Clin Endocrinol Metab. 1999; 84: 4185-90.

CHAPTER 4

Microvascular Dysfunction: Potential Role in the Pathogenesis of Obesity-Associated Hypertension and Insulin Resistance

Erik H Serné[1], Rick I Meijer[1], Michiel P de Boer[1], Renate T de Jongh[1], Richard G IJzerman[1], Wineke Bakker[2] and Etto C Eringa[2]

[1]*Department of Internal Medicine and* [2]*Laboratory for Physiology, Institute for Cardiovascular Research, VU Medical Centre, Amsterdam, The Netherlands*

Abstract: The intertwined epidemics of obesity and related disorders such as hypertension, insulin resistance, type 2 diabetes, and subsequent cardiovascular disease pose a major public health challenge. To meet this challenge, we must understand the interplay between adipose tissue and the vasculature. Microvascular dysfunction is important not only in the development of obesity-related target-organ damage, but also in the development of cardiovascular risk factors such as hypertension and insulin resistance. The present chapter examines the role of microvascular dysfunction as an explanation for the associations among obesity, hypertension and impaired insulin-mediated glucose disposal. We also discuss communicative pathways from adipose tissue to the microcirculation.

Keywords: Obesity, hypertension, insulin resistance, microcirculation.

1. INTRODUCTION

The global epidemic of obesity is bringing in its wake a catastrophic increase in the prevalence of metabolic diseases. Obesity has been implicated in the rising prevalence of the metabolic syndrome, a cluster of risk factors including, hypertension, insulin resistance and dyslipidemia, which confers an increased risk for type 2 diabetes and cardiovascular disease (CVD) [1]. Although this is well recognized, the underlying mechanisms are poorly understood. Obesity-associated microvascular dysfunction is hypothesized to explain part of this clustering and predispose obese subjects to CVD [2]. Microvascular dysfunction, by affecting both flow resistance and tissue perfusion, seems important not only in the development of obesity-related target-organ damage in the heart and kidney, but also in the development of hypertension and insulin resistance [2-5].

We will discuss the role of microvascular dysfunction as an explanation for the associations among obesity, hypertension and impaired insulin-mediated glucose disposal. Subsequently, we will examine communicative pathways from adipose tissue to the microcirculation.

2. MICROVASCULAR DYSFUNCTION IN OBESITY, HYPERTENSION AND INSULIN RESISTANCE

Morphologically, the microcirculation is widely taken to encompass vessels < 150 μm in diameter. It therefore includes arterioles, capillaries, and venules. Alternatively, a definition based on arterial vessel physiology rather than diameter or structure has been proposed [3]. By this definition, all arterial vessels that respond to increasing pressure by a myogenic reduction in lumen diameter are included in the microcirculation. Such a definition would include the smallest arteries and arterioles in the microcirculation in addition to capillaries and venules. Small arterial and arteriolar components should, therefore, be considered a continuum rather than distinct sites of resistance control. A primary function of the microcirculation is to optimise nutrient and oxygen supply within the tissue in response to variations in demand. Adequate perfusion via the microcirculatory network is essential for the integrity of tissue and organ function. In addition, it is at the level of the microcirculation that a substantial proportion of the drop in hydrostatic pressure occurs. The microcirculation is therefore extremely important in determining overall peripheral vascular resistance.

Obesity, hypertension and insulin resistance are characterized by microvascular dysfunction. [3, 6-8] Dysfunction of the microvasculature at the level of both resistance vessels and the nutritive capillary beds develops progressively along with an increase in adiposity, even in children [9-11]. Impaired microvascular endothelium-dependent vasodilatation occurs in response to various vasodilators, including insulin [10,12,13]. Obese individuals demonstrate diminished capillary recruitment to reactive hyperaemia [10], which is inversely associated with visceral adiposity as measured with MRI and truncal subcutaneous adipose tissue using skinfold measurements [9].

In hypertension, the structure and function of the microcirculation are altered [3,14]. The mechanisms regulating vasomotor tone are abnormal, leading to enhanced vasoconstriction or reduced vasodilator responses to various vasodilators, including insulin [3,14,15]. Moreover, there are anatomic alterations in the structure of individual precapillary resistance vessels, such as an increase in their wall-to-lumen ratio. Finally, there are changes at the level of the microvascular network involving a reduction in the number of arterioles or capillaries within vascular beds of various tissues (e.g. muscle and skin), so called vascular rarefaction [3, 14, 16].

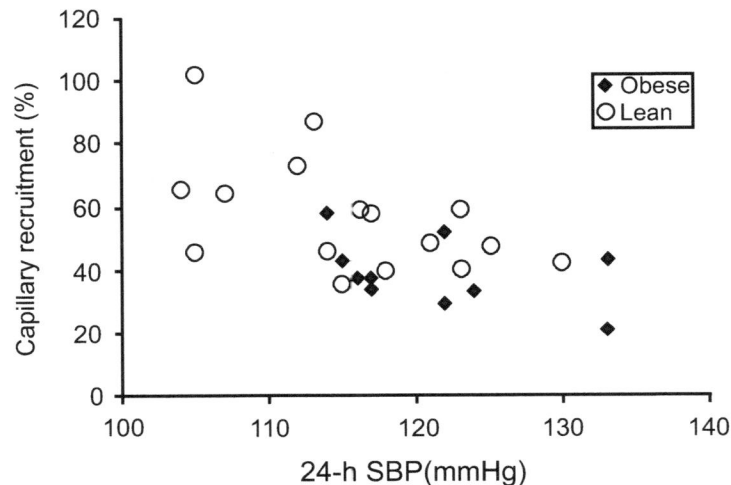

Figure 1: Inverse relationship between skin capillary recruitment and 24-hour systolic blood pressure (SBP) in lean and obese women. (Circulation. 2004; 109:2529)

Similar defects in microvascular function and structure are associated with insulin resistance, defined as decreased sensitivity and/or responsiveness to metabolic actions of insulin that promote glucose disposal. Capillary rarefaction is associated with insulin resistance [17]. In non-diabetic obese subjects as well as non-diabetic, overweight hypertensive patients endothelium-dependent vasodilatation and capillary recruitment to reactive hyperaemia are inversely associated with insulin sensitivity [10, 12, 16]. Even in healthy, normotensive non-obese subjects a direct relationship between insulin sensitivity and microvascular function can be discerned [2].

Taken together, microvascular dysfunction at the level of both resistance vessels and the nutritive capillary beds has been established in obesity, hypertension and insulin resistance. Importantly, microvascular abnormalities that lead to impaired tissue perfusion in obesity, hypertension and insulin resistance appear to represent a generalized condition that affects multiple tissues and organs. Not only peripheral microvascular function in skin and muscle, but also coronary, retinal and renal microvascular function is affected [3, 18, 19]. Therefore, impaired tissue perfusion may be involved in target-organ damage and complications that involve several vascular beds (e.g. retinopathy, lacunar stroke, microalbuminuria en heart failure) [3]. Microvascular abnormality is also a predictor of prognosis and an increased incidence of cardiovascular events [3, 18]. Overall Framingham risk score is inversely correlated with skin capillary recruitment [20], maximal skin capillary density [21], and coronary flow reserve [22].

Interestingly, epidemiological [23-26] and experimental [4-6] data suggest that obesity-related microvascular dysfunction may also contribute to the development of hypertension and insulin resistance.

3. MICROVASCULAR DYSFUNCTION AS A CAUSE OF HYPERTENSION

In most forms of experimental and clinical hypertension, cardiac output is close to normal and the peripheral vascular resistance is increased in proportion to the increase in blood pressure [3]. The increase in total peripheral vascular resistance is likely to reflect changes in the microcirculation. In several tissues both microvascular endothelium-dependent vasodilatation and capillary density has been found to correlate inversely with blood pressure in hypertensive and normotensive subjects Fig. **(1)** [2, 10, 14, 16].

Whereas it has been known for many years that increased wall-to-lumen ratio and microvascular rarefaction can be secondary to sustained elevation of blood pressure [3], there is also evidence that abnormalities in the microcirculation precede and thus may be a causal component of high blood pressure. Microvascular rarefaction, similar in magnitude to the rarefaction observed in patients with established hypertension, can already be demonstrated in subjects with mild intermittent hypertension and in normotensive subjects with a genetic predisposition to high blood pressure [27, 28]. Moreover, in hypertensive subjects, capillary rarefaction in muscle has been shown to predict the increase in mean arterial pressure over two decades [29]. More recently, a smaller retinal arteriolar diameter has been shown to predict the occurrence and development of hypertension in a prospective, population-based study of normotensive middle-aged persons [23, 24]. Other, indirect, evidence comes from studies demonstrating that inhibitors of angiogenesis and especially inhibitors of vascular endothelial growth factor (VEGF)/VEGFR-2 signalling cause arterial hypertension, which in severity is paralleled by microvascular rarefaction [30]. In addition, calculations by mathematical modelling of in vivo microvascular networks predict an exponential relationship between capillary and arteriolar number and vascular resistance [31, 32]. Total vessel rarefaction up to 42% (within the range observed in hypertensive humans) can increase tissue vascular resistance by 21%.

Our understanding of the role of obesity-associated microvascular abnormalities in the development of hypertension has been enhanced by studies in the obese Zucker rat, in which a defective leptin receptor gene causes excessive food intake and leads to obesity, hypertension, and type 2 diabetes. The obese Zucker rat show microvascular remodelling and rarefaction in skeletal muscle before any elevation of blood pressure has occurred, and rarefaction is not prevented if the increase in blood pressure is prevented by treatment with hydralazine [33]. Rarefaction in this situation, therefore, is not a consequence of hypertension. Thus, it seems likely that microvascular abnormalities in obesity can both result from and contribute to hypertension, and a "vicious cycle" may exist in which the microcirculation maintains or even amplifies an initial increase in blood pressure [34]. However, according to the Borst-Guyton concept, chronic hypertension can occur only if renal function is abnormal with a shift in the renal pressure-natriuresis relationship [35]. In the absence of the latter, increased peripheral resistance only temporarily raises blood pressure, to be followed by an increase in renal sodium excretion restoring blood pressure towards normal. Importantly, therefore, subtle renal microvascular disease [36] as well as a reduced number of nephrons [37] may reconcile the Borst-Guyton concept with the putative role of vessel rarefaction in the aetiology of high blood pressure [35, 38]. This may also explain the observed salt sensitivity of blood pressure in insulin resistant subjects [39]. In agreement with a central role for generalized microvascular dysfunction as a link between salt sensitivity, insulin resistance and hypertension recent data suggest an association between salt sensitivity and microvascular dysfunction independent of hypertensive status. More importantly, microvascular function, at least statistically, largely explained associations of salt sensitivity with both insulin resistance and elevated blood pressure [38].

In summary, microvascular dysfunction, by affecting peripheral vascular resistance and renal function, may initiate the pathogenic sequence and subsequently maintain or amplify the initial increase in blood pressure. It may also explain salt-sensitivity of blood pressure, associated with insulin resistance.

It is important to realize that microvascular rarefaction also affects the spatial pattern of flow in the microvascular bed, causing a non-uniform distribution of blood flow among exchange vessels. This non-uniform distribution of flow among vessels, which can be defined as some vessels receiving more and some less of their appropriate fraction of total flow, has been invoked to explain phenomena such as flow-limited muscular performance [40] and sub-optimal capillary transport of small solutes [41], which potentially may affect glucose metabolism.

4. MICROVASCULAR DYSFUNCTION AS A CAUSE OF INSULIN RESISTANCE

Insulin resistance is typically defined as decreased sensitivity and/or responsiveness to metabolic actions of insulin that promote glucose disposal. A major action of insulin in muscle tissue involves translocation of glucose transporters to the plasma membrane and activation of downstream pathways of glucose metabolism [42]. The glucose transporter protein is considered to be rate-limiting for insulin-stimulated glucose uptake in the muscle [42]. However, before insulin interacts with the receptor on the plasma membrane, insulin and glucose must be delivered to the muscle cells in normal amount and time-course. Since evidence suggests that insulin delivery to skeletal muscle interstitium is yet another rate-limiting step in insulin-stimulated muscle glucose, there has been an increasing interest in these pre-cellular steps, in particular with regard to the possible contribution of insulin's vascular actions to insulin-mediated glucose uptake [4-6]. Insulin acts on the vasculature at three discrete steps which may potentially regulate its own delivery to muscle interstitium [4-6]: (1) relaxation of resistance vessels to increase total blood flow; (2) relaxation of pre-capillary arterioles to increase the microvascular exchange surface perfused within skeletal muscle (microvascular recruitment); and (3) the trans-endothelial transport of insulin.

Insulin increases total blood flow and blood volume in skeletal muscle [4, 43]. Mainly because the ability of insulin to dilate skeletal muscle vasculature is impaired in a wide range of insulin-resistant states (e.g. obesity, hypertension, type 2 diabetes), Baron *et al.* [43] introduced the novel concept that insulin's vasodilatory and metabolic actions (i.e. glucose disposal) are functionally coupled. However, despite the compelling nature of these findings, the concept that insulin might control its own access and that of other substances, particularly glucose, has been vigorously challenged [44]. In experiments with lower doses of insulin and shorter time courses of insulin infusion, it was shown that insulin-mediated changes in total blood flow appear to have time kinetics and a dose dependence on insulin different from those for the effect on glucose uptake. In addition, studies in which glucose uptake has been measured during hyperinsulinemia and manipulation of total limb blood flow with different vasodilators have shown that total limb blood flow could be increased in either normal or insulin-resistant individuals, yet there was no increase in insulin-mediated glucose uptake [4-6]. Induction of endothelial dysfunction with subsequent impairment of insulin-induced increases in total limb blood flow also does not decrease insulin-mediated glucose uptake [45]. These discrepant findings have been ascribed to the fact that various vasoactive agents may change total flow but have distinct effects on the distribution of perfusion within the microcirculation. In addition, it should be appreciated that increasing total blood flow will have little or no impact on total glucose uptake by the tissue in the absence of an appreciable arterial–venous concentration gradient, as is the case in insulin resistance states [5]. However, expansion of the endothelial surface area available for exchange of insulin, glucose or other nutrients through the recruitment of additional microvasculature within muscle can enhance nutrient delivery to the tissue, even under circumstances where the extraction ratio is small, provided there is a demonstrable intravascular–interstitial gradient [5, 46].

Clark *et al.* [4] have introduced the concept that distribution of blood flow in nutritive compared to non-nutritive vessels, independent of total muscle flow, may affect insulin-mediated glucose uptake. By elegant studies in rats, applying different techniques to measure capillary recruitment (1-methylxanthine metabolism) and microvascular perfusion (contrast-enhanced ultrasound (CEU) and laser Doppler flowmetry, they could demonstrate that insulin mediates changes in muscle microvascular perfusion consistent with capillary recruitment [4]. This capillary recruitment is associated with changes in skeletal muscle glucose uptake independently of changes in total blood flow, requires lower insulin concentrations than necessary for changes in total blood flow, and precedes muscle glucose disposal [4, 46]. Moreover, insulin-mediated capillary recruitment is impaired in obese zucker rats [47]. Other indirect evidence also supports the concept that the in vivo effect of insulin is determined, at least in part, by insulin's own effect to reach metabolically active tissues by changing local blood flow distribution patterns. Recently, the effects of systemic insulin infusion on transport and distribution kinetics of the extracellular marker [14C] insulin were studied in an animal model that allowed access to hind limb lymph, a surrogate for interstitial fluid [48]. Insulin, at physiological concentrations, augments the access of the labeled inulin to insulin-sensitive tissues. In addition, they demonstrated that access of macromolecules to insulin-sensitive tissues is impaired during diet-induced insulin resistance [49]. The presented data suggests that insulin redirects blood flow from non-nutritive vessels to nutritive capillary beds, resulting in an increased and more homogeneous overall capillary perfusion termed "functional capillary recruitment". The latter would enhance the access of insulin and glucose to a greater mass of muscle for metabolism. Consistent with such a mechanism in humans, insulin increases microvascular blood volume as measured with CEU or positron emission tomography and concomitantly enhances the distribution volume of glucose in human muscle [4, 5, 50]. Subsequently, capillary recruitment was reported in the forearm of healthy humans following a mixed meal and was found to follow closely the time-dependent rise in plasma insulin [51]. In addition, insulin-mediated microvascular recruitment in the forearm was shown to be impaired in obese women when they were exposed to a physiological insulin clamp [52]. By directly visualizing capillaries in human skin, it has been demonstrated that systemic hyperinsulinemia is capable of increasing the number of perfused capillaries [10, 53]. Comparable to insulin-mediated microvascular recruitment in the forearm [52], the action of insulin on capillary recruitment is impaired in obese subjects [10, 54].

Further insight into the complex relationships among vasodilatation, blood flow velocity, and capillary recruitment was gained through measurement of the capillary permeability-surface area product (PS) for glucose and insulin. PS for a substance describes its capacity to reach the interstitial fluid. This depends on the permeability and the capillary surface area, which in turn depends on the amount of perfused capillaries. A recent investigation employing direct measurements of muscle capillary permeability showed that PS for glucose increased after an oral glucose load, and a further increase was demonstrated during an insulin infusion [55]. The increase of PS was exerted without any concomitant change in total blood flow. It was concluded that the insulin-mediated increase in PS seen after oral glucose is important for the glucose uptake rate in normal muscle [55]. Interestingly, the transcapillary delivery of insulin to the muscle interstitium and the onset of insulin action to stimulate glucose uptake are equally delayed among obese, insulin-resistant individuals [56]. In a recent study, using the same technique, the metabolic and vascular effects of the nitric oxide vasodilator metacholine were investigated in a group of obese, insulin resistant and insulin sensitive individuals during glucose-stimulated physiological hyperinsulinemia [57]. The results demonstrated that, in obesity, even in the absence of measurable increments in total forearm blood flow, capillary recruitment (i.e. PSglucose) and forearm glucose disposal increased in response to a glucose challenge, which effect was expectedly blunted in the insulin resistant individuals. Subsequently, it was demonstrated that in the obese, insulin-resistant subjects, an intrabrachial metacholine infusion attenuated the impairment of muscle microvascular recruitment and the kinetic defects in insulin action.

Yet another indirect approach to assess change in microvascular perfusion of muscle was used by Ellmerer and colleagues [58]. During hyperinsulinemic euglycemic clamps, transport parameters and distribution volumes of [14C]inulin (a polymer of D-fructose of similar molecular size to insulin) were determined in healthy, non-obese subjects. The results suggest that, in contrast to earlier findings of the same group performed in a canine model [48, 49], physiological hyperinsulinemia does not augment access of macromolecules to insulin-sensitive tissues in healthy humans. To date, this is the only study where the notion that insulin increases delivery to muscle has been challenged. The study is somewhat hampered by the fact that microvascular perfusion was not assessed at the same time, in contrast to earlier mentioned studies [55-57].

Insulin's effect on capillary recruitment is considered to be caused by insulin-mediated effects on precapillary arteriolar tone and/or on arteriolar vasomotion [4-6]. These effects can be studied by laser Doppler flowmetry. It has been shown that laser Doppler flow measurements in the constant-flow, erythrocyte-perfused rat hindlimb correlate with changes in muscle metabolism, indicating the ability of this technology to measure erythrocyte movement both proportional to nutritive flow and separate from total flow [59]. In rat muscle in vivo, physiological hyperinsulinemia induced an increase in the laser Doppler signal that is consistent with nutritive flow recruitment without a change in total flow [60]. Making use of cathodal iontophoresis and laser Doppler flowmetry, it has been demonstrated that locally applied insulin induces microvascular vasodilatation in human skin independently of insulin's systemic effects [53, 61, 62]. In obesity, this local effect of insulin on the microcirculation is impaired compared to healthy controls [62]. In addition, systemic hyperinsulinemia influences microvascular vasomotion in human skin [53] and muscle [63]. Vasomotion is a spontaneous rhythmic change of arteriolar diameter that almost certainly plays an important role in ensuring that tissue such as muscle is perfused sufficiently to sustain the prevailing metabolic demand [64] by periodically redistributing blood from one region of the muscle to another. It is an important determinant of the spatial and temporal heterogeneity of microvascular perfusion and, therefore, of the number of perfused capillaries [63, 64]. The origin and control of microvascular vasomotion is still a matter of debate. A central neurogenic regulatory mechanism is suggested by synchronicity on contralateral limbs and by the suppressive effect of central sympathectomy. However, local administration of vasoactive substances such as acetylcholine and sodium nitroprusside directly influences vasomotion. Furthermore, vasomotion has been shown in isolated small arteries, indicating a local regulatory mechanism. In view of these considerations, it can be suggested that vasomotion is regulated by both local vasoactive substances and influences of the central nervous system. The contribution of different regulatory mechanisms can be investigated by analysing the contribution of different frequency intervals to the variability of the laser Doppler signal. A number of very useful papers from Stefanovska *et al.* have analyzed the reflected laser Doppler signal from skin to provide indirect assessment of vasomotion [65, 66]. In humans they have interpreted the spectrum as follows: (1) 0.01–0.02 Hz, which is thought to contain local endothelial activity; (2) 0.02–0.06 Hz, which is thought to contain neurogenic activity; (3) 0.06–0.15 Hz, which is associated with the myogenic response of the smooth muscle cells in the vessel wall; (4) 0.15–0.4 Hz, which is the frequency interval of respiratory function; and (5) 0.4–1.6 Hz, which contains the heart beat frequency. It has been shown that systemic hyperinsulinemia affects microvascular vasomotion by increasing endothelial and neurogenic activity [53, 63] in skin and muscle, and that particularly the contribution of endothelial and neurogenic activity to microvascular vasomotion is impaired in insulin-resistant obese individuals [62]. Local hyperinsulinemia during cathodal ionophoresis of insulin, on the other hand, affects microvascular vasomotion by increasing myogenic activity [67]. Similarly, rat muscle studies showed the main increase due to insulin to be myogenic at 0.1 Hz [68].

Insulin trans-endothelial transport (TET) is a third potential site for regulating insulin delivery [5]. This is underscored by the consistent finding that steady-state insulin concentrations in plasma are approximately twice those in muscle interstitium. Recent in vivo and in vitro findings suggest that insulin traverses the vascular endothelium via a trans-cellular, receptor-mediated pathway, and emerging data indicate that insulin acts on the endothelium to facilitate its own TET.

All together, these data illustrate the importance of the microcirculation in regulating nutrient and hormone access to muscle, and raise the possibility that any impairment in capillary recruitment may cause an impairment in glucose uptake by muscle.

5. IMPAIRMENT OF INSULIN-MEDIATED MICROVASCULAR RECRUITMENT: POSSIBLE MECHANISMS

5.1. Vascular Insulin Resistance

The metabolic action of insulin to stimulate glucose uptake in skeletal muscle and adipose tissue is mediated through stimulation of PI3-kinase-dependent signalling pathways. These pathways involve the insulin receptor, insulin receptor substrate 1 (IRS-1), PI3- kinase, phosphoinositide-dependent kinase 1 (PDK-1), and protein kinase B (Akt) [69]. Elucidation of insulin-signalling pathways regulating endothelial production of NO reveals striking parallels with metabolic insulin-signalling pathways in skeletal muscle and adipose tissue. Insulin-induced stimulation of Akt directly increases endothelial NO synthase (eNOS) activity, leading to increased NO production [69].

In addition to its vasodilator actions, insulin also has vasoconstrictor effects. These vasoconstrictor effects are mainly mediated by the vasoconstrictor peptide endothelin-1 (ET-1) [69]. ET-1 is produced in the vascular endothelium through stimulation of the intracellular MAP-kinase signalling pathway and the extracellular signal-regulated kinase-1/2 (ERK1/2) [70]. Thus insulin has opposing endothelial derived vasodilator and vasoconstrictor effects, with the net effect being dependent on the balance between these two. Normally, the net result is either neutral or vasodilatory [71, 72].

Key to understanding decreased nutritive blood flow in obesity may be the dual effects of insulin on vascular tone and its differential impairment in obesity. In obese rats, these signalling pathways are selectively impaired: insulin-mediated activation of PI3-kinase, Akt and eNOS is impaired, but insulin-mediated activation of ERK1/2 is intact [73,74]. Notably, during obesity induced by high fat feeding, inflammation and insulin resistance developed in the vasculature well before these responses were detected in muscle, liver, or adipose tissue. This observation suggests that the vasculature is more susceptible than other tissues to the deleterious effects of nutrient overload and may play a pathophysiological role in inducing insulin resistance and increases in vascular resistance [75]. Recent experimental studies in rats demonstrate that ET-1 infusion in vivo severely blunted the increased capillary recruitment and limb blood flow caused by insulin [76]. These effects of ET-1 were accompanied by increased blood pressure and reduced muscle glucose uptake. In addition, insulin resistance in spontaneously hypertensive rats is associated with endothelial dysfunction characterized by imbalance between NO and ET-1 production [77].

In healthy humans, this balance of NO- and ET-1-dependent effects has also been demonstrated at the level of the resistance vessels of forearm [78]. Moreover, obese, hypertensive humans show an insulin-induced vasoconstriction [79] as well as increased ET-1-dependent vasoconstrictor tone and decreased NO-dependent vasodilator tone at the level of the resistance arteries [80]. Increased circulating levels of endothelin have been described in obesity and increased endogenous endothelin activity contribute to the impaired endothelium-dependent vasodilatation that characterizes this state [81, 82]. Furthermore, increased endogenous endothelin action contributes to insulin resistance in skeletal muscle of obese humans, likely through both vascular and tissue effects [82, 83]. However, endothelin-antagonism alone seems not sufficient to normalize vascular insulin sensitivity in obese subjects, suggesting that endothelin alone does not account for vascular insulin resistance in humans [84]. On the other hand, metacholine, a nitric oxide vasodilator, seems to improve muscle capillary recruitment and forearm glucose uptake to physiological hyperinsulinemia in obese, insulin resistant individuals [57].

Taken together, shared insulin-signalling pathways in metabolic and vascular target tissues with complementary functions seem to provide a mechanism to couple the regulation of glucose with hemodynamic homeostasis.

5.2. Obesity-Related Signalling

Obesity-related vascular dysfunction and insulin resistance may well be caused by altered signalling from adipose tissue to blood vessels, which impairs the balance of NO- and ET-1 production. (Vascular) insulin resistance in obesity is manifested through complex, heterogeneous mechanisms that can involve increased fatty acid flux, microhypoxia in adipose tissue, ER stress, secretion of adipocyte-derived cytokines and chronic tissue inflammation [85,86,87]. A discussion of all of these factors in detail is beyond the constraints of this chapter, and below we focus largely on the interactive role of nutrients (particularly fatty acids) and inflammation (particularly tumour necrosis factor- α (TNF-α)) on the pathogenesis of (vascular) insulin resistance.

5.3. Free Fatty Acids (FFA)

Obese individuals are characterized by a greater rate of breakdown and uptake (i.e. flux) of fatty acids as compared with lean individuals, and it is likely that this higher flux is an important mediator of insulin resistance. By use of magnetic resonance spectroscopy, FFA-induced insulin resistance in humans has been shown to result from a significant reduction in the intramyocellular glucose concentration, suggestive of glucose transport as the affected rate-limiting step [42]. The current hypothesis, supported by data from protein kinase theta (PKC-θ) knock out mice, proposes that fatty acids upon entering the muscle cell activate PKC-θ as either fatty acyl-CoA or diacylglycerol. PKC-θ activates a serine kinase cascade leading to the phosphorylation and inactivation of IRS-1 by preventing its activation by tyrosine phosphorylation [69]. Since the technique of magnetic resonance spectroscopy only identifies a gradient from extracellular to intracellular glucose in muscle cells, it remains to be proven that the gradient did not occur between the plasma and interstitial glucose and thus reflects a rate-limiting step of glucose delivery induced by fatty acids. Interestingly, studies suggest that glucose delivery contributes to sustaining the transmembrane glucose gradient and, therefore, is a determinant of glucose transport [88]. This would be consistent with the finding in rats that FFA elevation concomitantly impairs insulin-mediated muscle capillary recruitment and glucose uptake [89]. In addition, in lean individuals, FFA elevation induces skin microvascular dysfunction and reduces whole body glucose uptake, while in obese individuals FFA lowering has the opposite effect Fig. (**2**) [54]. Moreover, changes in capillary recruitment statistically explained ~29% of the association between changes in FFA levels and insulin-mediated glucose uptake.

A defect involving fatty-acid–induced impaired insulin signalling through the same PKC-θ mechanism in endothelial cells, which in turn may negatively influence the balance between insulin-mediated vasodilatation and vasoconstriction, may be responsible for the impaired capillary recruitment. In support of such a mechanism, PKC-θ has been shown to be present in the endothelium of muscle resistance arteries of both mice and humans and to be activated by physiological levels of insulin and pathophysiological levels of palmitic acid. By genetic and pharmacological inhibition of PKC-θ activity in mice, it was demonstrated that activated PKC-θ induces insulin-mediated vasoconstriction by the inhibition of insulin-mediated Akt activation, which results in a reduction of vasodilatation, and by the stimulation of insulin-mediated ERK1/2 activation, resulting in enhanced ET-1–dependent vasoconstriction Fig. (**2**) [90]. These data are consistent with a role for FFA-induced microvascular dysfunction in the development of obesity-associated disorders [54].

5.4. Inflammation

In parallel with the perturbations in fatty acid metabolism, adipocyte microhypoxia and ER stress precipitate a series of events that result in the recruitment of a specific population of pro-inflammatory, M1-like macrophages into adipose tissue [87]. Activation of these macrophages leads to the release of a variety of chemokines (which recruit additional macrophages) and pro-inflammatory cytokines by the adipocytes. In turn, these cytokines change the milieu of secreted circulating adipokines, which then have endocrine or paracrine effects on the vasculature [85]. In the past years, several adipokines have been shown to alter vascular tone and vessel wall inflammation. These effects may be achieved by direct interaction with vascular endothelium, or indirectly, by enhancing monocyte infiltration into the vessel wall. Adipokines that act directly on vascular endothelium include TNF-α, IL-6, leptin and adiponectin, while MCP-1, IL-8 and resistin increase monocyte adhesion to vascular endothelium [85].

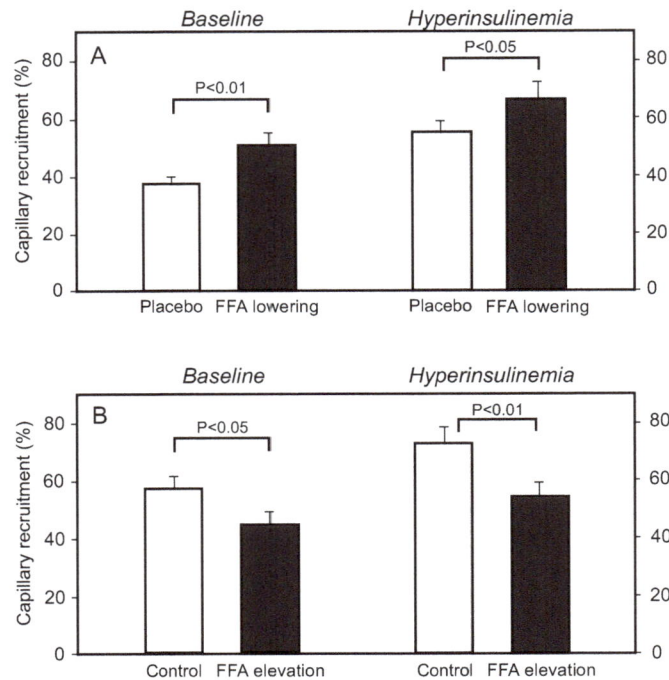

Figure 2: Capillary recruitment (%) before and during hyperinsulinemia in obese women (A): effects of FFA lowering versus placebo. Capillary recruitment before and during hyperinsulinemia in lean women (B): effects of FFA elevation versus saline infusion (control). (Diabetes. 2004; 53:2873).

Of the adipokines, TNF-α has been best characterised for its action in inducing metabolic insulin resistance through inflammatory pathways, with consequent effects on IRS-1 and Akt phosphorylation [91] and on AMP-kinase signalling [92]. TNF-α can certainly produce local and downstream endothelial activation and inhibition of nitric oxide production in small vessels. In rats, TNF-α elevation concomitantly impairs insulin-mediated muscle capillary recruitment and glucose uptake [93]. Moreover, in isolated skeletal muscle resistance arteries, TNF-α impairs the vasodilator effects but not the vasoconstrictor effects of insulin through activation of intracellular enzyme c-Jun N-terminal kinase (JNK) and impairment of insulin-mediated activation of Akt Fig. (**3**) [94]. This selective inhibition of the vasodilator effects of insulin results in insulin-mediated vasoconstriction in the presence of TNF-α. JNK has been shown to regulate whole-body insulin sensitivity as well as insulin-mediated cell

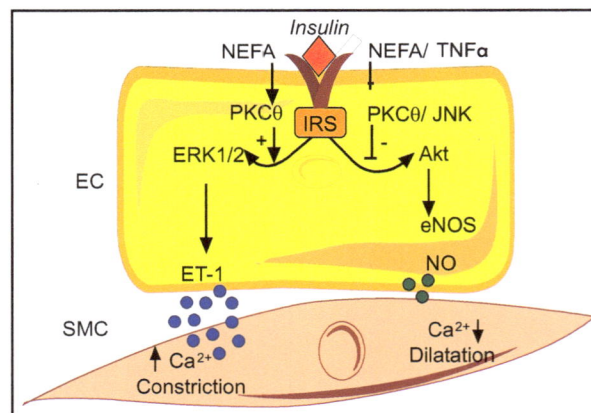

Figure 3: Effect on insulin signaling by TNF-α or non-esterified fatty acids (NEFA). Normal insulin signaling is mediated by either insulin receptor substrate (IRS), Akt, eNOS, and NO production leading to vasodilation or by ERK1/2 and ET-1 production leading to vasoconstriction. TNF-α and NEFA affect the insulin signaling pathway by the activation of JNK or PKCθ, leading to impaired Akt activation induced by TNFα and NEFA, and increase in ERK1/2 activation by NEFA, both of which lead to insulin-mediated vasoconstriction in muscle resistance arteries (Cell Tissue Res. 2009;335:165).

signalling [95]. In cultured bovine Aortic Endothelial Cells, TNF-α induces insulin resistance in the phosphatidylinositol 3-kinase/Akt/eNOS pathway via a p38 MAPK-dependent mechanism and enhances ERK1/2 and AMPK phosphorylation independent of the p38 MAPK pathway [96]. This differential modulation of TNF-α's actions by p38 MAPK suggests that p38MAPK plays a key role in TNF-α - mediated vascular insulin resistance and may contribute to the generalized endothelial dysfunction seen obesity. In humans, the TNF-α gene locus contributes to the determination of obesity and obesity-associated hypertension [97]. Recent interesting evidence is that insulin sensitivity is improved by treatment through neutralizing TNF-α with the monoclonal antibody, infliximab, in patients with ankylosing spondylitis [98], indicating that TNF-α is indeed an important adipokine that may be at least partially responsible for an insulin resistant state. Notably, compared to healthy controls, patients with ankylosing spondylitis had impaired microvascular endothelium-dependent vasodilatation and capillary recruitment, which was normalized following anti-TNF-α treatment [99]. Morphological studies reveal substantial differences in inflammation between subcutaneous and intra-abdominal (visceral) fat depots. Abdominal adipose tissue contains more monocytes and macrophages and expresses more TNF-α than subcutaneous adipose tissue in obesity [100,101]. In accordance, increased visceral adipose tissue and trunk/extremity skinfold ratio were shown to be associated with an increased inflammation score, which combined information on concentrations of C-reactive protein, IL-6, and TNF-α. The inflammation score was inversely associated with capillary recruitment and statistically explained 41% of the association between visceral adipose tissue and capillary recruitment. Circulating TNF-α levels are associated with capillary recruitment in some [102], but not all studies [9]. This may be explained by the fact that TNF-α may not be a good candidate as a systemic fat-derived signal, due to its low circulating concentration [103]. A new source of TNF-α which has recently been identified is perivascular adipose tissue around coronary arteries [104,105]. This implies that TNF-α is produced in the vicinity of the vascular endothelium and may mean that circulating levels of TNF-α underestimate the biologically relevant concentrations of this cytokine. In this context, we have suggested a regulatory role for local production of adipokines in deposits of fat around arterioles, so called muscle periarteriolar adipose tissue (mPAT) Fig. (**4**) [85,106]. We have demonstrated that there is a cuff of adipose tissue around the origin of nutrient arterioles, isolated from cremaster muscles from obese Zucker rats [85,106]. Using a variety of insulin signalling pathway inhibitors, we have shown that in these animals, the PI3-kinase insulin signalling pathway is impaired, and nitric oxide production is suppressed [85]. This has led us to propose that in states of obesity, perivascular fat may signal to the vessel wall, both locally

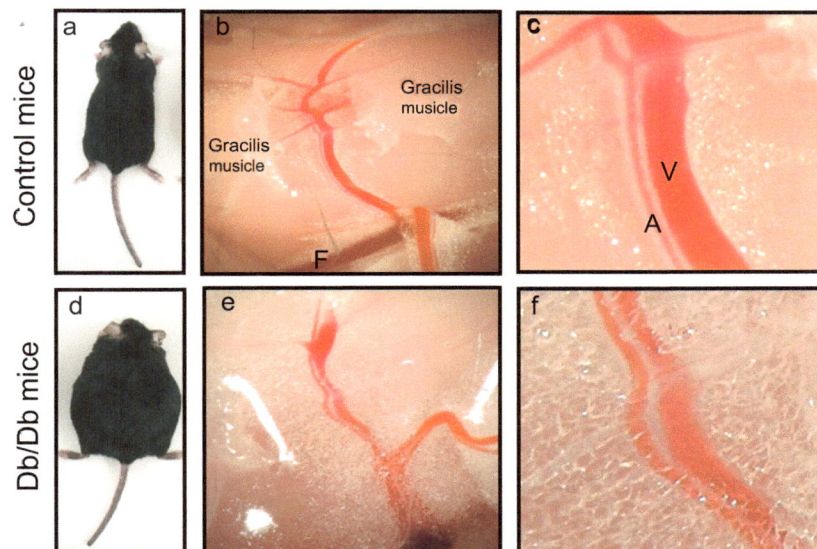

Figure 4: Increased local perivascular adipose tissue in skeletal muscle arterioles of Db/Db mice. After dissection of the gracilis muscle, the vasculature of the corresponding muscle in the control and Db/Db mice (b, e) becomes visible (A artery, V vein, F femoral artery). At higher magnification, the artery and vein can be distinguished (c, f). The Db/Db mice (d-f) possess more and larger fat cells surrounding the gracilis artery compared with control mice (a-c). Bars 1 mm (b, e), 0.25 mm (c, f). (Cell Tissue Res. 2009; 335:165.)

('paracrine') and downstream ('vasocrine'), through outside-to-inside signalling, with TNF-α being a likely mediator [106]. Perivascular fat around nutrient arterioles may inhibit the effects of systemic insulin on local vasodilatation, with consequent inhibition of nutritive blood flow and insulin action. Recently, some evidence has been published in support of the hypothesis that obesity-related changes in adipose tissue have direct effects on the vasoactive properties of perivascular adipose tissue [107]. Small arteries with and without perivascular adipose tissue were taken from subcutaneous gluteal fat biopsy samples and studied with wire myography and immunohistochemistry. It was demonstrated that healthy adipose tissue around human small arteries secrete adiponectin that influence vasodilatation by increasing nitric oxide bioavailability. However, in perivascular fat from obese subjects with metabolic syndrome the loss of this dilator effect was accompanied by an increase in adipocyte area and immunohistochemical evidence of inflammation, with increased activity of TNF-α. Application of the cytokines TNF-α and interleukin-6 to perivascular fat around healthy blood vessels reduced dilator activity, resulting in the obese phenotype. Similarly, induction of hypoxia stimulated inflammation and resulted in loss of anticontractile capacity.

In conclusion, both FFA and TNF-α are likely candidates to link visceral adipose tissue with defects in microvascular function, at least in part by influencing insulin signalling and thereby insulin's vascular effects.

6. CONCLUSION

Obesity has been implicated in the rising prevalence of the metabolic syndrome, a cluster of risk factors including, hypertension, insulin resistance, which confers an increased risk for type 2 diabetes and cardiovascular disease. In the present chapter we have reviewed the complex interaction between microvascular function, intracellular insulin signalling pathways and obesity-related endocrine and paracrine signalling molecules explaining the associations among obesity, hypertension and impaired insulin-mediated glucose uptake. A better understanding of the pathophysiology underlying the clustering of risk factors may lead to new therapeutic approaches that specifically target underlying causes of obesity-related disorders. We have provided evidence that microvascular abnormalities such as vascular rarefaction can cause an increase in peripheral resistance and might initiate the pathogenic sequence in hypertension. In addition, shared insulin-signalling pathways in metabolic and vascular target tissues may provide a mechanism to couple the regulation of glucose and hemodynamic homeostasis. Metabolic insulin resistance is characterized by pathway-specific impairment in PI3-kinase–dependent signalling, which in endothelium may cause imbalance between production of NO and secretion of ET-1, liming nutritive blood flow, and thus insulin and substrate delivery to target tissues. FFAs and pro-inflammatory cytokines including TNF-α may contribute to impairment of insulin's metabolic and vascular actions by modulating insulin signalling and transcription. Perivascular and truncal fat adipose tissue act as an integrated organ responsible for generating local and systemic inflammatory signals.

7. REFERENCES

[1]   Grundy SM, Brewer HB, Jr., Cleeman JI, Smith SC, Jr., Lenfant C. Definition of metabolic syndrome: Report of the National Heart, Lung, and Blood Institute/American Heart Association conference on scientific issues related to definition. Circulation. 2004; 109: 433-38.

[2]   Serné EH, Stehouwer CD, ter Maaten JC, *et al.* Microvascular function relates to insulin sensitivity and blood pressure in normal subjects. Circulation. 1999; 99: 896-902.

[3]   Levy BI, Schiffrin EL, Mourad JJ, *et al.* Impaired tissue perfusion: a pathology common to hypertension, obesity, and diabetes mellitus. Circulation 2008; 118: 968-76.

[4]   Clark MG. Impaired microvascular perfusion: a consequence of vascular dysfunction and a potential cause of insulin resistance in muscle. Am J Physiol Endocrinol Metab. 2008; 295: E732-50.

[5]   Barrett EJ, Eggleston EM, Inyard AC, *et al.* The vascular actions of insulin control its delivery to muscle and regulate the rate-limiting step in skeletal muscle insulin action. Diabetologia. 2009; 52: 752-64.

[6]   Serné EH, de Jongh RT, Eringa EC, IJzerman RG, Stehouwer CD. Microvascular dysfunction: a potential pathophysiological role in the metabolic syndrome. Hypertension. 2007; 50: 204-11.

[7]   Jonk AM, Houben AJ, de Jongh RT, Serné EH, Schaper NC, Stehouwer CD. Microvascular dysfunction in obesity: a potential mechanism in the pathogenesis of obesity-associated insulin resistance and hypertension. Physiology (Bethesda). 2007; 22: 252-60.

[8]   Wiernsperger N, Nivoit P, De Aguiar LG, Bouskela E. Microcirculation and the metabolic syndrome. Microcirculation. 2007; 14: 403-38.

[9]   De Jongh RT, IJzerman RG, Serné EH, *et al.* Visceral and truncal subcutaneous adipose tissue are associated with impaired capillary recruitment in healthy individuals. J Clin Endocrinol Metab. 2006; 91: 5100-6.

[10]   de Jongh RT, Serne EH, IJzerman RG, de Vries G, Stehouwer CD. Impaired microvascular function in obesity: implications for obesity-associated microangiopathy, hypertension, and insulin resistance. Circulation. 2004; 109: 2529-35.

[11]   Khan F, Green FC, Forsyth JS, Greene SA, Morris AD, Belch JJ. Impaired microvascular function in normal children: effects of adiposity and poor glucose handling. J Physiol. 2003; 551: 705-11

[12]　Steinberg HO, Chaker H, Leaming R, Johnson A, Brechtel G, Baron AD. Obesity/insulin resistance is associated with endothelial dysfunction. Implications for the syndrome of insulin resistance. J Clin Invest. 1996; 97: 2601-10.

[13]　Ketel IJ, Stehouwer CD, Serné EH, *et al.* Obese but not normal-weight women with polycystic ovary syndrome are characterized by metabolic and microvascular insulin resistance. J Clin Endocrinol Metab. 2008; 93: 3365-72.

[14]　Serné EH, Gans RO, ter Maaten JC, Tangelder GJ, Donker AJ, Stehouwer CD. Impaired skin capillary recruitment in essential hypertension is caused by both functional and structural capillary rarefaction. Hypertension. 2001; 38: 238-42.

[15]　Laine H, Knuuti MJ, Ruotsalainen U, *et al.* Preserved relative dispersion but blunted stimulation of mean flow, absolute dispersion, and blood volume by insulin in skeletal muscle of patients with essential hypertension. Circulation. 1998; 97: 2146-53.

[16]　Serné EH, Gans RO, ter Maaten JC, ter Wee PM, Donker AJ, Stehouwer CD. Capillary recruitment is impaired in essential hypertension and relates to insulin's metabolic and vascular actions. Cardiovasc Res. 2001; 49: 161-68.

[17]　Lillioja S, Young AA, Culter CL, *et al.* Skeletal muscle capillary density and fiber type are possible determinants of in vivo insulin resistance in man. J Clin Invest. 1987; 80: 415-24.

[18]　Schelbert HR. Coronary Circulatory Function Abnormalities in Insulin Resistance. Insights From Positron Emission Tomography. J Am Coll Cardiol 2009; 53: S3–8.

[19]　Wong TY, Duncan BB, Golden SH, *et al.* Associations between the metabolic syndrome and retinal microvascular signs: the Atherosclerosis Risk In Communities study. Invest Ophthalmol Vis Sci. 2004; 45: 2949-54.

[20]　IJzerman RG, de Jongh RT, Beijk MA, *et al.* Individuals at increased coronary heart disease risk are characterized by an impaired microvascular function in skin. Eur J Clin Invest. 2003; 33: 536-42.

[21]　Debbabi H, Uzan L, Mourad JJ, Safar M, Levy BI, Tibiriçà E. Increased skin capillary density in treated essential hypertensive patients. Am J Hypertens. 2006; 19: 477-83.

[22]　Wang L, Jerosch-Herold M, Jacobs DR Jr, Shahar E, Folsom AR. Coronary risk factors and myocardial perfusion in asymptomatic adults: the Multi-Ethnic Study of Atherosclerosis (MESA). J Am Coll Cardiol. 2006; 47: 565-72.

[23]　Wong TY, Klein R, Sharrett AR, Duncan BB, Couper DJ, Klein BE, Hubbard LD, Nieto FJ. Retinal arteriolar diameter and risk for hypertension. Ann Intern Med. 2004; 140: 248-55.

[24]　Ikram MK, Witteman JC, Vingerling JR, Breteler MM, Hofman A, de Jong PT. Retinal vessel diameters and risk of hypertension: the Rotterdam Study. Hypertension. 2006; 47: 189-94.

[25]　Nguyen TT, Wang JJ, Islam FM, *et al.* Retinal arteriolar narrowing predicts incidence of diabetes: the Australian Diabetes, Obesity and Lifestyle (AusDiab) Study. Diabetes. 2008; 57: 536-9.

[26]　Wong TY, Klein R, Sharrett AR, *et al.* Retinal arteriolar narrowing and risk of diabetes mellitus in middle-aged persons. JAMA. 2002; 287: 2528-33.

[27]　Antonios T.F.T., Singer D.R.J., Markandu N.D., Mortimer P.S., MacGregor G.A. Rarefaction of skin capillaries in borderline essential hypertension suggest an early structural abnormality. Hypertension. 1999; 34: 655–658.

[28]　Noon J.P., Walker B.R., Webb D.J., *et al.* Impaired microvascular dilatation and capillary rarefaction in young adults with a predisposition to high blood pressure. J Clin Invest. 1997; 99: 1873–1879.

[29]　Hedman A, Reneland R, Lithell HO. Alterations in skeletal muscle morphology in glucose-tolerant elderly hypertensive men: relationship to development of hypertension and heart rate. J Hypertens. 2000; 18: 559-565.

[30]　Lévy BI. Blood pressure as a potential biomarker of the efficacy angiogenesis inhibitor. Ann Oncol. 2009; 20: 200-3.

[31]　Greene AS., Tonellato P.J., Lui J., Lombard J.H., Cowly A.W. Microvascular rarefaction and tissue vascular resistance in hypertension. Am J Physiol. 1989; 256: H126–31.

[32]　Hudetz AG. Percolation phenomenon: the effect of capillary network rarefaction. Microvasc Res. 1993; 45: 1–10.

[33]　Frisbee JC. Hypertension-independent microvascular rarefaction in the obese Zucker rat model of the metabolic syndrome. Microcirculation. 2005; 12: 383-92.

[34]　Levy, BI., Ambrosio, G., Pries, AR., Struijker-Boudier, HA. Microcirculation in hypertension: A new target for treatment? Circulation. 2001; 104, 736-41.

[35]　De Boer MP, IJzerman RG, de Jongh RT, *et al.* Birth weight relates to salt sensitivity of blood pressure in healthy adults. Hypertension. 2008; 51: 928-32.

[36]　Johnson RJ, Herrera-Acosta J, Schreiner GF, Rodriguez-Iturbe B. Subtle acquired renal injury as a mechanism of salt-sensitive hypertension. N Engl J Med. 2002; 346: 913-23.

[37]　Le Noble FA, Stassen FR, Hacking WJ, Struijker Boudier HA. Angiogenesis and hypertension. J Hypertens. 1998; 16: 1563-72.

[38]　De Jongh RT, Serné EH, IJzerman RG, Stehouwer CD. Microvascular function: a potential link between salt sensitivity, insulin resistance and hypertension. J Hypertens. 2007; 25: 1887-93.

[39]　Galletti F, Strazzullo P, Ferrara I, Annuzzi G, Rivellese AA, Gatto S, Mancini M. NaCl sensitivity of essential hypertensive patients is related to insulin resistance. J Hypertens. 1997; 15: 1485-91.

[40]　Wright DL, Sonnenschein RR. Relations among activity, blood flow, and vascular state in skeletal muscle. Am J Physiol. 1965; 208: 782-89.

[41] Ellis CG, Wrigley SM, Groom AC. Heterogeneity of red blood cell perfusion in capillary networks supplied by a single arteriole in resting skeletal muscle. Circ Res. 1994; 75: 357-68.

[42] Shulman GI. Unraveling the cellular mechanism of insulin resistance in humans: new insights from magnetic resonance spectroscopy. Physiology (Bethesda). 2004; 19: 183-90.

[43] Baron AD. Hemodynamic actions of insulin. Am J Physiol. 1994; 267: E187-E202.

[44] Yki-Järvinen H, Utriainen T. Insulin-induced vasodilatation: physiology or pharmacology? Diabetologia. 1998; 41: 369-79.

[45] Shankar SS, Considine RV, Gorski JC, Steinberg HO. Insulin sensitivity is preserved despite disrupted endothelial function. Am J Physiol Endocrinol Metab. 2006; 291: E691-E696.

[46] Vincent MA, Clerk LH, Rattigan S, Clark MG, Barrett EJ. Active role for the vasculature in the delivery of insulin to skeletal muscle. Clin Exp Pharmacol Physiol. 2005; 32: 302-7.

[47] Wallis MG, Wheatley CM, Rattigan S, Barrett EJ, Clark AD, Clark MG. Insulin-mediated hemodynamic changes are impaired in muscle of Zucker obese rats. Diabetes. 2002; 51: 3492-8.

[48] Ellmerer M, Kim SP, Hamilton-Wessler M, Hucking K, Kirkman E, Bergman RN. Physiological hyperinsulinemia in dogs augments access of macromolecules to insulin-sensitive tissues. Diabetes. 2004; 53: 2741-47.

[49] Ellmerer M, Hamilton-Wessler M, Kim SP, Huecking K, Kirkman E, Chiu J, Richey J, Bergman RN. Reduced access to insulin-sensitive tissues in dogs with obesity secondary to increased fat intake. Diabetes. 2006; 55: 1769-75.

[50] Bonadonna RC, Saccomani MP, Del Prato S, Bonora E, DeFronzo RA, Cobelli C. Role of tissue-specific blood flow and tissue recruitment in insulin- mediated glucose uptake of human skeletal muscle. Circulation. 1998; 98: 234-41.

[51] Vincent MA, Clerk LH, Lindner JR, *et al.* Mixed meal and light exercise each recruit muscle capillaries in healthy humans. Am J Physiol Endocrinol Metab. 2006; 290: E1191-7.

[52] Clerk LH, Vincent MA, Jahn LA, Liu Z, Lindner JR, Barrett EJ. Obesity blunts insulin-mediated microvascular recruitment in human forearm muscle. Diabetes. 2006; 55: 1436-42.

[53] Serné EH, IJzerman RG, Gans RO, *et al.* Direct evidence for insulin-induced capillary recruitment in skin of healthy subjects during physiological hyperinsulinemia. Diabetes. 2002; 51: 1515-22.

[54] De Jongh RT, Serné EH, IJzerman RG, de Vries G, Stehouwer CD. Free fatty acid levels modulate microvascular function: relevance for obesity-associated insulin resistance, hypertension, and microangiopathy. Diabetes. 2004; 53: 2873-82.

[55] Gudbjornsdottir S, Sjöstrand M, Strindberg L, Lonnroth P. Decreased muscle capillary permeability surface area in type 2 diabetic subjects. J Clin Endocrinol Metab. 2005; 90: 1078-82.

[56] Sjöstrand M, Gudbjörnsdottir S, Holmäng A, Lönn L, Strindberg L, Lönnroth P. Delayed transcapillary transport of insulin to muscle interstitial fluid in obese subjects. Diabetes. 2002 ; 51: 2742-8.

[57] Murdolo G, Sjöstrand M, Strindberg L, *et al.* Effects of Intrabrachial metacholine infusion on muscle capillary recruitment and forearm glucose uptake during physiological hyperinsulinemia in obese, insulin-resistant individuals. J Clin Endocrinol Metab. 2008; 93: 2764-73.

[58] Weinhandl H, Pachler C, Mader JK, *et al.* Physiological hyperinsulinemia has no detectable effect on access of macromolecules to insulin-sensitive tissues in healthy humans. Diabetes. 2007; 56: 2213-7.

[59] Clark AD, Youd JM, Rattigan S, Barrett EJ, Clark MG. Heterogeneity of laser Doppler flowmetry in perfused muscle indicative of nutritive and nonnutritive flow. Am J Physiol Heart Circ Physiol. 2001; 280: H1324-H1333.

[60] Clark AD, Barrett EJ, Rattigan S, Wallis MG, Clark MG. Insulin stimulates laser Doppler signal by rat muscle in vivo, consistent with nutritive flow recruitment. Clin Sci. 2001; 100: 283-90.

[61] Rossi M, Cupisti A, Ricco R, Santoro G, Pentimone F, Carpi A. Skin vasoreactivity to insulin iontophoresis is reduced in elderly subjects and is absent in treated non-insulin-dependent diabetes patients. Biomed Pharmacother. 2004; 58: 560-5.

[62] De Jongh RT, Serné EH, IJzerman RG, Jørstad HT, Stehouwer CD. Impaired local microvascular vasodilatory effects of insulin and reduced skin microvascular vasomotion in obese women. Microvasc Res. 2008; 75: 256-62.

[63] De Jongh RT, Clark AD, IJzerman RG, Serne EH, de Vries G, Stehouwer CD. Physiological hyperinsulinaemia increases intramuscular microvascular reactive hyperaemia and vasomotion in healthy volunteers. Diabetologia. 2004; 47: 978-86.

[64] Rücker M, Strobel O, Vollmar B, Roesken F, Menger MD. Vasomotion in critically perfused muscle protects adjacent tissues from capillary perfusion failure. Am J Physiol Heart Circ Physiol. 2000; 279: H550-8.

[65] Stefanovska A, Bracic M, Kvernmo HD. Wavelet analysis of oscillations in the peripheral blood circulation measured by laser Doppler technique. IEEE Trans Biomed Eng. 1999; 46: 1230-9.

[66] Kvernmo HD, Stefanovska A, Kirkeboen KA, Kvernebo K. Oscillations in the human cutaneous blood perfusion signal modified by endothelium-dependent and endothelium-independent vasodilators. Microvasc Res. 1999; 57: 298-309.

[67] Rossi M, Maurizio S, Carpi A. Skin blood flowmotion response to insulin iontophoresis in normal subjects. Microvasc Res. 2005; 70: 17-22.

[68] Newman JMB, Ross RM, Richards SM, Clark MG, Rattigan S. Acute insulin resistance results in altered vasomotion in rat muscle (Abstract). Proc Eur Soc Microcirc. In press.

[69]   Kim JA, Montagnani M, Koh KK, Quon MJ. Reciprocal relationships between insulin resistance and endothelial dysfunction: molecular and pathophysiological mechanisms. Circulation. 2006; 113: 1888-1904.

[70]   Eringa EC, Stehouwer CD, Nieuw Amerongen GP, Ouwehand L, Westerhof N, Sipkema P. Vasoconstrictor effects of insulin in skeletal muscle arterioles are mediated by ERK1/2 activation in endothelium. Am J Physiol Heart Circ Physiol. 2004; 287: H2043-H2048.

[71]   Eringa EC, Stehouwer CD, Merlijn T, Westerhof N, Sipkema P. Physiological concentrations of insulin induce endothelin-mediated vasoconstriction during inhibition of NOS or PI3-kinase in skeletal muscle arterioles. Cardiovasc Res. 2002; 56: 464-471.

[72]   Verma S, Yao L, Stewart DJ, Dumont AS, Anderson TJ, McNeill JH. Endothelin antagonism uncovers insulin-mediated vasorelaxation in vitro and in vivo. Hypertension. 2001; 37: 328-33.

[73]   Eringa EC, Stehouwer CD, Roos MH, Westerhof N, Sipkema P. Selective resistance to vasoactive effects of insulin in muscle resistance arteries of obese Zucker (fa/fa) rats. Am J Physiol Endocrinol Metab. 2007; 293: E1134-9.

[74]   Jiang ZY, Lin YW, Clemont A, Feener EP, Hein KD, Igarashi M, Yamauchi T, White MF, King GL. Characterization of selective resistance to insulin signaling in the vasculature of obese Zucker (fa/fa) rats. J Clin Invest. 1999; 104: 447-57.

[75]   Kim F, Pham M, Maloney E, *et al.* Vascular inflammation, insulin resistance, and reduced nitric oxide production precede the onset of peripheral insulin resistance. Arterioscler Thromb Vasc Biol. 2008; 28: 1982-8.

[76]   Ross RM, Kolka CM, Rattigan S, Clark MG. Acute blockade by endothelin-1 of haemodynamic insulin action in rats. Diabetologia. 2007; 50: 443-451.

[77]   Potenza MA, Marasciulo FL, Chieppa DM, Brigiani GS, Formoso G, Quon MJ, Montagnani M. Insulin resistance in spontaneously hypertensive rats is associated with endothelial dysfunction characterized by imbalance between NO and ET-1 production. Am J Physiol Heart Circ Physiol. 2005; 289: H813-H822.

[78]   Cardillo C, Nambi SS, Kilcoyne CM, Insulin stimulates both endothelin and nitric oxide activity in the human forearm. Circulation. 1999; 100: 820-5.

[79]   Gudbjornsdottir S, Elam M, Sellgren J, Anderson EA. Insulin increases forearm vascular resistance in obese, insulin-resistant hypertensives. J Hypertens. 1996; 14: 91-97.

[80]   Cardillo C, Campia U, Iantorno M, Panza JA. Enhanced vascular activity of endogenous endothelin-1 in obese hypertensive patients. Hypertension. 2004; 43: 36-40.

[81]   Mather KJ, Mirzamohammadi B, Lteif A, Steinberg HO, Baron AD. Endothelin contributes to basal vascular tone and endothelial dysfunction in human obesity and type 2 diabetes. Diabetes. 2002; 51: 3517-23.

[82]   Lteif A, Vaishnava P, Baron AD, Mather KJ. Endothelin limits insulin action in obese/insulin-resistant humans. Diabetes. 2007; 56: 728-34.

[83]   Ahlborg G, Shemyakin A, Böhm F, Gonon A, Pernow J. Dual endothelin receptor blockade acutely improves insulin sensitivity in obese patients with insulin resistance and coronary artery disease. Diabetes Care. 2007; 30: 591-6.

[84]   Lteif AA, Fulford AD, Considine RV, Gelfand I, Baron AD, Mather KJ. Hyperinsulinemia fails to augment ET-1 action in the skeletal muscle vascular bed in vivo in humans. Am J Physiol Endocrinol Metab. 2008; 295: E1510-7.

[85]   Eringa EC, Bakker W, Smulders YM, Serné EH, Yudkin JS, Stehouwer CD. Regulation of vascular function and insulin sensitivity by adipose tissue: focus on perivascular adipose tissue. Microcirculation. 2007; 14: 389-402.

[86]   Lee DE, Kehlenbrink S, Lee H, Hawkins MA, Yudkin JS. Getting the Message Across- Mechanisms of Physiological Cross-Talk by Adipose Tissue. Am J Physiol Endocrinol Metab. 2009 Mar 3. [Epub ahead of print].

[87]   Schenk S, Saberi M, Olefsky JM. Insulin sensitivity: modulation by nutrients and inflammation. J Clin Invest. 2008; 118: 2992-3002.

[88]   Kelley DE, Williams KV, Price JC. Insulin regulation of glucose transport and phosphorylation in skeletal muscle assessed by PET. Am J Physiol. 1999; 277: E361-E369.

[89]   Clerk LH, Rattigan S, Clark MG. Lipid infusion impairs physiologic insulin-mediated capillary recruitment and muscle glucose uptake in vivo. Diabetes. 2002; 51: 1138-45.

[90]   Bakker W, Sipkema P, Stehouwer CD, *et al.* Protein kinase C theta activation induces insulin-mediated constriction of muscle resistance arteries. Diabetes. 2008; 57: 706-13.

[91]   Shoelson SE, Lee J, Goldfine AB. Inflammation and insulin resistance. Clin Invest. 2006; 116: 1793-801.

[92]   Steinberg GR, Michell BJ, van Denderen BJ, *et al.* Tumor necrosis factor alpha-induced skeletal muscle insulin resistance involves suppression of AMP-kinase signaling. Cell Metab. 2006; 4: 465-74.

[93]   Youd JM, Rattigan S, Clark MG. Acute impairment of insulin-mediated capillary recruitment and glucose uptake in rat skeletal muscle in vivo by TNF-alpha. Diabetes. 2000; 49: 1904-9.

[94]   Eringa EC, Stehouwer CD, Walburg K, Clark AD, Nieuw Amerongen GP, Westerhof N, Sipkema P. Physiological concentrations of insulin induce endothelin-dependent vasoconstriction of skeletal muscle resistance arteries in the presence of tumor necrosis factor-alpha dependence on c-Jun N-terminal kinase. Arterioscler Thromb Vasc Biol. 2006; 26: 274-80.

[95]   Hirosumi J, Tuncman G, Chang L, Gorgun CZ, Uysal KT, Maeda K, Karin M, Hotamisligil GS. A central role for JNK in obesity and insulin resistance. Nature. 2002; 420: 333-36.

[96]   Li G, Barrett EJ, Barrett MO, Cao W, Liu Z. Tumor necrosis factor-alpha induces insulin resistance in endothelial cells via a p38 mitogen-activated protein kinase-dependent pathway. Endocrinology. 2007; 148: 3356-63.

[97]   Pausova Z, Deslauriers B, Gaudet D, Tremblay J, Kotchen TA, Larochelle P, Cowley AW, Hamet P. Role of tumor necrosis factor-alpha gene locus in obesity and obesity-associated hypertension in French Canadians. Hypertension. 2000; 36: 14-19.

[98]   Kiortsis DN, Mavridis AK, Vasakos S, Nikas SN, Drosos AA. Effects of infliximab treatment on insulin resistance in patients with rheumatoid arthritis and ankylosing spondylitis. Ann Rheum Dis. 2005; 64: 765-6.

[99]   Van Eijk IC, Peters MJ, Serné EH, *et al.* Microvascular function is impaired in ankylosing spondylitis and improves after tumour necrosis factor alpha blockade. Ann Rheum Dis. 2009; 68: 362-6.

[100] Bruun JM, Lihn AS, Pedersen SB, Richelsen B. Monocyte chemoattractant protein-1 release is higher in visceral than subcutaneous human adipose tissue (AT): implication of macrophages resident in the AT. J Clin Endocrinol Metab. 2005; 90: 2282-9.

[101] Hotamisligil GS, Spiegelman BM. Tumor necrosis factor alpha: a key component of the obesity-diabetes link. Diabetes. 1994; 43: 1271-8.

[102] IJzerman RG, Voordouw JJ, van Weissenbruch MM, Yudkin JS, Serne EH, Delemarre-van de Waal HA, Stehouwer CD. TNF-alpha levels are associated with skin capillary recruitment in humans: a potential explanation for the relationship between TNF-alpha and insulin resistance. Clin Sci. 2006; 110: 361-68.

[103] Hotamisligil GS, Arner P, Caro JF, Atkinson RL, Spiegelman BM. Increased adipose tissue expression of tumor necrosis factor-alpha in human obesity and insulin resistance. J Clin Invest. 1995; 95: 2409-15.

[104] Mazurek T, Zhang L, Zalewski A, *et al.* Human epicardial adipose tissue is a source of inflammatory mediators. Circulation. 2003; 108: 2460-6.

[105] Chatterjee TK, Stoll LL, Denning GM, *et al.* Proinflammatory phenotype of perivascular adipocytes: influence of high-fat feeding. Circ Res. 2009; 104: 541-9.

[106] Yudkin JS, Eringa E, Stehouwer CD. "Vasocrine" signalling from perivascular fat: a mechanism linking insulin resistance to vascular disease. Lancet. 2005; 365: 1817-20.

[107] Greenstein AS, Khavandi K, Withers SB, *et al.* Local inflammation and hypoxia abolish the protective anticontractile properties of perivascular fat in obese patients. Circulation. 2009; 119: 1661-70.

CHAPTER 5

Inflammatory Responses to Obesity and Insulin Resistance

Georg Singer[1] and D. Neil Granger[2]

[1]Department of Pediatric Surgery, Medical University of Graz, Graz, Austria; [2]Department of Molecular and Cellular Physiology, LSU Health Sciences Center, Shreveport, LA 71130

Address correspondence to: D. Neil Granger, PhD. Department of Molecular and Cellular Physiology LSU Health Sciences Center1501 Kings Highway Shreveport, Louisiana, 71130-3932; Tel: 318-675-6011; Fax: 318-675-6005; e-mail: dgrang@lsuhsc.edu
Dr. Granger is supported by a grant from the National Heart Lung and Blood Institute (HL26441)

Abstract: Obesity is likely to become a major worldwide epidemic in the 21st century. Clinical evidence demonstrates exaggerated inflammatory responses and an enhanced tissue injury in obese subjects with cardiovascular disease, sepsis, thrombosis and allergic diseases. Emerging evidence suggests that obesity per *se* is associated with a systemic inflammatory response that is characterized by endothelial cell dysfunction, oxidative stress, and the activation of circulating immune cells. A large number of cytokine-like substances (adipokines) produced by adipose tissue have been implicated in the systemic inflammatory response associated with obesity. Insulin resistance also appears to contribute to the inflammatory phenotype observed in obesity. There is emerging evidence from experimental and clinical studies that implicate the microvasculature as a major target for the deleterious effects of obesity-induced inflammation, and that the altered microvascular responses underlie the exaggerated injury responses to cardiovascular disease, sepsis, thrombosis and allergic diseases in obese subjects.

1. INTRODUCTION

Obesity is likely to become a major worldwide epidemic in the 21st century. In 2005, the World Health Organization (WHO) estimated that more than 1.5 billion adults worldwide are overweight and more than 400 million adults are obese (defined as a body mass index > 30). The WHO further projects that by 2015, approximately 2.3 billion adults will be overweight and more than 700 million will be obese. Consequently being overweight or obese has become the norm in the western society [1].

The presence of obesity predisposes to the development of risk factors for cardiovascular disease, such as hypertension, hypercholesterolemia, coronary artery disease and diabetes. Moreover the mortality and morbidity of other diseases like sepsis, rheumatoid arthritis and thrombosis appear to be elevated in obese subjects. The pathophysiological mechanisms that mediate these effects are poorly defined. However, there is mounting evidence that obesity exerts these deleterious effects on the cardiovascular system by inducing an inflammatory state in both large and small vessels. Endothelial cell activation/dysfunction appears to be an early and rate-determining response to these risk factors that accounts for the inflammatory phenotype that is assumed by the vasculature. The development of atherosclerosis in large arteries, impaired capacity for dilation of arterioles, and enhanced recruitment of inflammatory cells in postcapillary venules all result from this endothelial cell activation Fig. (**1**).

In 1993, it was first described that adipocytes in rodents secrete the proinflammatory protein TNF-α [2]. This observation laid the foundation for the current concept that adipose tissue is not merely an inert storage site for fat, but is a highly active secretory organ. In obesity, this secretory organ can create a chronic state of low-grade inflammation that results from increased insulin resistance and the presence of increased levels of proinflammatory mediators. This condition leads the vasculature to assume an inflammatory phenotype that results in a functionally impaired microvasculature that exhibits an increased vulnerability to additional inflammatory stimuli that yields more tissue injury and organ dysfunction in response to an acute inflammatory insult.

In the first part of this article we will summarize evidence that implicates factors derived from adipocytes and insulin resistance in the development of the microvascular inflammation and vessel

Nicolas Wiernsperger (Ed.)

dysfunction associated with obesity. In the second part, we address the clinical consequences of obesity-associated inflammation.

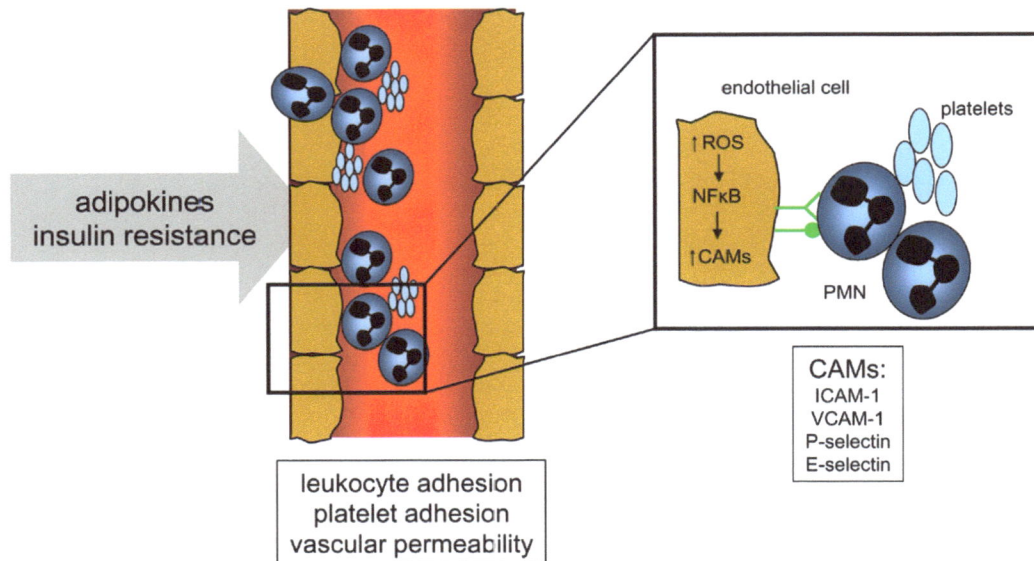

Figure 1: Mechanism that underlies the inflammatory phenotype assumed by the microvasculature during sepsis. Adipokines that are secreted as a consequence of obesity as well as insulin resistance act on endothelial cells and/or on circulating immune cells. A major consequence of the adipocyte-derived products is oxidative stress (i.e. increases of reactive oxidative species) in endothelial cells. This oxidative stress upregulates NFκB and subsequently proinflammatory genes including CAMs get upregulated thereby facilitating leukocyte and platelet adhesion and leukocyte extravasation.

2. HOW DOES OBESITY PROMOTE INFLAMMATION?

A decade ago, adipose tissue was viewed as an organ with the sole role of energy storage and the provision of thermal and mechanical insulation. Current research, however, has led to the concept of adipocytes as highly active and reactive endocrine cells that generate and react to signals that serve to maintain a relatively constant rate of energy expenditure in the body. These cells also participate in a variety of physiological and pathophysiological processes, such as insulin sensitivity, vascular sclerotic processes and immunity and inflammation [3]. Following the discovery that adipose tissue secretes TNF-α, many more proinflammatory cytokines that are linked to adipose tissue have been described. For instance, leptin and the pro-inflammatory protein IL-6, acute phase proteins like CRP and the anti-inflammatory cytokine adiponectin have been linked to adiposity [4]. To date more than fifty obesity-related inflammatory proteins have been identified, many of which are referred to as adipocytokines or adipokines [5, 6]. The blood levels of most of these adipokines are elevated in both obese humans and experimental animals, although not to same extent as observed in classic inflammatory conditions [7]. The elevated systemic adipokine concentrations, coupled to changes in different markers of inflammation, have contributed to the view that obesity represents a systemic state of chronic low-grade inflammation Fig. (**2**) [8].

The exact mechanisms that underlie the enhanced secretion of adipokines during obesity remain unclear. An imbalance between energy intake and energy expenditure causes an accumulation of triglycerides in hypertrophied adipocytes subsequently leading to overweight or obesity. One might expect that this increase of adipose tissue is accompanied with an increase in vascularization thereby providing oxygen and nutrients [9]. However, it has been shown that obese mice have a lower adipose tissue capillary density due to rarefication (Figure 2), with an accompanying reduction in the level of vascular endothelial growth factor (VEGF), one of the most potent angiogenic factors [10, 11]. Therefore, an imbalance between growth of adipose tissue and vascularization seems to exist. This may, at least partially, explain why obesity is associated with a decreased partial pressure of oxygen in both subcutaneous and visceral fat in both humans and experimental animals [12, 13].

Although the exact mechanisms of the recruitment of macrophages into adipose tissue are not fully understood, hypoxia may play a role [14]. Macrophages are thought to represent a major source of the inflammatory mediators secreted from adipose tissue. While obesity is associated with an increased number of macrophages in adipose tissue Fig. (**2**), weight loss does not reduce macrophage density in subcutaneous white adipose tissue [15, 16].

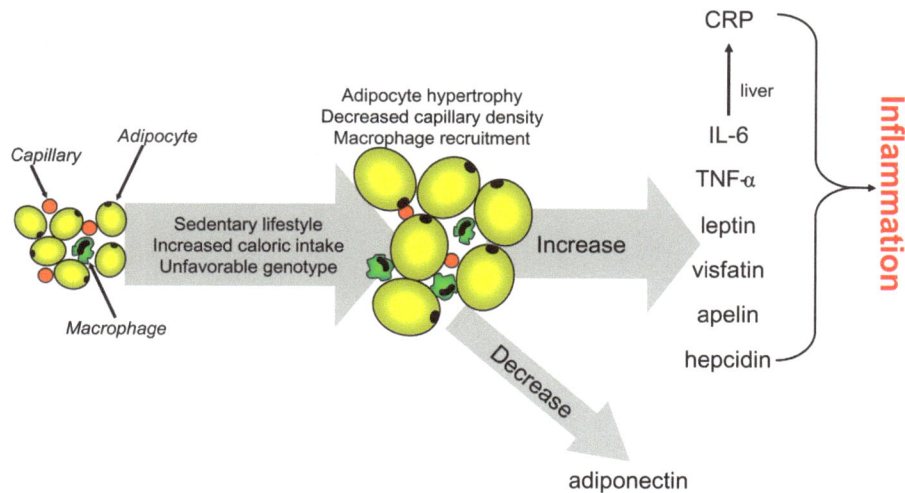

Figure 2: The link between obesity and inflammation. Obesity results from a sedentary lifestyle, increased calorie intake, and/or unfavorable genetic phenotype. Obesity is associated with the adipocyte hypertrophy, recruitment of macrophages and a reduction of capillary density in adipose tissue. Within this hypoxic environment, the activated adipocytes and infiltrated macrophages produce a variety of adipokines that contribute to the chronic low-grade inflammatory state that accompanies obesity.

While most of the studies concentrate on visceral adipose tissue, recent findings suggest that perivascular adipose tissue (PAT) is critically involved in the regulation of vasomotor function. Virtually all arteries are surrounded by PAT which has long been overlooked and thought to only serve a mechanical purpose [17]. However, there is a growing body of evidence that invokes a physiological and pathophysiological role of VAT, led by the observation that when PAT is left on the vessel during *ex vivo* vascular constriction studies, the responses of aortic rings to norepinephrine is significantly attenuated [18]. These findings have been confirmed by more recent studies describing an inhibitory action of perivascular fat on aortic and mesenteric contractile responses to a variety of vasoconstrictors. Moreover, the anti-contractile effects of PAT are directly dependent on the amount of adipose tissue [19]. While these findings suggest a potential protective effect of PAT in maintaining vascular function, peripheral adipose tissue may also cause severe vascular dysfunction. Henrichot et al have shown that human PAT exerts chemotactic properties through the secretion of different chemokines. The supernatant from PAT strongly induced the chemotaxis of peripheral blood leukocytes. This migration was mostly mediated by IL-8 and MCP-1 which also are produced by PAT [20]. An involvement of PAT in the vasomotor dysfunction associated angiotensin II-induced hypertension in mice has also been demonstrated. Chronic angiotensin II infusion leads to hypertension, enhanced superoxide formation and an infiltration of TNF-α producing T-lymphocytes into PAT surrounding these vessels. Supporting the role of angiotensin II, these responses were not observed in angiotension II treated mice either lacking T-cells or treated with a TNF-α antagonist [21].

The available evidence that implicates key adipokines in inflammatory responses, including the microvascular responses to inflammation is summarized below.

Leptin (from the Greek 'leptos' meaning thin) is a 16-kDa protein encoded by the obese (ob) gene located on chromosomes 7 and 6 in humans and mice, respectively [22, 23]. The primary role of leptin is to decrease food intake and increase energy consumption by acting on hypothalamic cells to induce anorexigenic factors and inhibit orexigenic factors [3]. Reductions in leptin signaling or receptor function has been shown to increase energy intake and lower energy expenditure [24]. But leptin has also been shown to influence a myriad of other biological functions like inflammation and immunity, lipid and glucose metabolism, insulin secretion, hematopoiesis, angiogenesis and gastrointestinal function [25-27].

Two distinct genetic abnormalities related to leptin are known to result in severe obesity in humans and experimental animals. Mutations of the leptin-encoding gene that result in leptin deficiency cause obesity in mice (ob/ob model), rats and humans [23, 28]. Similarly, mutations of the long isoform of the leptin receptor – encoded by the diabetes (db) gene – also result in obesity (db/db model, leptin receptor deficiency) [29, 30]. While these mutations are rare in humans there are cases occurring in families with a high prevalence of obesity. The vast majority of cases of human obesity are associated with elevated levels of leptin (leptinemia) rather than leptin deficiency; implicating a role for leptin resistance and therefore making administration of leptin not an effective therapy for this condition [24]. Adipose tissue is the major source of leptin, and both leptin expression and plasma levels of leptin correlate directly with the mass of adipose tissue in humans. Hence, leptin levels are reduced after weight reduction [31-34].

Leptin receptors are found on a variety of cells, including vascular endothelial cells and endothelial progenitor cells [35-37]. Early obesity is characterized with vascular oxidative stress and endothelial dysfunction in association with increased levels of leptin [38]. In human umbilical vein endothelia cells (HUVEC) exposed to leptin, there is an increased expression of eNOS and a dramatic increase in the production of reactive oxygen species [39]. Bovine aortic endothelial cells also respond to leptin with a concentration-dependent increase in the formation of ROS [40]. Oxidative stress is generally associated with an increased expression of endothelial cell adhesion molecules like vascular cell adhesion molecule-1 [41] and intercellular adhesion molecule-1 [42] and the subsequent recruitment of inflammatory cells [43]. The enhanced production of reactive oxygen species (ROS) elicited by leptin may therefore contribute to the induction of the inflammatory phenotype that is assumed by endothelial cells in obesity.

Circulating immune system cells such as monocytes and T-lymphocytes also express leptin receptors and there is emerging evidence that engagement of these receptors by leptin activates the immune cells to promote an inflammatory phenotype [44-46]. Leptin shifts Th-cells towards a Th-1 phenotype, thereby favoring the production of the proinflammatory cytokines IL-2 and IFN-γ; while it also suppresses the production of anti-inflammatory cytokines such as IL-10 in both human and animal studies [47]. Moreover, leptin increases the production of CRP in endothelial cells [36]. In turn, it has also been shown that both TNF-α and IL-1 can induce leptin production [48]. The close association between proinflammatory cytokines and leptin is supported by the obsevation that leptin receptor deficient mice (ob/ob) are resistant to chronic inflammatory diseases like atherosclerosis, inflammatory bowel disease and arthritis [7, 49, 50].

Adiponectin (APO) normally circulates at the highest level among all adipokines [7]. The adiponectin protein consists of a collagenous and a globular domain, with the latter exhibiting structural similarities with TNF-α [51]. Although APO is synthesized by adipocytes, serum levels of this adipokine are negatively correlated to body weight. Obese subjects have decreased APO levels while anorectic patients present with increased levels [51, 52]. APO levels increase with weight loss and with the application of thiazolidinediones, which enhance insulin sensitivity [53]. Additionally there is a negative correlation between waist circumference and adiponectin levels in adolescents, preceding a correlation between insulin sensitivity and waist circumference [54].

The anti-inflammatory properties of APO include its ability to suppress cytokine-induced up-regulation of endothelial cell adhesion molecules. It has been demonstrated that APO deficient mice elicit an increased expression of E-selectin and VCAM-1 in vascular endothelium. Moreover, systemic administration of recombinant adiponectin to those mice significantly attenuated leukocyte-endothelium interactions and adhesion molecule expression providing evidence that loss of adiponectin induces a primary state of endothelial dysfunction with increased leukocyte-endothelium adhesiveness [55]. This effect on endothelial cell adhesion molecules may reflect the ability of APO to inhibit the activity of nuclear factor kappa-B (NFkB), a transcription factor that modulates the biosynthesis of endothelial cell adhesion molecules. This may be due in part to the anti-oxidant properties of APO, which decreases reactive oxygen species and augments endothelial nitric oxide production [56, 57].

APO also appears to decrease the expression of pro-inflammatory cytokines like IL-8 as well as tissue factor, which plays a pivotal role in thrombus formation and atherogenesis [58, 59]. APO also reduces the production and activity of pro-inflammatory cytokines TNF-α [60] and IL-6, while increasing the levels of the anti-inflammatory cytokines IL-10 and IL-1R-antagonist [61-63]. Support for an association between APO and inflammation is derived from the observation that its secretion by adipocytes is inhibited by proinflammatory cytokines like IL-6 and TNF-α [64, 65].

Resistin This adipose tissue-derived protein belongs to the resistin-like molecule family (RELM), along with RELM-α, -β and -γ [66]. Resistin is almost exclusively expressed in adipocytes of mice and was suggested to be associated with insulin resistance [67]. In human (unlike rodents) fat, resistin level is low to undetectable and it is produced by inflammatory cells, mainly macrophages [68]. However, the relationship between resistin levels and obesity is still unclear, with some reports describing a positive correlation [69] and others showing no correlation [70-72]. Elevated levels of circulating resistin are significantly related to an increased risk of development of type 2 diabetes [73].

Resistin was first reported to contribute to insulin resistance. However, there is a growing body of evidence that resistin also has proinflammatory properties. In humans with severe inflammation, a significant correlation between resistin and inflammatory markers has been demonstrated [74]. In an *in vitro* study performed in fully differentiated adipocytes, resistin caused an increased production of TNF-α, IL-6 and MCP-1, while decreasing the production of IL-10 [75]. In human peripheral blood mononuclear cells, resistin strongly upregulates IL-6 and TNF-α via a NF-κB dependent pathway [76]. The addition of recombinant human resistin to macrophages (both murine and human) results in an enhanced secretion of pro-inflammatory cytokines, TNF-α and IL-12 [77]. In turn, TNF-α and IL-6 are capable of inducing resistin gene expression in peripheral blood mononuclear cells [78].

Resistin also causes endothelial cell dysfunction via the induction of oxidative stress and downregulation of eNOS [79]. Resistin has been shown to directly act on vascular endothelial cells to induce endothelin-1 release, and increase the expression of the chemokine MCP-1 [80]. Pathophysiologically relevant concentrations of resistin cause an upregulation of VCAM-1 and ICAM-1 [81, 82]. Even though evidence suggests a clear involvement of resistin in inflammatory conditions its exact role in obesity-related inflammation remains unclear.

IL-6 and CRP Another cytokine that has received considerable attention for its association with obesity-induced inflammation is IL-6. It is secreted by a wide variety of different cells, including adipocytes, from which it can exert both local and distant actions [83]. Both plasma levels and mRNA levels of IL-6 in adipose tissue are elevated in obesity [6]. IL-6 secretion in adipose tissue from obese subjects is 10-fold higher than that from lean individuals, if normalized for the number of adipocytes present [84].

IL-6 increases the expression of adhesion molecules and angiotensin II (AT1) receptors on endothelial cells, both of which favor vascular inflammation [85]. The endothelial cell dysfunction induced by IL-6 is also manifested as changes in vascular permeability resulting from alterations in endothelial cell junctions and changes in cell shape [86]. In addition to its direct proinflammatory effects, IL-6 alters the expression of other inflammatory proteins. For example, both IL-6 increases resistin mRNA expression in human peripheral blood mononuclear cells [87].

IL-6 is best known for its ability to increase the production of C-reactive protein (CRP) by the liver. While this acute phase protein has been widely used as a systemic marker of inflammation, there is emerging evidence that it can directly mediate inflammation and cause endothelial cell dysfunction, in part due to its ability to activate the complement system [88, 89]. Moreover, CRP exerts many proatherogenic effects on vascular endothelium such as upregulating adhesion molecules and MCP-1, while downregulating eNOS activity [90]. Like IL-6, plasma levels of CRP are elevated in obese subjects. Supporting a role for IL-6 and CRP in obesity-induced inflammation is the observation that weight loss significantly reduces these inflammatory markers [91].

TNF-α Tumor necrosis factor-α (TNF-α) is a well-known and extensively characterized proinflammatory cytokine that can profoundly alter endothelial cell and microvascular function. Its effects on endothelium include enhanced formation of ROS (via NADPH oxidase), upregulation of endothelial cell adhesion molecules, increased production of chemokines and cytokines, and decreased barrier function [92]. Moreover, mice lacking TNF-α or TNF-α receptors are resistant to the development of obesity induced insulin resistance [93].

While TNF-α is secreted by a variety of different cells, in adipose tissue the majority of TNF-α is secreted by macrophages [94]. Of relevance to obesity-associated inflammation is the observation that the TNF-α levels are positively correlated with the amount of adipose tissue [95, 96]. TNF-α plays a pivotal role in the upregulation of other cytokines and adipokines while suppressing adiponectin production [97, 98] The elevated circulating levels of TNF-α detected in obese women are accompanied by endothelial dysfunction (impaired endothelium-dependent vasodilation) and elevated blood levels of soluble endothelial cell adhesion molecules such as P-selectin, ICAM-1 and VCAM-1, which reflects endothelial cell activation [99]. All of these effects were ameliorated by weight loss.

Visfatin, Hepcidin, and Apelin A variety of novel adipokines including visfatin, hepcidin, apelin and vaspin have been implicated to the development of the chronic low-grade inflammatory state seen in obesity. Visfatin is expressed in many cells and tissues but it is predominantly found in visceral adipose tissue [98]. Therefore, it is considered to be an adipose tissue-derived hormone that correlates with visceral fat mass in obese patients. A positive correlation between visceral adipose tissue gene expression and BMI along with a negative correlation between BMI and subcutaneous visfatin has been described, while other studies could not demonstrate a clear relationship [100]. However, CRP, TNF-α and waist circumference do show a positive correlation with visfatin [101]. In endothelial cells, visfatin induces MCP-1 and IL-6 production [102].

Hepcidin was originally described as a urinary antimicrobial peptide [103]. Recent studies have demonstrated a positive correlation between this peptide and obesity. An association of the peptide with CRP and IL-6 has also been shown [104]. Hepcidin mRNA expression is upregulated in human heptoma cells by leptin [105].

Originally identified from bovine stomach extracts, apelin is an adipokine that is produced in white adipose tissue, but also expressed in the kidney and heart. Although relatively little is known about the physiological role of apelin, it is known to be upregulated in obese and hyperinsulinemic humans and mice [106, 107]. Apelin synthesis in adipocytes is stimulated by insulin [108] and positive hemodynamic effects of apelin have been reported [109]. A TNF-α-dependent up-regulation of apelin expression has been demonstrated in human and mouse adipose tissue [110]. Visfatin, hepcidin, and apelin increase the complexity of the inflammatory state associated with obesity and further studies are warranted to shed more light on the association between inflammation and these newly designated adipokines.

3. INFLAMMATION AND INSULIN RESISTANCE

Obesity is associated with a variety of adverse health outcomes such as high blood pressure, insulin resistance and type 2 diabetes. Insulin resistance is defined as an inadequate response of target organs like the liver, adipose tissue and skeletal muscle to physiologic levels of insulin. Insulin resistance represents a hallmark of the metabolic syndrome. Even though there are genetic predispositions for insulin resistance, one of the most common acquired factors causing insulin resistance is obesity [111]. The association between obesity and insulin resistance has raised the issue of whether insulin resistance is a cause or a consequence of obesity-related inflammation.

A link between adipocyte-derived cytokines and insulin resistance is suggested by reports describing an improved insulin resistance following the administration of adiponectin in rodents [112]. While adiponectin transgenic mice exhibit partial amelioration of insulin resistance [113], increases in insulin resistance has been shown in adiponectin knockout mice [114, 115]. Further support for a role of adipokines in obesity-associated insulin resistance is provided by the observation that plasma levels of adiponectin in humans are negatively correlated with insulin resistance and positively correlated with markers of insulin sensitivity [116-118]. More support for such a cause-effect relationship in human type II diabetes is provided by epidemiological studies demonstrating that the inflammation (assessed using systemic markers such as plasma CRP, IL-6, etc) precedes and predicts the development of type II diabetes [119]. While the dependence of insulin resistance on obesity-related inflammatory mediators remains an unresolved issue, there is a growing body of evidence that supports the possibility that insulin resistance may contribute to the inflammatory phenotype that is assumed by the microvasculature in obesity. This possibility relates, in part, to the fact that insulin normally acts as an anti-inflammatory molecule. Hence, disruption of insulin signaling mechanisms may result in an exacerbation of the inflammatory phenotype that is induced by mediators released from adipocytes.

Insulin resistance is associated with endothelial dysfunction [120]. This dysfunction is manifested as an increased production of reactive oxygen species, an increased expression of adhesion molecules and chemokines, and an impaired capacity of arterioles/arteries to relax in response to endothelium-dependent vasodilators, such as acetycholine [121]. The increased adhesion molecule expression appears to sustain the binding of both leukocytes and platelets [122]. There is evidence that insulin administration, either in vivo or in vitro, can attenuate these responses as well as suppress NFkB activation and the activation of genes for a variety of inflammatory cytokines [123, 124]. Support for an anti-inflammatory action of insulin is provided by reports describing a reduction in the plasma concentrations of TNF-α, ICAM-1, MCP-1 and CRP, with an increased level of IL-10, in patients treated with thiazolidinediones (insulin sensitizers) [125, 126]. These effects may partially reflect an action of the thiazolidinediones on adipokine production, since rosiglitazone has been shown to elevate adiponectin and reduce resistin levels in humans [127].

Insulin may also exert an influence on the activity of circulating immune cells and platelets. Significantly higher amounts of CD36, CD14 and CD18 are expressed on monocytes isolated from obese subjects with type II diabetes and they appear to be functionally activated [128]. This may explain why mononuclear cells isolated from diabetic animals bind with enhanced avidity to the endothelium [129]. Since monocytes have been implicated in atherogenesis, the activation of these cells in type II diabetics may explain why this condition is a major risk factor for atherosclerosis [130]. Platelets, which have also been implicated in atherogenesis, similarly exhibit signs of activation in type II diabetes. The expression of P-selectin is increased on the surface of circulating platelets and there is evidence of increased platelet aggregation in patients suffering from type II diabetes [131].

While the pro-inflammatory phenotype exhibited by vascular endothelium and circulating immune cells in type II diabetes may well result specifically from the insulin insensitivity exhibited by these cells, it is also possible that metabolic consequences secondary to insulin resistance, such as hyperglycemia, may contribute to the induction of this phenotype. Glucose, at concentrations that are detected in plasma of type II diabetics, can result in endothelial cell activation with an accompanying increase in the expression of adhesion molecules, increased superoxide production, and diminished barrier function (increased vascular permeability) [132]. In vitro and in vivo studies have revealed that these detrimental responses of endothelial cells to hyperglycemia may result from ligation of the endothelial receptor (RAGE) for advanced glycolation end-products (AGEs). It is also noteworthy that RAGE may function as an endothelial adhesion receptor that binds to the leukocyte beta2-integrin to promote leukocyte-endothelial cell adhesion [133]. Whether these hyperglycemia-induced pathways contribute to the inflammatory phenotype associated with obesity remains unclear and is worthy of further attention.

4.   CLINICAL   CONSEQUENCES   OF   OBESITY-ASSOCIATED INFLAMMATION

The epidemiological evidence linking inflammation to obesity has led to the proposal that immune dysfunction is a major factor contributing to the increased morbidity associated with obesity. Even though organs other than adipose tissue do not exhibit the enhanced inflammatory state they are still exposed to elevated levels of adipokines that are secreted from an overly activated pool of adipocytes and inflammatory cells within the adipose tissue. These adipokine responses, coupled to the accompanying insulin resistance, appear to enhance the vulnerability of the microvasculature in different organ systems of obese animals to additional inflammatory stimuli. This is supported by clinical evidence that also demonstrates exaggerated inflammatory responses and an enhanced tissue injury in obese subjects with cardiovascular disease, sepsis, thrombosis and allergic diseases (Table **1**).

Ischemia/Reperfusion: A variety of studies indicate that obesity represents an independent risk factor for cardiovascular diseases (CVD) such as stroke and myocardial infarction. In an animal study performed in obese Zucker rats, it was demonstrated that brain infarcts are approximately 58% larger in obese rats after ischemic stroke compared to their lean counterparts [134]. Despite the strong epidemiological evidence linking obesity to ischemic tissue diseases, there has been relatively little effort to address this issue in animal models and to address the mechanisms by which obesity increases the risk for ischemic tissue disease. There is evidence however that links leptin and CRP to CVD [135]. In a large prospective clinical study, leptin was independently associated with an increased risk of coronary artery disease [136] and leptin proved to be a significant and independent predictor of recurrent cardiovascular events (cardiovascular death, nonfatal myocardial infarction and stroke) in men [137].

Table 1: Examples of the clinical consequences of obesity in different inflammatory diseases.

Disease	Consequences of obesity
Stroke	- brain infarcts are larger in obese rats - more apoptosis in adiponectin deficient mice - increase of leukocyte and platelet adhesion in ob/ob mice - increase of blood-brain barrier permeability and infarct volume in ob/ob mice
Sepsis	- increased mortality in obese patients - increased rate of complications in obese patients - enhanced expression of inflammatory genes of ob/ob mice - increase of leukocyte and platelet adhesion in brain and small intestine of ob/ob and db/db mice - enhanced intestinal permeability of obese mice
Thrombosis	- increase of blood fibrinogen in obese subjects - correlation of BMI and levels of plasminogen-activator-inhibitor-1 - higher platelet concentration in obese subjects
Allergic Diseases	- increased risk for asthma and bronchial hyperreactivity of obese patients - positive association of obesity with atopic dermatitis

Experimentally, it has been shown that adiponectin knockout mice exhibit larger infarct sizes with more apoptosis that their wild type counterparts and that the administration of adiponectin blunts these injury responses to ischemia-reperfusion in both stains of mice [138]. It has also been reported that ob/ob exhibit larger increases in leukocyte and platelet adhesion, blood-brain barrier permeability and infarct volume, and elevated plasma levels of MCP-1 and IL-6 following ischemia/reperfusion compared with wild-type mice. While reconstitution of leptin in ob/ob mice tends to further enhance all reperfusion-induced responses, immunoneutralization of MCP-1 reduced infarct volume in ob/ob mice [139], implicating a role for this chemokine in the obesity-associated enhanced tissue injury. Finally, a recent report demonstrates that leptin administration during reperfusion significantly reduces myocardial infarct size in perfused hearts from C57Bl/6 mice [140]. If leptin resistance does accompany obesity in humans (as discussed above), then these studies in mice would suggest that an exacerbation of the myocardial ischemic injury response in human obesity could result from an inability of leptin to exert its normal protective effect on the heart.

Sepsis: is the leading cause of death in non-coronary intensive care units in the US and has a mortality rate as high as that of myocardial infarction [141]. The annualized incidence of sepsis cases in the United States has increased more than 3-fold over the past two decades, and sepsis in general is associated with a high cost of medical care [142]. The management of sepsis in obese patients is a growing concern. There are several reports demonstrating that the overall mortality of sepsis is significantly higher in obese patients compared to their lean counterparts [143]. Furthermore, the rates of intensive care unit complications such as pneumonia, ARDS and acute renal failure are higher in obese patients [144]. The mechanisms that underlie the enhanced organ injury/failure during sepsis in obese patients remain poorly understood, but may relate to the low-grade systemic inflammatory response that is associated with obesity.

Animal studies show an enhanced inflammatory response of different organs to sepsis in obese animals compared to their lean counterparts. Enhanced expression of inflammatory genes in different tissues of endotoxin-challenged obese (ob/ob) mice (compared to lean mice) [145, 146], and an exacerbation of these sepsis-induced blood cell-endothelial cell interactions in the cerebral microvasculature of obese (ob/ob) mice have been reported [147]. We demonstrated similar exaggerated responses of leukocyte and platelet adhesion in the intestinal microcirculation following polymicrobial sepsis in two strains of prediabetic obese mice, i.e., ob/ob and db/db mice, (compared to their septic lean counterparts) [148]. In addition, it has been shown that genetically obese mice display enhanced intestinal permeability leading to increased portal endotoxemia [149]. Moreover, the sensitivity to LPS-induced mortality is significantly greater in ob/ob mice compared with their own lean littermates [150].

Thrombosis: Excess body weight is a risk factor for first and recurrent venous thromboembolic events [151]. Similarly, the metabolic syndrome is associated with a two-fold increase of development of venous thromboembolism [152]. The link between obesity and thromboembolism may result from the increased plasma factor VII activity that is associated with increased plasma triglyceride levels, as well as the increased hepatic synthesis of fibrinogen and an enhanced synthesis and release of von Willebrand factor in response to cytokines originating in visceral adipose tissue [153]. A 40% increase in blood fibrinogen – an acute phase protein that affects haemostasis, blood rheology, platelet aggregation and endothelial function –has been detected in obese subjects compared to age- and gender-matched non-obese individuals [154]). BMI also correlates with the levels of the anti-fibrinolytic and pro-thrombotic molecule plasminogen-activator-inhibitor 1 [155]).

There is a growing body of evidence that implicates adipokines in the hypercoagulopathy associated with obesity. For instance, increased leptin is independently associated with significant increases in coagulation factor VIII, von Willebrand factor, tissue plasminogen activator, and fibrin D-dimer levels [156]). Moreover, the long isoform of the leptin receptor has been detected in human platelets and high concentrations of leptin promote platelet aggregation in vitro [157]. Additionally, obese adolescents present with a higher platelet concentration when compared to a non-obese control group [158]. It has been demonstrated that leptin deficiency elicits an antithrombotic effect. Further confirming an integral role of leptin in the development of thrombosis, inhibition of endogenous leptin using a neutralizing antibody provides protection from thrombosis [159].

Allergic Diseases: A recent meta-analysis of prospective epidemiological studies of asthma incidence in overweight and obese subjects has revealed that being overweigh or obese confers an increased risk for asthma, with disease risk exhibiting a positive relation to BMI [160]. A study including lung function measurements has shown an increased risk of bronchial hyper-reactivity in obese subjects [161]. Childhood obesity also exhibits positive associations with bronchial asthma prevalence and atopic dermatitis severity [162]. TNF-α, a cytokine produced by adipocytes and which has been implicated into the development of allergic diseases [163] may provide a link between obesity and increased asthma risk. It is known that TNF-α increases the production of Th-2 cytokines, such as IL-4 and IL-5, by bronchial epithelial cells as well as other pro-inflammatory cytokines like IL-6.

There is a growing body of evidence showing that leptin may play a crucial immunopathophysiological role in allergic inflammation via the activation of eosinophils. Human eosinophils express leptin receptors [164]. In a recent study performed by Wong, it was demonstrated that leptin induced an increased cell surface expression of ICAM-1 and CD18 on eosinophils. Leptin also stimulates the chemokinesis of eosinophils by inducing the release of inflammatory cytokines IL-1beta and IL-6, and chemokines IL-8, and MCP-1 [165]. Of potential relevance to this mechanism is the observation that significantly higher serum leptin levels are detected in female patients with pollen-induced allergic rhinitis outside the pollen season, compared to a healthy control group [166].

Supporting a close relationship between allergic diseases and obesity is the observation that obesity is associated with decreased levels of IL-10, an anti-inflammatory cytokine that can deactivate the inflammatory host response by macrophages and lymphocytes. IL-10 inhibits eosinophilia by suppressing IL-5 and GM-CSF, by direct effects on eosinophil apoptosis, and via effects on cell proliferation by downregulating IL-1. IL-10 is also a suppressor of nitric oxide (NO) production, which has also been implicated in the pathophysiology of airway inflammatory diseases [167].

5. CONCLUSIONS

Over the last two decades a large amount of compelling evidence has accumulated that links inflammation to obesity. Consequently, obesity is now considered to represent a state of chronic low-grade inflammation. This contention is based on epidemiological studies that demonstrate 1) increased levels of inflammatory mediators (including adipokines) in obese humans compared to their lean counterparts and 2) a strong link between obesity and inflammatory diseases such as cardiovascular disease, sepsis, thrombosis and allergic diseases. The growing list of adipokines that are thought to participate in obesity-associated inflammation now exceeds 50. Animal studies on genetically obese laboratory animals are generally consistent with the view of a chronic low-grade inflammatory state. However, the extent to which the inflammatory phenotype assumed by these animal models mimic the human condition remains poorly defined. More work is needed to determine whether/how diet- and exercise-induced weight loss will reverse the inflammatory responses in animal models of obesity, as predicted by clinical evidence. Similarly, there is a need for animal studies that are designed to distinguish the inflammatory effects that result from adipocyte-derived factors (e.g. adipokines) from those directly related to the metabolic consequences of the insulin resistance, a challenge made all the more difficult by the possibility that adipokines may cause insulin resistance. By addressing these unresolved issues, progress will be made towards the development of novel therapeutic strategies that will reduce the inflammation that accompanies obesity and renders this condition a risk factor for life-threatening diseases.

6. REFERENCES

[1]   Wardle J, Boniface D. Changes in the distributions of body mass index and waist circumference in English adults, 1993/1994 to 2002/2003. Int J Obes (Lond) 2008; 32: 527-32.

[2]   Hotamisligil GS, Shargill NS, Spiegelman BM. Adipose expression of tumor necrosis factor-alpha: direct role in obesity-linked insulin resistance. Science 1993; 259: 87-91.

[3]   Lago F, Dieguez C, Gomez-Reino J, Gualillo O. The emerging role of adipokines as mediators of inflammation and immune responses. Cytokine Growth Factor Rev 2007; 18: 313-25.

[4]   Lyon CJ, Law RE, Hsueh WA. Minireview: adiposity, inflammation, and atherogenesis. Endocrinology 2003; 144: 2195-200.

[5]   Greenberg AS, Obin MS. Obesity and the role of adipose tissue in inflammation and metabolism. Am J Clin Nutr 2006; 83: 461S-465S.

[6]   Trayhurn P, Wood IS. Adipokines: inflammation and the pleiotropic role of white adipose tissue. Br J Nutr 2004; 92: 347-55.

[7]   Fantuzzi G. Adipose tissue, adipokines, and inflammation. J Allergy Clin Immunol 2005; 115: 911-9; quiz 920.

[8]   Lee YH, Pratley RE. The evolving role of inflammation in obesity and the metabolic syndrome. Curr Diab Rep 2005; 5: 70-5.

[9]   Nishimura S, Manabe I, Nagasaki M, et al. Adipogenesis in obesity requires close interplay between differentiating adipocytes, stromal cells, and blood vessels. Diabetes 2007; 56: 1517-26.

[10]   Hausman GJ, Richardson RL. Adipose tissue angiogenesis. J Anim Sci 2004; 82: 925-34.

[11]   Lijnen HR, Christiaens V, Scroyen I, et al. Impaired adipose tissue development in mice with inactivation of placental growth factor function. Diabetes 2006; 55: 2698-704.

[12]   Pasarica M, Sereda OR, Redman LM, et al. Reduced Adipose Tissue Oxygenation in Human Obesity - Evidence for Rarefaction, Macrophage Chemotaxis and Inflammation without an Angiogenic Response. Diabetes 2008;

[13]   Ye J, Gao Z, Yin J, He Q. Hypoxia is a potential risk factor for chronic inflammation and adiponectin reduction in adipose tissue of ob/ob and dietary obese mice. Am J Physiol Endocrinol Metab 2007; 293: E1118-28.

[14]   Trayhurn P, Wang B, Wood IS. Hypoxia in adipose tissue: a basis for the dysregulation of tissue function in obesity? Br J Nutr 2008; 100: 227-35.

[15]   Cancello R, Henegar C, Viguerie N, et al. Reduction of macrophage infiltration and chemoattractant gene expression changes in white adipose tissue of morbidly obese subjects after surgery-induced weight loss. Diabetes 2005; 54: 2277-86.

[16]   Ortega E, Xu X, Koska J, et al. Macrophage content in subcutaneous adipose tissue: associations with adiposity, age, inflammatory markers, and whole-body insulin action in healthy Pima Indians. Diabetes 2008;

[17]   Guzik TJ, Marvar PJ, Czesnikiewicz-Guzik M, Korbut R. Perivascular adipose tissue as a messenger of the brain-vessel axis: role in vascular inflammation and dysfunction. J Physiol Pharmacol 2007; 58: 591-610.

[18]   Soltis EE, Cassis LA. Influence of perivascular adipose tissue on rat aortic smooth muscle responsiveness. Clin Exp Hypertens A 1991; 13: 277-96.

[19]   Gollasch M, Dubrovska G. Paracrine role for periadventitial adipose tissue in the regulation of arterial tone. Trends Pharmacol Sci 2004; 25: 647-53.

[20]   Henrichot E, Juge-Aubry CE, Pernin A, et al. Production of chemokines by perivascular adipose tissue: a role in the pathogenesis of atherosclerosis? Arterioscler Thromb Vasc Biol 2005; 25: 2594-9.

[21]   Guzik TJ, Hoch NE, Brown KA, et al. Role of the T cell in the genesis of angiotensin II induced hypertension and vascular dysfunction. J Exp Med 2007; 204: 2449-60.

[22]   Otero M, Lago R, Lago F, et al. Leptin, from fat to inflammation: old questions and new insights. FEBS Lett 2005; 579: 295-301.

[23]   Zhang Y, Proenca R, Maffei M, et al. Positional cloning of the mouse obese gene and its human homologue. Nature 1994; 372: 425-32.

[24]   Friedman JM, Halaas JL. Leptin and the regulation of body weight in mammals. Nature 1998; 395: 763-

[25]   Lord GM, Matarese G, Howard JK, *et al.* Leptin modulates the T-cell immune response and reverses starvation-induced immunosuppression. Nature 1998; 394: 897-901.

[26]   Unger RH, Zhou YT, Orci L. Regulation of fatty acid homeostasis in cells: novel role of leptin. Proc Natl Acad Sci U S A 1999; 96: 2327-32.

[27]   Wozniak SE, Gee LL, Wachtel MS, Frezza EE. Adipose Tissue: The New Endocrine Organ? A Review Article. Dig Dis Sci 2008;

[28]   Montague CT, Farooqi IS, Whitehead JP, *et al.* Congenital leptin deficiency is associated with severe early-onset obesity in humans. Nature 1997; 387: 903-8.

[29]   Lee GH, Proenca R, Montez JM, *et al.* Abnormal splicing of the leptin receptor in diabetic mice. Nature 1996; 379: 632-5.

[30]   Wu-Peng XS, Chua SC, Jr., Okada N, *et al.* Phenotype of the obese Koletsky (f) rat due to Tyr763Stop mutation in the extracellular domain of the leptin receptor (Lepr): evidence for deficient plasma-to-CSF transport of leptin in both the Zucker and Koletsky obese rat. Diabetes 1997; 46: 513-8.

[31]   Arvidsson E, Viguerie N, Andersson I, *et al.* Effects of different hypocaloric diets on protein secretion from adipose tissue of obese women. Diabetes 2004; 53: 1966-71.

[32]   Considine RV, Sinha MK, Heiman ML, *et al.* Serum immunoreactive-leptin concentrations in normal-weight and obese humans. N Engl J Med 1996; 334: 292-5.

[33]   Dencker M, Thorsson O, Karlsson MK, *et al.* Leptin is closely related to body fat in prepubertal children aged 8-11 years. Acta Paediatr 2006; 95: 975-9.

[34]   Viguerie N, Vidal H, Arner P, *et al.* Adipose tissue gene expression in obese subjects during low-fat and high-fat hypocaloric diets. Diabetologia 2005; 48: 123-31.

[35]   Lollmann B, Gruninger S, Stricker-Krongrad A, Chiesi M. Detection and quantification of the leptin receptor splice variants Ob-Ra, b, and, e in different mouse tissues. Biochem Biophys Res Commun 1997; 238: 648-52.

[36]   Singh P, Hoffmann M, Wolk R, Shamsuzzaman AS, Somers VK. Leptin induces C-reactive protein expression in vascular endothelial cells. Arterioscler Thromb Vasc Biol 2007; 27: e302-7.

[37]   Wolk R, Deb A, Caplice NM, Somers VK. Leptin receptor and functional effects of leptin in human endothelial progenitor cells. Atherosclerosis 2005; 183: 131-9.

[38]   Galili O, Versari D, Sattler KJ, *et al.* Early experimental obesity is associated with coronary endothelial dysfunction and oxidative stress. Am J Physiol Heart Circ Physiol 2007; 292: H904-11.

[39]   Korda M, Kubant R, Patton S, Malinski T. Leptin-induced endothelial dysfunction in obesity. Am J Physiol Heart Circ Physiol 2008; 295: H1514-21.

[40]   Yamagishi SI, Edelstein D, Du XL, *et al.* Leptin induces mitochondrial superoxide production and monocyte chemoattractant protein-1 expression in aortic endothelial cells by increasing fatty acid oxidation via protein kinase A. J Biol Chem 2001; 276: 25096-100.

[41]   Marui N, Offermann MK, Swerlick R, *et al.* Vascular cell adhesion molecule-1 (VCAM-1) gene transcription and expression are regulated through an antioxidant-sensitive mechanism in human vascular endothelial cells. J Clin Invest 1993; 92: 1866-74.

[42]   Cominacini L, Garbin U, Pasini AF, *et al.* Antioxidants inhibit the expression of intercellular cell adhesion molecule-1 and vascular cell adhesion molecule-1 induced by oxidized LDL on human umbilical vein endothelial cells. Free Radic Biol Med 1997; 22: 117-27.

[43]   Couillard C, Ruel G, Archer WR, *et al.* Circulating levels of oxidative stress markers and endothelial adhesion molecules in men with abdominal obesity. J Clin Endocrinol Metab 2005; 90: 6454-9.

[44]   Lord GM, Matarese G, Howard JK, Bloom SR, Lechler RI. Leptin inhibits the anti-CD3-driven proliferation of peripheral blood T cells but enhances the production of proinflammatory cytokines. J Leukoc Biol 2002; 72: 330-8.

[45]   Maruyama I, Nakata M, Yamaji K. Effect of leptin in platelet and endothelial cells. Obesity and arterial thrombosis. Ann N Y Acad Sci 2000; 902: 315-9.

[46]   Otero M, Lago R, Gomez R, *et al.* Towards a pro-inflammatory and immunomodulatory emerging role of leptin. Rheumatology (Oxford) 2006; 45: 944-50.

[47]   Dubey L, Hesong Z. Role of leptin in atherogenesis. Exp Clin Cardiol 2006; 11: 269-75.

[48]   Gualillo O, Eiras S, Lago F, Dieguez C, Casanueva FF. Elevated serum leptin concentrations induced by experimental acute inflammation. Life Sci 2000; 67: 2433-41.

[49]   de Boer OJ, van der Wal AC, Becker AE. Atherosclerosis, inflammation, and infection. J Pathol 2000; 190: 237-43.

[50]   Nishina PM, Naggert JK, Verstuyft J, Paigen B. Atherosclerosis in genetically obese mice: the mutants obese, diabetes, fat, tubby, and lethal yellow. Metabolism 1994; 43: 554-8.

[51]   Chandran M, Phillips SA, Ciaraldi T, Henry RR. Adiponectin: more than just another fat cell hormone? Diabetes Care 2003; 26: 2442-50.

[52]   Pannacciulli N, Vettor R, Milan G, *et al.* Anorexia nervosa is characterized by increased adiponectin plasma levels and reduced nonoxidative glucose metabolism. J Clin Endocrinol Metab 2003; 88: 1748-52.

[53]   Maeda N, Takahashi M, Funahashi T, *et al.* PPARgamma ligands increase expression and plasma concentrations of adiponectin, an adipose-derived protein. Diabetes 2001; 50: 2094-9.

[54]   Rasmussen-Torvik LJ, Pankow JS, Jacobs DR, Jr., *et al.* Influence of waist on adiponectin and insulin sensitivity in adolescence. Obesity (Silver Spring) 2009; 17: 156-61.

[55]   Ouedraogo R, Gong Y, Berzins B, *et al.* Adiponectin deficiency increases leukocyte-endothelium interactions via upregulation of endothelial cell adhesion molecules in vivo. J Clin Invest 2007; 117: 1718-26.

[56]   Matsuo Y, Imanishi T, Kuroi A, *et al.* Effects of plasma adiponectin levels on the number and function of endothelial progenitor cells in patients with coronary artery disease. Circ J 2007; 71: 1376-82.

[57]   Ouedraogo R, Wu X, Xu SQ, *et al.* Adiponectin suppression of high-glucose-induced reactive oxygen species in vascular endothelial cells: evidence for involvement of a cAMP signaling pathway. Diabetes 2006; 55: 1840-6.

[58]   Chen YJ, Zhang LQ, Wang GP, *et al.* Adiponectin inhibits tissue factor expression and enhances tissue factor pathway inhibitor expression in human endothelial cells. Thromb Haemost 2008; 100: 291-300.

[59]   Kobashi C, Urakaze M, Kishida M, *et al.* Adiponectin inhibits endothelial synthesis of interleukin-8. Circ Res 2005; 97: 1245-52.

[60]   Masaki T, Chiba S, Tatsukawa H, *et al.* Adiponectin protects LPS-induced liver injury through modulation of TNF-alpha in KK-Ay obese mice. Hepatology 2004; 40: 177-84.

[61]   Kumada M, Kihara S, Ouchi N, *et al.* Adiponectin specifically increased tissue inhibitor of metalloproteinase-1 through interleukin-10 expression in human macrophages. Circulation 2004; 109: 2046-9.

[62]   Wolf AM, Wolf D, Rumpold H, Enrich B, Tilg H. Adiponectin induces the anti-inflammatory cytokines IL-10 and IL-1RA in human leukocytes. Biochem Biophys Res Commun 2004; 323: 630-5.

[63]   Wulster-Radcliffe MC, Ajuwon KM, Wang J, Christian JA, Spurlock ME. Adiponectin differentially regulates cytokines in porcine macrophages. Biochem Biophys Res Commun 2004; 316: 924-9.

[64]   Bruun JM, Lihn AS, Verdich C, *et al.* Regulation of adiponectin by adipose tissue-derived cytokines: in vivo and in vitro investigations in humans. Am J Physiol Endocrinol Metab 2003; 285: E527-33.

[65]   Fasshauer M, Kralisch S, Klier M, *et al.* Adiponectin gene expression and secretion is inhibited by interleukin-6 in 3T3-L1 adipocytes. Biochem Biophys Res Commun 2003; 301: 1045-50.

[66]   Steppan CM, Brown EJ, Wright CM, *et al.* A family of tissue-specific resistin-like molecules. Proc Natl Acad Sci U S A 2001; 98: 502-6.

[67]   Steppan CM, Bailey ST, Bhat S, *et al.* The hormone resistin links obesity to diabetes. Nature 2001; 409: 307-12.

[68]   Patel L, Buckels AC, Kinghorn IJ, *et al.* Resistin is expressed in human macrophages and directly regulated by PPAR gamma activators. Biochem Biophys Res Commun 2003; 300: 472-6.

[69]   Azuma K, Katsukawa F, Oguchi S, *et al.* Correlation between serum resistin level and adiposity in obese individuals. Obes Res 2003; 11: 997-1001.

[70]   Chen CC, Li TC, Li CI, *et al.* Serum resistin level among healthy subjects: relationship to anthropometric and metabolic parameters. Metabolism 2005; 54: 471-5.

[71]   Farvid MS, Ng TW, Chan DC, Barrett PH, Watts GF. Association of adiponectin and resistin with adipose tissue compartments, insulin resistance and dyslipidaemia. Diabetes Obes Metab 2005; 7: 406-13.

[72]   Guran T, Turan S, Bereket A, *et al.* The role of leptin, soluble leptin receptor, resistin, and insulin secretory dynamics in the pathogenesis of hypothalamic obesity in children. Eur J Pediatr 2008;

[73]   Chen BH, Song Y, Ding EL, *et al.* Circulating Levels of Resistin and Risk of Type 2 Diabetes in Men and Women: Results from Two Prospective Cohorts. Diabetes Care 2008;

[74]   Stejskal D, Adamovska S, Bartek J, Jurakova R, Proskova J. Resistin - concentrations in persons with type 2 diabetes mellitus and in individuals with acute inflammatory disease. Biomed Pap Med Fac Univ Palacky Olomouc Czech Repub 2003; 147: 63-9.

[75]   Fu Y, Luo L, Luo N, Garvey WT. Proinflammatory cytokine production and insulin sensitivity regulated by overexpression of resistin in 3T3-L1 adipocytes. Nutr Metab (Lond) 2006; 3: 28.

[76]   Bokarewa M, Nagaev I, Dahlberg L, Smith U, Tarkowski A. Resistin, an adipokine with potent proinflammatory properties. J Immunol 2005; 174: 5789-95.

[77]   Silswal N, Singh AK, Aruna B, *et al.* Human resistin stimulates the pro-inflammatory cytokines TNF-alpha and IL-12 in macrophages by NF-kappaB-dependent pathway. Biochem Biophys Res Commun 2005; 334: 1092-101.

[78]   Pang SS, Le YY. Role of resistin in inflammation and inflammation-related diseases. Cell Mol Immunol 2006; 3: 29-34.

[79]   Kougias P, Chai H, Lin PH, *et al.* Adipocyte-derived cytokine resistin causes endothelial dysfunction of porcine coronary arteries. J Vasc Surg 2005; 41: 691-8.

[80]   Verma S, Li SH, Wang CH, *et al.* Resistin promotes endothelial cell activation: further evidence of adipokine-endothelial interaction. Circulation 2003; 108: 736-40.

[81]   Kawanami D, Maemura K, Takeda N, *et al.* Direct reciprocal effects of resistin and adiponectin on vascular endothelial cells: a new insight into adipocytokine-endothelial cell interactions. Biochem Biophys Res Commun 2004; 314: 415-9.

[82]   Skilton MR, Nakhla S, Sieveking DP, Caterson ID, Celermajer DS. Pathophysiological levels of the obesity related peptides resistin and ghrelin increase adhesion molecule expression on human vascular endothelial cells. Clin Exp Pharmacol Physiol 2005; 32: 839-44.

[83]   Mohamed-Ali V, Goodrick S, Rawesh A, *et al.* Subcutaneous adipose tissue releases interleukin-6, but not tumor necrosis factor-alpha, in vivo. J Clin Endocrinol Metab 1997; 82: 4196-200.

[84]   Fried SK, Bunkin DA, Greenberg AS. Omental and subcutaneous adipose tissues of obese subjects release interleukin-6: depot difference and regulation by glucocorticoid. J Clin Endocrinol Metab 1998; 83: 847-50.

[85]   Wassmann S, Stumpf M, Strehlow K, *et al.* Interleukin-6 induces oxidative stress and endothelial dysfunction by overexpression of the angiotensin II type 1 receptor. Circ Res 2004; 94: 534-41.

[86]   Devaraj S, Venugopal SK, Singh U, Jialal I. Hyperglycemia induces monocytic release of interleukin-6 via induction of protein kinase c-{alpha} and -{beta}. Diabetes 2005; 54: 85-91.

[87]   Kaser S, Kaser A, Sandhofer A, *et al.* Resistin messenger-RNA expression is increased by proinflammatory cytokines in vitro. Biochem Biophys Res Commun 2003; 309: 286-90.

[88]   Pepys MB, Hirschfield GM. C-reactive protein: a critical update. J Clin Invest 2003; 111: 1805-12.

[89]   Pasceri V, Willerson JT, Yeh ET. Direct proinflammatory effect of C-reactive protein on human endothelial cells. Circulation 2000; 102: 2165-8.

[90]   Verma S, Devaraj S, Jialal I. Is C-reactive protein an innocent bystander or proatherogenic culprit? C-reactive protein promotes atherothrombosis. Circulation 2006; 113: 2135-50; discussion 2150.

[91]   Forsythe LK, Wallace JM, Livingstone MB. Obesity and inflammation: the effects of weight loss. Nutr Res Rev 2008; 21: 117-33.

[92]   Aggarwal BB, Natarajan K. Tumor necrosis factors: developments during the last decade. Eur Cytokine Netw 1996; 7: 93-124.

[93]   Uysal KT, Wiesbrock SM, Marino MW, Hotamisligil GS. Protection from obesity-induced insulin resistance in mice lacking TNF-alpha function. Nature 1997; 389: 610-4.

[94]   Uysal KT, Wiesbrock SM, Hotamisligil GS. Functional analysis of tumor necrosis factor (TNF) receptors in TNF-alpha-mediated insulin resistance in genetic obesity. Endocrinology 1998; 139: 4832-8.

[95]   Hotamisligil GS, Arner P, Caro JF, Atkinson RL, Spiegelman BM. Increased adipose tissue expression of tumor necrosis factor-alpha in human obesity and insulin resistance. J Clin Invest 1995; 95: 2409-15.

[96]   Ronti T, Lupattelli G, Mannarino E. The endocrine function of adipose tissue: an update. Clin Endocrinol (Oxf) 2006; 64: 355-65.

[97]   Coppack SW. Pro-inflammatory cytokines and adipose tissue. Proc Nutr Soc 2001; 60: 349-56.

[98]   Rabe K, Lehrke M, Parhofer KG, Broedl UC. Adipokines and insulin resistance. Mol Med 2008; 14: 741-

[99]   Ziccardi P, Nappo F, Giugliano G, *et al.* Reduction of inflammatory cytokine concentrations and improvement of endothelial functions in obese women after weight loss over one year. Circulation 2002; 105: 804-9.

[100] Rasouli N, Kern PA. Adipocytokines and the metabolic complications of obesity. J Clin Endocrinol Metab 2008; 93: S64-73.

[101] Bo S, Ciccone G, Baldi I, *et al.* Plasma visfatin concentrations after a lifestyle intervention were directly associated with inflammatory markers. Nutr Metab Cardiovasc Dis 2008;

[102] Liu SW, Qiao SB, Yuan JS, Liu DQ. Visfatin Stimulates Production of Monocyte Chemotactic Protein-1 and Interleukin-6 in Human Vein Umbilical Endothelial Cells. Horm Metab Res 2008;

[103] Park CH, Valore EV, Waring AJ, Ganz T. Hepcidin, a urinary antimicrobial peptide synthesized in the liver. J Biol Chem 2001; 276: 7806-10.

[104] Bekri S, Gual P, Anty R, *et al.* Increased adipose tissue expression of hepcidin in severe obesity is independent from diabetes and NASH. Gastroenterology 2006; 131: 788-96.

[105] Chung B, Matak P, McKie AT, Sharp P. Leptin increases the expression of the iron regulatory hormone hepcidin in HuH7 human hepatoma cells. J Nutr 2007; 137: 2366-70.

[106] Boucher J, Masri B, Daviaud D, *et al.* Apelin, a newly identified adipokine up-regulated by insulin and obesity. Endocrinology 2005; 146: 1764-71.

[107] Garcia-Diaz D, Campion J, Milagro FI, Martinez JA. Adiposity dependent apelin gene expression: relationships with oxidative and inflammation markers. Mol Cell Biochem 2007; 305: 87-94.

[108] Beltowski J. Apelin and visfatin: unique "beneficial" adipokines upregulated in obesity? Med Sci Monit 2006; 12: RA112-9.

[109] Grisk O. Apelin and vascular dysfunction in type 2 diabetes. Cardiovasc Res 2007; 74: 339-40.

[110] Daviaud D, Boucher J, Gesta S, *et al.* TNFalpha up-regulates apelin expression in human and mouse adipose tissue. Faseb J 2006; 20: 1528-30.

[111] Schenk S, Saberi M, Olefsky JM. Insulin sensitivity: modulation by nutrients and inflammation. J Clin Invest 2008; 118: 2992-3002.

[112] Yamauchi T, Kamon J, Waki H, *et al.* The fat-derived hormone adiponectin reverses insulin resistance associated with both lipoatrophy and obesity. Nat Med 2001; 7: 941-6.

[113] Yamauchi T, Kamon J, Waki H, *et al.* Globular adiponectin protected ob/ob mice from diabetes and ApoE-deficient mice from atherosclerosis. J Biol Chem 2003; 278: 2461-8.

[114] Kubota N, Terauchi Y, Yamauchi T, *et al.* Disruption of adiponectin causes insulin resistance and neointimal formation. J Biol Chem 2002; 277: 25863-6.

[115] Maeda N, Shimomura I, Kishida K, *et al.* Diet-induced insulin resistance in mice lacking adiponectin/ACRP30. Nat Med 2002; 8: 731-7.

[116] Bacha F, Saad R, Gungor N, Arslanian SA. Adiponectin in youth: relationship to visceral adiposity, insulin sensitivity, and beta-cell function. Diabetes Care 2004; 27: 547-52.

[117] Hivert MF, Sullivan LM, Fox CS, *et al.* Associations of adiponectin, resistin, and tumor necrosis factor-alpha with insulin resistance. J Clin Endocrinol Metab 2008; 93: 3165-72.

[118] Pellme F, Smith U, Funahashi T, *et al.* Circulating adiponectin levels are reduced in nonobese but insulin-resistant first-degree relatives of type 2 diabetic patients. Diabetes 2003; 52: 1182-6.

[119] Dandona P, Aljada A, Bandyopadhyay A. Inflammation: the link between insulin resistance, obesity and diabetes. Trends Immunol 2004; 25: 4-7.

[120] Steinberg HO, Chaker H, Leaming R, *et al.* Obesity/insulin resistance is associated with endothelial dysfunction. Implications for the syndrome of insulin resistance. J Clin Invest 1996; 97: 2601-10.

[121] Ingelsson E, Hulthe J, Lind L. Inflammatory markers in relation to insulin resistance and the metabolic syndrome. Eur J Clin Invest 2008; 38: 502-9.

[122] Tschoepe D, Roesen P, Schwippert B, Gries FA. Platelets in diabetes: the role in the hemostatic regulation in atherosclerosis. Semin Thromb Hemost 1993; 19: 122-8.

[123] Aljada A, Ghanim H, Mohanty P, Kapur N, Dandona P. Insulin inhibits the pro-inflammatory transcription factor early growth response gene-1 (Egr)-1 expression in mononuclear cells (MNC) and reduces plasma tissue factor (TF) and plasminogen activator inhibitor-1 (PAI-1) concentrations. J Clin Endocrinol Metab 2002; 87: 1419-22.

[124] Dandona P, Aljada A, Mohanty P, *et al.* Insulin inhibits intranuclear nuclear factor kappaB and stimulates IkappaB in mononuclear cells in obese subjects: evidence for an anti-inflammatory effect? J Clin Endocrinol Metab 2001; 86: 3257-65.

[125] Dandona P, Aljada A, Mohanty P. The anti-inflammatory and potential anti-atherogenic effect of insulin: a new paradigm. Diabetologia 2002; 45: 924-30.

[126] Ghanim H, Garg R, Aljada A, *et al.* Suppression of nuclear factor-kappaB and stimulation of inhibitor kappaB by troglitazone: evidence for an anti-inflammatory effect and a potential antiatherosclerotic effect in the obese. J Clin Endocrinol Metab 2001; 86: 1306-12.

[127] Ghanim H, Dhindsa S, Aljada A, *et al.* Low-dose rosiglitazone exerts an antiinflammatory effect with an increase in adiponectin independently of free fatty acid fall and insulin sensitization in obese type 2 diabetics. J Clin Endocrinol Metab 2006; 91: 3553-8.

[128] Fogelstrand L, Hulthe J, Hulten LM, Wiklund O, Fagerberg B. Monocytic expression of CD14 and CD18, circulating adhesion molecules and inflammatory markers in women with diabetes mellitus and impaired glucose tolerance. Diabetologia 2004; 47: 1948-52.

[129] Tsao PS, Niebauer J, Buitrago R, *et al.* Interaction of diabetes and hypertension on determinants of endothelial adhesiveness. Arterioscler Thromb Vasc Biol 1998; 18: 947-53.

[130] Cipolletta C, Ryan KE, Hanna EV, Trimble ER. Activation of peripheral blood CD14+ monocytes occurs in diabetes. Diabetes 2005; 54: 2779-86.

[131] Ouvina SM, La Greca RD, Zanaro NL, Palmer L, Sassetti B. Endothelial dysfunction, nitric oxide and platelet activation in hypertensive and diabetic type II patients. Thromb Res 2001; 102: 107-14.

[132] Wautier JL, Schmidt AM. Protein glycation: a firm link to endothelial cell dysfunction. Circ Res 2004; 95: 233-8.

[133] Chavakis T, Bierhaus A, Al-Fakhri N, *et al.* The pattern recognition receptor (RAGE) is a counterreceptor for leukocyte integrins: a novel pathway for inflammatory cell recruitment. J Exp Med 2003; 198: 1507-15.

[134] Osmond JM, Mintz JD, Dalton B, Stepp DW. Obesity Increases Blood Pressure, Cerebral Vascular Remodeling, and Severity of Stroke in the Zucker Rat. Hypertension 2008;

[135] Romero-Corral A, Sierra-Johnson J, Lopez-Jimenez F, *et al.* Relationships between leptin and C-reactive protein with cardiovascular disease in the adult general population. Nat Clin Pract Cardiovasc Med 2008; 5: 418-25.

[136] Wallace AM, McMahon AD, Packard CJ, *et al.* Plasma leptin and the risk of cardiovascular disease in the west of Scotland coronary prevention study (WOSCOPS). Circulation 2001; 104: 3052-6.

[137] Soderberg S, Colquhoun D, Keech A, *et al.* Leptin, but not adiponectin, is a predictor of recurrent cardiovascular events in men: results from the LIPID study. Int J Obes (Lond) 2009; 33: 123-30.

[138] Shibata R, Sato K, Pimentel DR, *et al.* Adiponectin protects against myocardial ischemia-reperfusion injury through AMPK- and COX-2-dependent mechanisms. Nat Med 2005; 11: 1096-103.

[139] Terao S, Yilmaz G, Stokes KY, *et al.* Inflammatory and injury responses to ischemic stroke in obese mice. Stroke 2008; 39: 943-50.

[140] Smith CC, Mocanu MM, Davidson SM, *et al.* Leptin, the obesity-associated hormone, exhibits direct cardioprotective effects. Br J Pharmacol 2006; 149: 5-13.

[141] Angus DC, Linde-Zwirble WT, Lidicker J, *et al.* Epidemiology of severe sepsis in the United States: analysis of incidence, outcome, and associated costs of care. Crit Care Med 2001; 29: 1303-10.

[142] Martin GS, Mannino DM, Eaton S, Moss M. The epidemiology of sepsis in the United States from 1979 through 2000. N Engl J Med 2003; 348: 1546-54.

[143] El-Solh A, Sikka P, Bozkanat E, Jaafar W, Davies J. Morbid obesity in the medical ICU. Chest 2001; 120: 1989-97.

[144] Yaegashi M, Jean R, Zuriqat M, Noack S, Homel P. Outcome of morbid obesity in the intensive care unit. J Intensive Care Med 2005; 20: 147-54.

[145] Scott LK, Vachharajani V, Minagar A, Mynatt RL, Conrad SA. Differential RNA expression of hepatic tissue in lean and obese mice after LPS-induced systemic inflammation. Front Biosci 2005; 10: 1828-34.

[146] Scott LK, Vachharajani V, Mynatt RL, Minagar A, Conrad SA. Brain RNA expression in obese vs lean mice after LPS-induced systemic inflammation. Front Biosci 2004; 9: 2686-96.

[147] Vachharajani V, Russell JM, Scott KL, *et al.* Obesity exacerbates sepsis-induced inflammation and microvascular dysfunction in mouse brain. Microcirculation 2005; 12: 183-94.

[148] Singer G, Stokes KY, Terao S, Granger DN. Sepsis-Induced Intestinal Microvascular and Inflammatory Responses in Obese Mice. Shock 2008;

[149] Brun P, Castagliuolo I, Di Leo V, *et al.* Increased intestinal permeability in obese mice: new evidence in the pathogenesis of nonalcoholic steatohepatitis. Am J Physiol Gastrointest Liver Physiol 2007; 292: G518-25.

[150]   Faggioni R, Fantuzzi G, Gabay C, *et al.* Leptin deficiency enhances sensitivity to endotoxin-induced lethality. Am J Physiol 1999; 276: R136-42.

[151]   Eichinger S, Hron G, Bialonczyk C, *et al.* Overweight, obesity, and the risk of recurrent venous thromboembolism. Arch Intern Med 2008; 168: 1678-83.

[152]   Ay C, Tengler T, Vormittag R, *et al.* Venous thromboembolism--a manifestation of the metabolic syndrome. Haematologica 2007; 92: 374-80.

[153]   Coca M, Cucuianu M, Hancu N. Effect of abdominal obesity on prothrombotic tendency in type 2 diabetes. Behavior of clotting factors VII and VIII, fibrinogen and von Willebrand Factor. Rom J Intern Med 2005; 43: 115-26.

[154]   Rillaerts E, van Gaal L, Xiang DZ, Vansant G, De Leeuw I. Blood viscosity in human obesity: relation to glucose tolerance and insulin status. Int J Obes 1989; 13: 739-45.

[155]   Mertens I, Van Gaal LF. Obesity, haemostasis and the fibrinolytic system. Obes Rev 2002; 3: 85-101.

[156]   Wannamethee SG, Tchernova J, Whincup P, *et al.* Plasma leptin: associations with metabolic, inflammatory and haemostatic risk factors for cardiovascular disease. Atherosclerosis 2007; 191: 418-26.

[157]   Konstantinides S, Schafer K, Koschnick S, Loskutoff DJ. Leptin-dependent platelet aggregation and arterial thrombosis suggests a mechanism for atherothrombotic disease in obesity. J Clin Invest 2001; 108: 1533-40.

[158]   Foschini D, Dos Santos RV, Prado WL, *et al.* Platelet and leptin in obese adolescents. J Pediatr (Rio J) 2008; 84: 516-21.

[159]   Konstantinides S, Schafer K, Neels JG, Dellas C, Loskutoff DJ. Inhibition of endogenous leptin protects mice from arterial and venous thrombosis. Arterioscler Thromb Vasc Biol 2004; 24: 2196-201.

[160]   Beuther DA, Sutherland ER. Overweight, obesity, and incident asthma: a meta-analysis of prospective epidemiologic studies. Am J Respir Crit Care Med 2007; 175: 661-6.

[161]   Chinn S, Jarvis D, Burney P. Relation of bronchial responsiveness to body mass index in the ECRHS. European Community Respiratory Health Survey. Thorax 2002; 57: 1028-33.

[162]   Kusunoki T, Morimoto T, Nishikomori R, *et al.* Obesity and the prevalence of allergic diseases in schoolchildren. Pediatr Allergy Immunol 2008; 19: 527-34.

[163]   Hersoug LG, Linneberg A. The link between the epidemics of obesity and allergic diseases: does obesity induce decreased immune tolerance? Allergy 2007; 62: 1205-13.

[164]   Conus S, Bruno A, Simon HU. Leptin is an eosinophil survival factor. J Allergy Clin Immunol 2005; 116: 1228-34.

[165]   Wong CK, Cheung PF, Lam CW. Leptin-mediated cytokine release and migration of eosinophils: implications for immunopathophysiology of allergic inflammation. Eur J Immunol 2007; 37: 2337-48.

[166]   Ciprandi G, Filaci G, Negrini S, *et al.* Serum Leptin Levels in Patients with Pollen-Induced Allergic Rhinitis. Int Arch Allergy Immunol 2008; 148: 211-218.

[167]   Ogawa Y, Duru EA, Ameredes BT. Role of IL-10 in the resolution of airway inflammation. Curr Mol Med 2008; 8: 437-45.

CHAPTER 6

Oxidative Stress and Microvascular Function in Insulin-Resistant States

P. Rösen and R. Rösen*

*German Diabetes Research Centre, Düsseldorf, and *Institute of Pharmacology at the University of Cologne, Federal Republic of Germany*

Address correspondence to: Prof. Dr. Peter Rösen, Auf'm Hennekamp 65, D-40225 Düsseldorf, FRG, Germany; E-mail: roesen@uni-duesseldorf.de

Abstract: It became evident in the last years that an increased vascular risk is not only associated with frank diabetes, but also already with states of insulin resistance. This risk does not only affect the large vessels contributing to the augmented cardiovascular risk often observed in insulin resistant patients, but also various functions of the microvasculature. Here we present some evidence that insulin resistant states are clearly associated with an increased formation of reactive oxygen species (ROS) and linked to a state often called "oxidative stress". Various mechanisms (NADPH-oxidase, disturbed mitochondrial function, uncoupling of nitric oxide synthase) may contribute to oxidative stress, but may also aggravate insulin resistance. It is discussed whether both oxidative stress and insulin resistance are causally linked and why oxidative stress leads to various defects of microvascular function (changes in vasomotion, permeability, reduced capillary bed, induction of apoptosis, changes in gene expression by activation of transcription factors (NFkappB, AP-1, STAT).

1. INTRODUCTION

There is a lot of evidence showing that in type 2 diabetic patients the vasculature is early disturbed and it is widely accepted that endothelial dysfunction precedes the onset of frank diabetes and diabetes. [1-3]. Therefore it has been suggested that the endothelial dysfunction is the trigger which initiates the vascular complications observed in diabetes. However microvascular dysfunction is not only a typical feature in frank diabetes, but it is also a cardinal feature of the metabolic syndrome and more generally of insulin resistant states that affects pressure and flow patterns, increasing peripheral resistance and decreasing sensitivity for insulin mediated glucose disposal [4].

Here we have to focus on the question whether the formation of reactive oxygen species (ROS) or the so-called "oxidative stress" plays a relevant role in the history of those microvascular defects typically seen in states of insulin resistance.

2. OXIDATIVE STRESS

Oxidative stress is a phenomenon often cited and regarded to, but still not well defined. Even in healthy individuals, many if not all cells of the body produce reactive oxygen and nitrogen derived radicals (Tab.1) by mitochondria, by nitric oxide synthases and various other enzyme systems which contribute to regulation and maintenance of various functions in the body [5-7] :

- Enzyme-catalyzed reactions
- Electron transport in mitochondria
- Signal transduction and gene expression
- Activation of nuclear transcription factors
- Regulation of vascular perfusion (NO)
- Regulation of growth and induction of apoptosis

Table1: Reactive oxygen and nitrogen species

Reactive oxygen species		*Reactive nitrogen species*	
- Superoxide	O_2^-	Nitric oxide	$NO^.$
- Hydroxyl	$OH^.$	Nitrogen oxide	$NO_2^.$
- Peroxyl	$RO_2.$		
- Alkoxyl	RO^-		
- Hydroperoxyl	$HO_2^.$		

Under most conditions, the formation of ROS/RNS is strictly controlled and the activity is temporally and locally restricted by various anti-oxidative mechanisms. Taking into account the physiological formation and activity of ROS, oxidative stress would indicate a pathophysiological event in states of illness, in which the strict control mechanisms are overrun and the activity of ROS/RNS is not any longer restricted to the site of its origin. In general, the reducing environment inside cells helps to prevent such an oxidative damage which is maintained by the oxidative metabolism and by action of anti-oxidative enzymes and substances such as glutathione, thioredoxin, the vitamins E and C, and enzymes as superoxide dismutase, catalase and the selenium-dependent glutathione and thioredoxin hydroperoxidase. These enzymes and substances serve to remove reactive oxygen species. As a typical example for a state of oxidative stress, the formation of ROS by activated neutrophiles or macrophages can be taken which nevertheless play an important role to defense the body in inflammatory states [5,7].

Thus, oxidative stress may arise, if the formation of ROS/RNS is excessive or alternatively if the activity of the anti-oxidative mechanisms such as anti-oxidative vitamins or anti-oxidative enzymes are not working sufficiently to restrict the production of ROS/RNS. Only under those conditions the generation of ROS/RNS become harmful and may justify the term oxidative stress.

At present, oxidative stress is assumed to be an underlying factor in health and disease. More and more evidence is accumulating that a proper balance between oxidants and anti-oxidants is involved in maintaining health and longevity, and that altering the balance in favor of oxidants may result in pathophysiological responses causing functional disorders and disease. Especially oxidative stress is claimed to be involved, casually or concomitantly, as an important factor in the development of diseases such as atherosclerosis, diabetes mellitus, arthritis, but presumably also in development of microangiopathic complications. Even the process of aging is discussed to be related to the loss of control in the formation of ROS [5].

3. IS OXIDATIVE STRESS ALREADY ASSOCIATED OR A FUNCTIONAL CONSEQUENCE OF INSULIN RESISTANCE?

There is evidence that oxidative stress is enhanced in manifest diabetes and may contribute to the loss of β-cells as well as to vascular complications generally observed in diabetic patients [6,8-10]. Less is known whether the generation of ROS is already enhanced in pre-diabetic patients, patients with an impaired glucose-tolerance, but not yet elevated levels of fasting glucose. These patients are resistant to the action of insulin and are known to carry a high risk to develop frank diabetes. The insulin resistance developing in those patients is a complex phenomenon and may be caused by different mechanisms [11-14].

That the formation of ROS is strongly enhanced in manifest diabetes and importantly contributes to the development of vascular and neurological disorders as consequence of long-acting diabetes is supported by a considerable amount of clinical and experimental data [6,8,9,15,16]. However recent data suggest that oxidative stress is a more general phenomenon strongly associated with various diseases and states of metabolic stress [5]. Especially, the formation of ROS has been shown to be enhanced in pathophysiological conditions characteristic for the so-called "metabolic syndrome": a complex disorder characterized by insulin resistance, dyslipidemia, hypertension, a chronically pro-inflammatory state and often obesity, especially expansion of the visceral fat compartment. It has been shown that the metabolic syndrome is strictly associated with the degree of oxidative stress [17] and it has been hypothesized that the visceral adipose tissue contributes to malfunction of endothelium by releasing pro-inflammatory adipokines (leptin, TNFa, Il-6, angiotensin II, NEFA) which provoke oxidative stress, increased insulin resistance and eventually hypertension [18]. It is estimated that approximately one third of the apparanetly healthy population is sufficiently insulin resistant to develop significant clinical disease

[19,20]. Insulin resistance is most often already present before the development of hyperglycemia [21,22]. That the generation of ROS measured by various parameters (hydroperoxides, malondialdehyde, isoprostanes) is in fact elevated has been shown in obese insulin resistant patients as well as in animals [23-28]. In addition, patients with dyslipidemia present signs of an accelerated generation of ROS [29-31]. The same feature has been proven in patients with essential hypertension[32-38]. All states of a chronically inflammatory state are generally associated with oxidative stress (for example abdominal obesity) [17]. Thus there is overwhelming evidence that the characteristic features of the metabolic syndrome such as dyslipidemia and especially abdominal obesity, insulin resistance, hypertension, and chronic inflammation are closely associated with an enhanced formation of ROS.

However, all these observations in patients and animals do not prove a causal relationship between the generation of ROS and the insulin resistant states. In addition, various parameters have been determined to quantify oxidative stress such as hydroperoxides, oxidized lipoproteins, malondialdehyde, nitrosylation of proteins, and formation of carbonyls by oxidation of proteins and isoprostanes as oxidation products of the arachidonic acid metabolism. It is, however, still a matter of discussion which of these factors mirrors the oxidative stress and is a valid parameter [39]. Furthermore it has to be taken into account that these various oxidation products arise from different metabolic pathways and may characterize parameters of different pathophysiological origins. In addition, taking into account the high anti-oxidant capacity of blood (albumin, proteins containing sulfhydryl groups the question remains as to what changes in the concentrations of ROS in blood really stand for. They indicate processes occurring elsewhere in the body and it has to be expected that the concentrations of ROS determined in blood simply represent the overflow of what runs elsewhere in the body.

That oxidative stress and states of insulin resistance are causally associated is suggested mainly by experimental observations. It is generally accepted and can be taken as proven that exposure of endothelial cells, smooth muscle cells, and nerve cells to high concentrations of glucose, even oscillating concentrations of glucose or fatty acids increase the generation of ROS [9,24,40-44]. This assumption is further supported by the in vitro observations that the generation of ROS can be inhibited by supplementation with antioxidants. Also the consequences of oxidative stress such as activation of nuclear factor kappa B (NFkB),induction of apoptosis, changes in gene expression such as elevated expression of adhesion molecules are nearly completely prevented by reducing the generation of ROS [8,43-45].In vitro studies using vascular or nervous cells have shown that those cells are very sensitive to high concentrations of glucose and fatty acids and react on those perturbations with an increase in generation of ROS. It is interesting to note that mostly cells which take up glucose in an insulin-independent manner are particularly affected and respond under conditions of metabolic stress with an increased formation of ROS. The same tissues and cells are typically involved in development of vascular defects. It has also to be mentioned that one of the earliest symptom of insulin resistant states is often the diminished response of the lipolytic system in adipose tissue to insulin with still maintained sensitivity of the effect of insulin on glucose uptake. As consequence increased concentrations of fatty acids in the blood and an enhanced supply of fatty acids to vascular and nervous cells are observed. Thus, hyperglycemic conditions and hyperlipidemic states are often strongly correlated, but alterations in the lipolytic system seem often to precede changes in glucose uptake. However, since similar results are obtained if those cells are incubated with fatty acids instead of glucose, it is likely that it is the metabolic overload of the cells which provokes the formation of ROS, rather than a specific metabolite.

A typical example is shown in Figs. (1-4). By staining endothelial cells with dichlorofluoresceine the formation of ROS can be directly seen. In these cells the generation of ROS is dependent on the concentration of glucose and fatty acids. Its formation is inhibited by vitamin E, but also by L-nitroarginine indicating that uncoupling of nitric oxide synthase plays an important role for the generation of ROS Fig. (2). A similar picture is obtained when porcine aortas are used. High glucose enhances the generation of ROS. Removal of endothelium dramatically reduces the generation of ROS showing that especially the endothelium is a primary source of ROS Fig. (3). In this experimental set-up nitric oxide synthesis seems to be of major importance. Similar results are obtained if the cells or the porcine aortas are incubated with fatty acids instead of glucose (data not shown) indicating that principally comparable mechanisms contribute to the generation of ROS in hyperglycemic or hyperlipidemic states. In parallel to the increased generation of ROS, the release of nitric oxide is clearly diminished if the tissue is incubated with fatty acids or high concentrations of glucose Fig. (4).

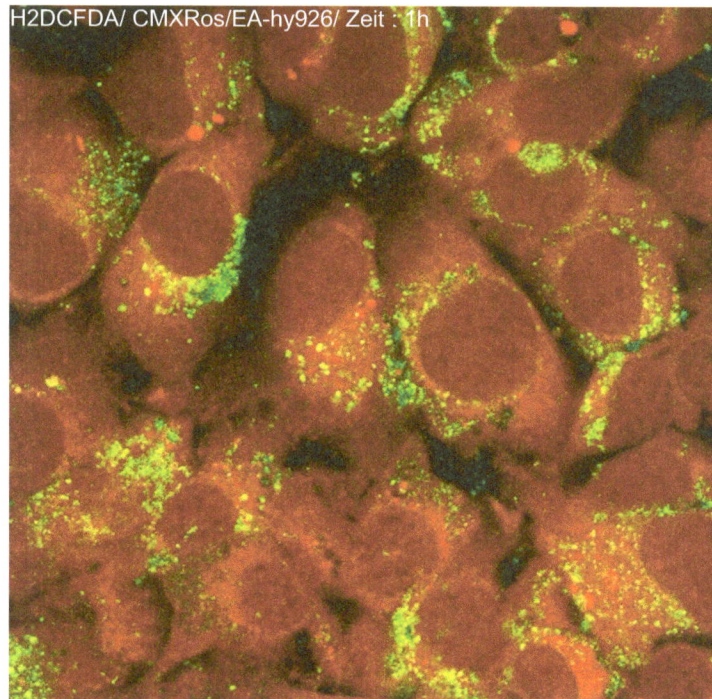

Figure 1: Localization of ROS generation in human endothelial cells. HUVECs were incubated with high glucose (30 mmol/L) and preloaded with the DCF-DA (1 μM) for 1 hr to determine the ROS generation (green). To visualize mitochondria, the cells were co-stained with MitoTracker Red CMXRos™ (red). The fluorescence was analyse by the confocal microscope (LSM Pascal, Zeiss, Jena, Germany, Plan-Apochromat 100x/1.4 Oil). Yellow spots indicate an overlapping of green and red fluorescence suggesting ROS generation by mitochondria.

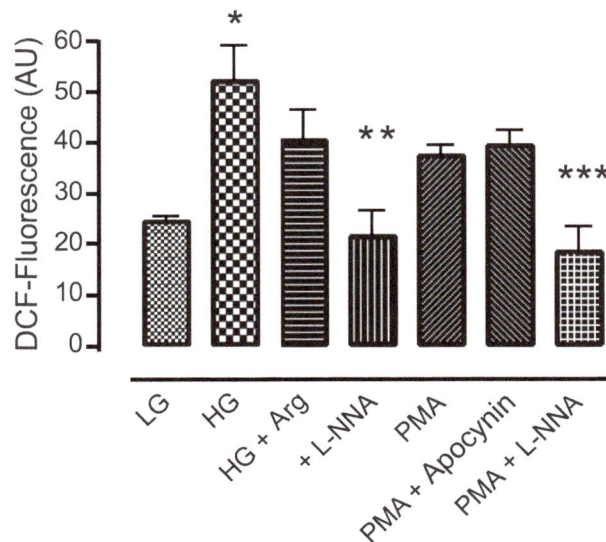

Figure 2: Inhibition of the formation of reactive oxygen intermediates by apocynin and L-nitroarginine. HUVECs were preloaded with the dichlorodihydrofluorescein ester (1 μM) for 45 min. After washing the cells were incubated with low (5 mmol/L: LG) and high D-glucose (30 mmol/L: HG) in the presence and absence of apocynin to inihibit NADPH-oxidase (1 μmol/L) and L-N-nitroarginine (100 μmol/L, L-NNA) to inhibit nitric oxide snthase. After incubation for 1 hr (37°C) the fluorescent was analysed as described by fluorescent microscopy. Mean $\pm$ SEM of 5 independent experiments are given. In each slide five fields were analysed. In another set of experiments HUVECs were incubated with 5 mmol/l glucose and stimulated by the phorbolester PMA (10 mmol/l) in the presence and absence of DPI (1 μmol/l) or L-NNA (100 μmol/l).

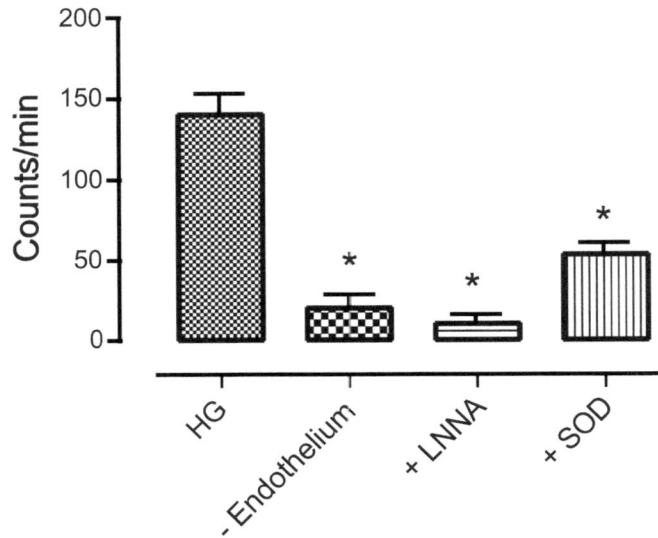

Figure 3: ROS generation by isolated porcine coronary arteries is dependent on nitric oxide synthase and the presence of endothelium. Porcine coronary arteries were isolated and then incubated with increasing concentrations of glucose for 3 hrs. The formation of superoxide anions was determined by Lucigenin as described in Methods. In a part of incubation superoxide dismutase (SOD, 10 U/ml) or nitric oxide synthase was inhibited L-NNA (100 μmol/L). Removal of endothelium by slight rubbing of the vessel surface abolished the generation of ROS. Mean ± SEM of 5 independent experiments are given.

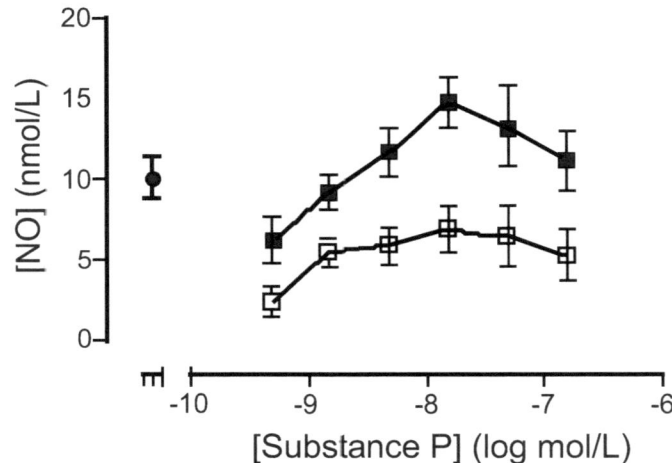

Figure 4: Release of nitric oxide by porcine coronary arteries after stimulation by substance P. Porcine coronary arteries were isolated and then incubated with either low (5 mmol/L, filled squares) or high (30 mmol/L, open squares) glucose for 3 hrs and then stimulated by addition of substance P. The formation of NO was followed by a NO specific electrode. The maximal concentrations are given. Mean ± SEM of 5 independent experiments are given.

In patients the evidence is not yet as univocal, but there are several observations in line with the experimental data. Ceriello has presented some evidence that a persistent hyperglycemia is not afforded to enhance the generation of ROS and reduction of anti-oxidant activity, but that hyperglycemic and hyperlipidemic "spikes" are sufficient to enhance the formation of ROS and to produce a state of oxidative stress [25,30,42,46-49]. The greater the increase in oxidative stress and the drop in the antioxidant activity the higher were the levels of hyperglycemia. These observations can also explain why in healthy subjects and in patients a single meal rich in glucose, fatty acids or advanced glycation end-products diminish the concentration of anti-oxidants and increase parameters of oxidative stress [23,30,31,42,49].In summary, these data and observations in non-diabetic human subjects indicate clearly that already in the pre-diabetic state an enhanced generation of ROS is a typical feature of cells and tissues which may develop later on complications generally seen in a late diabetic state.

4. HOW ARE THE ROS GENERATED IN PRE-DIABETIC STATES?

A variety of cellular enzyme systems are potential sources of ROS, including NAD(P)H-oxidase, xanthine oxidase, uncoupled endothelial nitric oxide (NO) synthase (eNOS), arachidonic acid metabolizing enzymes including cytochrome *P*-450 enzymes, lipoxygenase and cyclooxygenase. In addition, the mitochondrial respiratory chain may be a main source of ROS [50,51]}. However we have to take into account that the source may vary dependent on the tissues and cells involved. In vascular cells four enzyme systems seem to predominate: NAD(P)H-oxidase, xanthine oxidase, uncoupled eNOS, and mitochondrial electron leakage [6,8,9,43,44,50,51]. The functional significance of mitochondria derived ROS in vascular endothelial cells has received little attention for long time, since in general vascular cells exhibit low metabolic activity [52] and mitochondria-generated ROS seem to be less well regulated compared with other systems like NAD(P)H oxidase [53]. However, recently special attention is attributed to the mitochondrial respiratory chain as major source of ROS in most mammalian cells. Excess production of ROS from mitochondria has been implicated in aging, a range of degenerative diseases and manifestation of diabetes and its complications [8,54-56]. In our hand, uncoupling of nitric oxide synthase is of major relevance since we could prevent the formation of ROS in hyperglycemic conditions by inhibition of this enzyme in endothelial cells as well as in porcine aortas by L-arginine. Nitric oxide synthase and the insulin receptor are morphologically closely linked, since both are expressed in caveolae, tiny invaginations in the plasma membrane [57]. This colocalization suggests that defects in the function of nitric oxide synthase by producing ROS might directly interfere with the colocalized structure of the insulin receptor, of the glucose transporters and some caveolin isoforms affecting the permeability of the plasma membrane. It is an intriguing idea, which however remains to be proved. However, there is also considerable evidence for an important contribution of NADPH-oxidase to the generation of ROS in smooth muscle and endothelial cells. It has been shown very convincingly that the expression and the activity of NADPH-oxidase which transfers a single electron to molecular oxygen to produce superoxide is elevated in models of the metabolic syndrome, in rats after feeding a high or a high carbohydrate diet [40,58,59]. These observations suggest that various systems contribute to the generation of oxidative stress in states of insulin resistance and of the metabolic syndrome and that these ROS generating systems are likely linked together by a complex interrelationship; activation of one might cause the subsequent activation of the others without being quantitatively the major source. Ceriello et al. have pointed out that in humans even in the pre-diabetic state the capacity of the anti-oxidant activities is reduced [46]. Not only anti-oxidative enzymes as superoxide dismutase but also the concentrations of anti-oxidant vitamins were reduced in the pre-diabetic state. This conclusion is supported and expanded by experimental studies showing that the expression of various anti-oxidative enzymes such as the superoxide dismutase isoenzymes, the glutathione peroxidase and heme-oxagenase-2 is diminished by high fat and high carbohydrate feeding [58]. Thus the capacity to inactivate ROS seems to be generally hampered. The increased concentrations of reduced glutathione are presumably a consequence of the increase in the oxidative burden and of repeatedly occurring oxidative stress.

5. IS THERE AN INTERRELATIONSHIP BETWEEN ROS AND INSULIN RESISTANCE?

We know that smaller amounts of ROS facilitate the insulin signaling [60,61]. Low levels of ROS enhance the insulin mediated glucose uptake [62]. These small amounts of ROS may be generated by NADPH-oxidase activation since inhibition of the NADPH-oxidase isoforms reduces the insulin sensitivity of various cells. It has been suggested that the inhibition of protein-tyrosine-phosphatases by ROS may be involved which can stabilize the activated insulin receptor substrate complex and thereby prolong the activation induced by insulin after binding to its receptor. Thus ROS play an important, but yet incompletely understood role in insulin signaling.

In contrast to these small amounts of ROS enhancing insulin signaling, insulin resistance is the cause for the generation of deleterious amounts of ROS sustaining oxidative stress. We do not know in detail which mechanisms are causing insulin resistance, but because of the strong correlation between obesity and insulin resistance it has been suggested that an adipose derived factor plays a predominant role (TNFa, leptin, resistin, free fatty acids, [63-68]. An excess of caloric intake and low energy expenditure which are typically observed in subjects with the metabolic syndrome, are closely associated with an expansion of visceral adipose tissue and a change in the pattern of adipokines released by this tissue (less adiponectin, more TNFa, free fatty acids, resistin and others). We know also that increased levels of fatty acids are positively correlated with insulin resistance, [63,64]. Steinberg and Baron provided direct evidence that fatty acids directly reduce the activation of nitric oxide synthase, diminish the perfusion of skeletal muscle perfusion and cause some degree of insulin resistance (measured by the rate of uptake of glucose) [69,70]. Thus, it has intriguing to suggest that it is an adipose tissue derived factor which is causing insulin resistance. The resulting excessive supply of metabolites may be the cause for an enlargement of the mitochondrial membrane potential. It is known that if a critical value of this potential is overrun, electrons may escape from the mitochondrial electron transport chain. The escaping electrons can be transferred to molecular oxygen resulting in the formation of superoxide [8]. Such a conclusion is supported by various observations. Mitochondrial dysfunction is clearly associated with reduced insulin sensitivity [71,72]. Mitochondrial dysfunction and gene expression of mitochondrial OXPHOS genes are related to insulin resistance [73]. Mutations in mitochondrial genes not protected by histones caused by aging and cellular stress have also been proposed as mechanism to explain the reduction of insulin sensitivity with increasing age. It is interesting to note that in parallel the mitochondrial biogenesis is impaired in elderly human subjects and the rate of oxidative phosphorylation becomes reduced in strong association with developing insulin resistance. In addition to the mitochondrial dysfunction fatty acid and various lipid metabolites accumulate which may contribute further to deterioration of mitochondrial function and to ROS production resulting in defect in insulin signaling.

Thus on the one hand, the generation of ROS is the consequence of insulin resistance. On the other side, oxidative stress is known to impair insulin resistance with respect to glucose uptake. Independently from the mechanism of their generation, ROS have been shown to lead to inhibition of glycerolaldehyde dehydrogenase, to an impaired uptake of glucose, to accumulation of glucose metabolites and activation of alternative pathways to metabolize glucose (hexose pentose pathway) resulting in an inhibition of the glycolytic flux [8]. In addition, the formation of ROS might be aggravated by protein kinase C activated by mitochondrial ROS or dihydroxyacetone-phosphate which is able to activate of NADPH-oxidase [40,74]/id} leading to a burst of ROS formation. The group of Brownlee has presented evidence that such a burst of ROS may severely deteriorate β-cell function and thereby contribute to the developing metabolic defect [75]. Thus, ROS play a double role, in small amounts they facilitate insulin signaling, but in larger amounts they contribute to development of insulin resistance, which further reinforce the metabolic maladaptation [76].

Lastly inhibition of the branch of the insulin signaling via the PI3kinase/Akt is already often observed, whereas activation of the MAPKinase pathway is not yet affected or may be overstimulated by high insulin [61]; activation of MAPKinase further aggravates insulin resistance, but also the generation of ROS. A vicious, self-enhancing cycle may arise which does not only affect the insulin signaling, but also other signaling pathways involved in regulation of vascular flow properties, cell growth and apoptosis and may also affect other tissues close to the insulin sensitive tissue by dispreading of ROS. Interestingly, Yudkin [14] had proposed that specifically the perivascular fat produces pro-inflammatory cytokines such as TNFa which may act locally on the adjacent vascular tissue and thereby impair the endothelial dependent function by stimulating the formation of ROS.

6. IS THE OXIDATIVE STRESS A FACTOR RELEVANT FOR THE EARLY VASCULAR DYSFUNCTION SEEN IN PRE-DIABETIC PATIENTS?

That oxidative stress is a major pathogenic factor contributing to malfunction in various parts of the vascular tree has already been demonstrated and is extensively discussed elsewhere [77]. It influences not only the activation of ion channels, signal transduction pathways, the remodeling of cytoskeleton, but also pathways regulating the intercellular communication such as the expression of adhesion molecules, but contributes also to the loss of vascular cells by apoptosis and the formation of new vessels by angiogenesis [77].

The function of microcirculation is mainly determined by the activity of the endothelium which is able to release various mediators, either vasodilators such as nitric oxide, prostacyclin, bradykinin, and the endothelium derived hyperpolarizing factor (EDHT) or vasoconstrictors as endothelin-1, angiotensin II and thromboxane [26,78].

In small arteries and arterioles nitric oxide plays the dominant role in the regulation of vasomotor tone. In these vessels nitric oxide is mainly synthesized by the endothelial nitric oxide synthase (eNOS, NOS III)[79-81]. This enzyme converts L-arginine to nitric oxide transferring electrons from $NADPH_2$ on molecular oxygen.The nitric oxide released by the endothelium by eNOS in small amounts (in contrast to iNOS, NOS II, which synthesize nitric oxide in micromolar, toxic concentrations) activates guanylate cyclase, the generated cGMP results in activation of proteinkinase G which leads to a decrease in intracellular calcium, dephosphorylation of myosin light chains and subsequently relaxation of smooth muscle cells. For details see also [82,83].

In the presence of superoxide nitric oxide is, however, very rapidly inactivated to peroxides, since the reaction of nitric oxide with molecular oxygen is much faster that then desactivation of superoxide by superoxide dismutase and catalase [84] resulting in a reduced biovailability of nitric oxide in response to insulin, shear stress or other agonists. In addition, increasing concentrations of superoxide or hydroperoxides may cause severe defects in electron transport system of eNOS itself leading to a state of uncoupling. Electrons escape and are transferred to molecular oxygen to give superoxide further diminishing the bioavailability of nitric oxide without changes in its expression. A similar dysfunction arises in states of L-arginine deficiency and of loss of tetrahydrobiopterin, a necessary cofactor for eNOS activity[43,85-89]. In those situations eNOS itself becomes a dominant factor for the generation of ROS. It is also important to take into account that nitric oxide reacts very fast with superoxide to peroxynitrite which is a powerful prooxidant and exerts various effects on cell signaling [84]. Thus, two very reactive ROS are mainly formed under those conditions, superoxide and peroxynitrite. This can be nicely shown in endothelial cells or aortas incubated either with high concentrations of glucose or fatty acids: inhibition of eNOS by L-NAME does not only prevent the release of ROS, but also various defects following loss of nitric oxide and generation of ROS such as activation of NFkappaB, induction of apoptosis, increased expression of adhesion molecules VCAM-1 and ICAM-1 [43,44]. Similarly, the generation of ROS by aortas exposed to metabolic stress is totally abolished by removal of endothelium indicating that the endothelium is the main source of vascular ROS generation and partly by L-NAME again demonstrating the important role for ROS formation Fig. (**4**).

Endothelial dysfunction which is an important factor in initiating vascular dysfunction may develop as consequence of the reduced nitric oxide bioavailabilty. In line with these assumptions we assume that the bioavailability of nitric oxide is reduced in pre-diabetic, insulin-resistant state:

- As already outlined the production of nitric oxide is diminished in endothelial cells exposed to metabolic stress, whereas the generation of ROS is elevated.

- In obese Zucker rats the generation of nitric oxide by the endothelial nitric oxide synthase is decreased, but the formation of superoxide excessive. In addition the microvessel density is clearly diminished [90]. In other models of the metabolic syndrome such as the high fat fed Fischer rat, a similar endothelial dysfunction with an enhanced formation of superoxides has been described recently [58].

- In patients the response to acetylcholine is attenuated and the diminution of nitric oxide correlates with BMI, systolic blood pressure and triglycerides [91,92]. Infusion and uptake of fatty acids provokes a reduced endothelium dependent vasodilatation in response to insulin, insulin resistance with respect to glucose uptake [69]. There is also good evidence that the nitric oxide bioavailability is reduced in insulin resistant subjects and in particularly in obese, insulin resistant patients [69,93]. Not only the response to insulin, but also to the acetylcholine, NO mediated vasodilatation was clearly impaired [70,94]. The degree of insulin sensitivity correlates with the magnitude of endothelium dependent vasodilatation. The defect in nitric oxide mediated vasodilatation may contribute to aggravate insulin resistance by reducing the capillary network perfused in response to insulin and the delayed and diminished delivery of insulin to its target cells. A direct link between insulin resistance and endothelial dysfunction has been observed by Murdie et al.[95]

- In women with a history of gestational diabetes the endothelial dysfunction was even impaired, and was correlated with insulin resistance even if blood glucose levels were normal [96].

- The endothelopathy seems to precede the development of diabetes [97]. Even in relatives (first degree) of type 2 diabetic patients an endothelial dysfunction can be shown closely related to insulin resistance [98-101].

- It has also be shown that a low grade of inflammation is associated with insulin resistance and the metabolic syndrome [102,103] which is able to disturb endothelial dependent vasodilatation in large, but more so in small vessels (small arteries, arterioles).

It has to be noted that other factors than hyperglycemia itself are relevant for development of endothelial dysfunction, chronic inflammation, associated with oxidative stress. In line with this assumption, in early stages of type 1 diabetic patients endothelial function has been described to be slightly impaired, not affected or even increased [104]. Even a 24 h lasting hyperglycemia did not affect the vasoreactiviy of endothelium in humans [4,105]. Thus in these patients endothelial dysfunction occurs consistently only in advanced stages of the disease and is mostly associated with the presence of microalbuminuria [106-108]. Hyperglycemia itself seems therefore not to be a main factor for impaired endothelial function. This does, however, not exclude that hyperglycemia may contribute to development of vascular disturbances, but presumably later in the natural history of this disease.

The defective insulin mediated vasodilatation is assumed to be responsible for the following defects Figs. **(5, 6)**:

- the expansion of the capillary network is impaired [109,109];

- the ability of insulin to redirect blood flow in the microcirculation where the uptake of oxygen and the exchange of metabolites takes place, is hampered; the diffusion of insulin to the site of its need and action is delayed and diminished which aggravates the insulin resistance. It is important to note that the inability of insulin to recruit additional capillary beds as well as a diminished size of the capillary bed are most relevant mechanisms to inhibit the metabolic activity of insulin on the uptake of glucose by skeletal muscle [110]. Such an effect could be reinforced by adipokines released by the visceral adipose tissue. Less release of adiponectin is causally linked to an inadequate response of endothelial nitric oxide synthase to insulin; other pro-inflammatory cytokines (TNFa, IL-8.IL-1b) as well peroxynitrite will even worse the response.

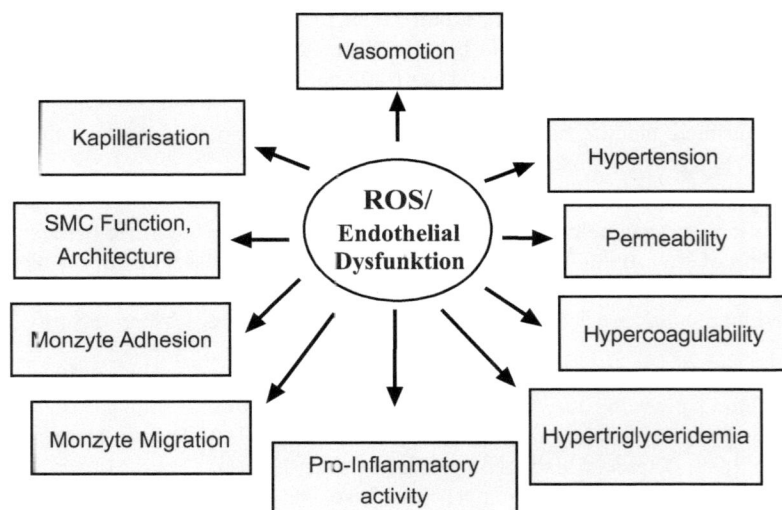

Figure 5: Established effects of ROS on vascular functions.

Beside an enhanced inactivation of nitric oxide by ROS, insulin resistance may directly contribute to an impaired nitric oxide release, since activation of eNOS by insulin is disturbed, because the insulin signaling pathway leading to its activation (PI3 kinase/Akt) is defect [3,111,112]. Activation of JNK/ERK1/2 in insulin resistance contributes significantly to impair this branch of the insulin signaling pathway, whereas MAPKinases are further activated by insulin [61].

In addition to the diminished bioavailability of nitric oxide oxidative stress, either by superoxide, hydroperoxide or peroxide, may have severe consequences for the properties and function of vascular cells (for review [113]:

- activation of transcription factors (NFkappaB. AP1, Stat [81,114,115]):

It has been shown that the activation of these transcription factors is depending on the redox state of the cells and can be prevented by treatment of the cells with antioxidants such as tocopherol, glutathione, lipoic acid, but in endothelial cells als by inhibition L-NAME suggesting an involvement of nitric oxide synthase [43,81]. However the exact mechanism of coupling between changes in the redox state and activation of the transcription factor is not yet clear.

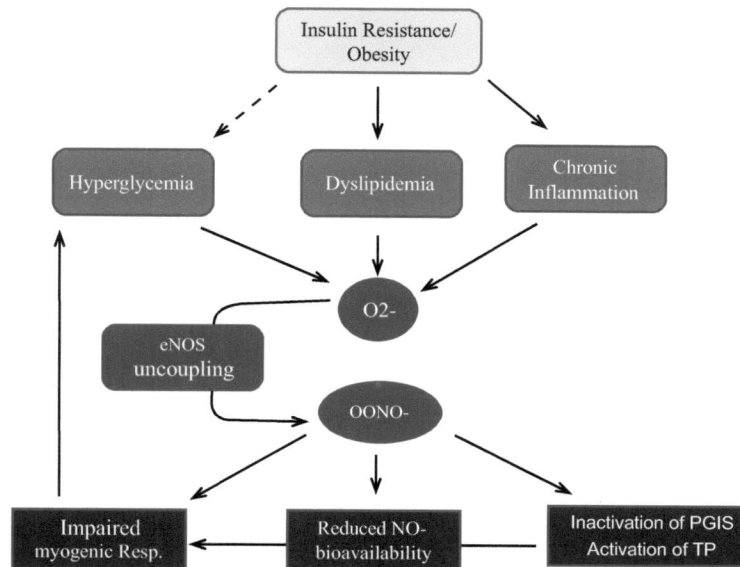

Figure 6: Schematic representation of the influence of insulin resistance on major pathophysiologically relevant pathways, on the production of ROS and subsequent effects on vascular motion.

NFkappaB, AP-1 and Stat control the expression of a range of genes involved in inflammation and proliferation [114-116]. Activation of these transcription factors plays an important role for activation of genes encoding TNFa, IL-1b, macrophage-colony stimulating factor, tissue factor, vascular adhesion molecule, intercellular adhesion molecule 1, activation of metallo-proteinase, and the inducible form of nitric oxide synthase (iNOS, NOSI) which generates nitric oxide in toxic, micromolar concentrations [81,117]. Activation of Stat has been shown to be specifically important in regulation of cytokine signaling and therefore in processes leading to inflammation and growth factor production [115]. From these data it follows that oxidative stress and activation of these transcriptions factors leads to a thrombogenic transformation of the endothelial surface and exerts a strong pro-inflammatory activity. An enhanced adhesion of leukocytes and thrombocytes at the vessel surface is favored as well as the proliferation of smooth muscle cells. Obstruction and narrowing of vessels by the formed leukocytes aggregates or the adhesion of leukocytes might severely contribute to disturbances of microvascular flow.

- activation of various isoforms of protein kinase C (especially β and δ-isoforms; for review [2,8,118,119]:

Activation of protein kinase C isoforms have been implicated in the activation of vascular endothelial growth factor, in the increased formation of TGF-b, collagen and fibronectin, the elevated levels of plasminogen activator-inhibitor 1 (PAI-1). Its activation may also contribute to activation of NADPH-oxidase [40,74] and to the augmented formation of endothelin-1.

- induction of apoptosis: There is some evidence that ROS play a relevant role for induction of apoptosis. A part of the reactions is dependent of the activation of NFkappaB which exerts a pro-apoptotic effect on endothelial cells and contributes to the loss of intact, antithrombotic vascular cells [43,44]. The loss of endothelial cells might contribute to the increased permeability which is a main mechanism for increased filtration. An increased interstitial fluid accumulation is one cause for obstruction and narrowing of vessels [77]. Disruption of microvasculature might be aggravated by contraction of pericytes by ROS. Such alterations might be of special importance for development of neuro-, nephro- and retinopathic defects seen in later states of insulin resistance, hypertension and diabetes.

Although the mechanisms are not yet elucidated in detail and a lot of questions remain open, there is at time convincing evidence that the formation of ROS represents an important factor for the development of changes in the microvascular flow and may link insulin resistance and early vascular disturbances. Since it has been shown that the commonly used antioxidants are not effective to prevent the development of those complications, it is time to develop mediators and pharmacological active compounds which more specifically interfere with the formation of ROS at the site of their generation.

7. REFERENCES

[1] Brunner, H.; Cockcroft, J. R.; Deanfield, J.; Donald, A.; Ferrannini, E.; Halcox, J.; Kiowski, W.; Luscher, T. F.; Mancia, G.; Natali, A.; Oliver, J. J.; Pessina, A. C.; Rizzoni, D.; Rossi, G. P.; Salvetti, A.; Spieker, L. E.; Taddei, S.; Webb, D. J. Endothelial function and dysfunction. Part II: Association with cardiovascular risk factors and diseases. A statement by the Working Group on Endothelins and Endothelial Factors of the European Society of Hypertension. J. Hypertens. 23:233-246; 2005.

[2] Rask-Madsen, C.; King, G. Mechanisms of disease: endothelial dysfunction in insulin resistance and diabetes. Nat. Clin. Pract. Endocrinol. Metab. 3:46-56; 2007.

[3] Andersen, K.; Pedersen, B. K. The role of inflammation in vascular insulin resistance with focus on IL-6. Horm Metab Res 40:635-639; 2008.

[4] Jonk, A. M.; Houben, A. J.; de Jongh, R. T.; Serne, E. H.; Schaper, N. C.; Stehouwer, C. D. Microvascular dysfunction in obesity: a potential mechanism in the pathogenesis of obesity-associated insulin resistance and hypertension. Physiology. (Bethesda.) 22:252-260; 2007.

[5] Packer, L.; Rösen, P.; Tritschler, H.; King, G. L.; Azzi, A. Antioxidants in diabetes management.: New York Marcel Dekker; 2000.

[6] Rosen, P.; Nawroth, P. P.; King, G.; Moller, W.; Tritschler, H. J.; Packer, L. The role of oxidative stress in the onset and progression of diabetes and its complications: a summary of a Congress Series sponsored by UNESCO-MCBN, the American Diabetes Association and the German Diabetes Society. Diabetes Metab Res Rev. 17:189-212; 2001.

[7] Sies, E. Antioxidants in disease: mechanisms and therapy: London Academic Press; 1997.

[8] Brownlee, M. Biochemistry and molecular cell biology of diabetic complications. Nature 414:813-820; 2001.

[9] Nishikawa, T.; Edelstein, D.; Brownlee, M. The missing link: a single unifying mechanism for diabetic complications. Kidney Int. Suppl 77:S26-S30; 2000.

[10] Baynes, J. W. Role of oxidative stress in development of complications in diabetes. Diabetes 40:405-412; 1991.

[11] Consitt, L. A.; Bell, J. A.; Houmard, J. A. Intramuscular lipid metabolism, insulin action, and obesity. IUBMB. Life 61:47-55; 2009.

[12] Karlsson, H. K.; Zierath, J. R. Insulin signaling and glucose transport in insulin resistant human skeletal muscle. Cell Biochem. Biophys. 48:103-113; 2007.

[13] Gallagher, E. J.; LeRoith, D.; Karnieli, E. The metabolic syndrome-from insulin resistance to obesity and diabetes. Endocrinol. Metab Clin. North Am. 37:559-79, vii; 2008.

[14] Yudkin, J. S. Inflammation, obesity, and the metabolic syndrome. Horm Metab Res 39:707-709; 2007.

[15] Ziegler, D.; Sohr, C. G.; Nourooz-Zadeh, J. Oxidative stress and antioxidant defense in relation to the severity of diabetic polyneuropathy and cardiovascular autonomic neuropathy. Diabetes Care 27:2178-2183; 2004.

[16] Stirban, A.; Rosen, P.; Tschoepe, D. Complications of type 1 diabetes: new molecular findings. Mt. Sinai J. Med. 75:328-351; 2008.

[17] Wellen, K. E.; Hotamisligil, G. S. Inflammation, stress, and diabetes. J. Clin. Invest 115:1111-1119; 2005.

[18] Katagiri, H.; Yamada, T.; Oka, Y. Adiposity and cardiovascular disorders: disturbance of the regulatory system consisting of humoral and neuronal signals. Circ. Res 101:27-39; 2007.

[19] Facchini, F. S.; Hua, N.; Abbasi, F.; Reaven, G. M. Insulin resistance as a predictor of age-related diseases. J. Clin. Endocrinol. Metab 86:3574-3578; 2001.

[20] Yip, J.; Facchini, F. S.; Reaven, G. M. Resistance to insulin-mediated glucose disposal as a predictor of cardiovascular disease. J. Clin. Endocrinol. Metab 83:2773-2776; 1998.

[21] DeFRonzo, RA. Pathogenesis of type 2 diabetes:metabolic and molecular implications for identifying diabetes genes. Diabetes Reviews 5, 177-269. 1997.

[22] Reaven, G. Insulin resistance and its consequences: type 2 diabetes and coronary heart disease. In LeRoith, D.; Taylor, S.; Olefsky, J. eds. Diabetes mellitus: A fundamental and clinical text. Philadelphia: Lippicott Williams & Wilkins; 2000:604-615.

[23] Natali, A.; Baldi, S.; Vittone, F.; Muscelli, E.; Casolaro, A.; Morgantini, C.; Palombo, C.; Ferrannini, E. Effects of glucose tolerance on the changes provoked by glucose ingestion in microvascular function. Diabetologia 51:862-871; 2008.

[24] Ceriello, A.; Esposito, K.; Piconi, L.; Ihnat, M. A.; Thorpe, J. E.; Testa, R.; Boemi, M.; Giugliano, D. Oscillating glucose is more deleterious to endothelial function and oxidative stress than mean glucose in normal and type 2 diabetic patients. Diabetes 57:1349-1354; 2008.

[25] Ceriello, A. Postprandial hyperglycemia and diabetes complications: is it time to treat? Diabetes 54:1-7; 2005.

[26] Frisbee, J. C. Obesity, insulin resistance, and microvessel density. Microcirculation. 14:289-298; 2007.

[27] Knudson, J. D.; Dincer, U. D.; Bratz, I. N.; Sturek, M.; Dick, G. M.; Tune, J. D. Mechanisms of coronary dysfunction in obesity and insulin resistance. Microcirculation. 14:317-338; 2007.

[28]　Rebolledo, OR, Marra, CA, Raschia, A, Rodriguez, S, and Gagliardino, JJ. Abdominal adipose tissue: early metabolic dysfunction associated to insulin resistance and oxidative stress induced by an unbalanced diet. Horm Metab Res 40, 794-800. 2008.

[29]　Ceriello, A.; Assaloni, R.; Da Ros, R.; Maier, A.; Piconi, L.; Quagliaro, L.; Esposito, K.; Giugliano, D. Effect of atorvastatin and irbesartan, alone and in combination, on postprandial endothelial dysfunction, oxidative stress, and inflammation in type 2 diabetic patients. Circulation 111:2518-2524; 2005.

[30]　Ceriello, A.; Quagliaro, L.; Piconi, L.; Assaloni, R.; Da Ros, R.; Maier, A.; Esposito, K.; Giugliano, D. Effect of postprandial hypertriglyceridemia and hyperglycemia on circulating adhesion molecules and oxidative stress generation and the possible role of simvastatin treatment. Diabetes 53:701-710; 2004.

[31]　Ceriello, A. Nitrotyrosine: new findings as a marker of postprandial oxidative stress. Int. J. Clin. Pract. Suppl 51-58; 2002.

[32]　Puddu, P.; Puddu, G. M.; Cravero, E.; Rosati, M.; Muscari, A. The molecular sources of reactive oxygen species in hypertension. Blood Press 17:70-77; 2008.

[33]　Holvoet, P. Relations between metabolic syndrome, oxidative stress and inflammation and cardiovascular disease. Verh. K. Acad. Geneeskd. Belg. 70:193-219; 2008.

[34]　Lavie, L. Oxidative stress--a unifying paradigm in obstructive sleep apnea and comorbidities. Prog. Cardiovasc. Dis. 51:303-312; 2009.

[35]　Thomas, S. R.; Witting, P. K.; Drummond, G. R. Redox control of endothelial function and dysfunction: molecular mechanisms and therapeutic opportunities. Antioxid. Redox. Signal. 10:1713-1765; 2008.

[36]　Schulz, E.; Jansen, T.; Wenzel, P.; Daiber, A.; Munzel, T. Nitric oxide, tetrahydrobiopterin, oxidative stress, and endothelial dysfunction in hypertension. Antioxid. Redox. Signal. 10:1115-1126; 2008.

[37]　Grossman, E. Does increased oxidative stress cause hypertension? Diabetes Care 31 Suppl 2:S185-S189; 2008.

[38]　Ceriello, A. Possible role of oxidative stress in the pathogenesis of hypertension. Diabetes Care 31 Suppl 2:S181-S184; 2008.

[39]　Halliwell, B. Antioxidants: the basics - what they are - how to evaluate them. In Sies, H. eds. Antioxidants in disease: mechanisms and therapy. London: Academic Press; 1997:3-20.

[40]　Inoguchi, T.; Li, P.; Umeda, F.; Yu, H. Y.; Kakimoto, M.; Imamura, M.; Aoki, T.; Etoh, T.; Hashimoto, T.; Naruse, M.; Sano, H.; Utsumi, H.; Nawata, H. High glucose level and free fatty acid stimulate reactive oxygen species production through protein kinase C--dependent activation of NAD(P)H oxidase in cultured vascular cells. Diabetes 49:1939-1945; 2000.

[41]　Christ, M.; Bauersachs, J.; Liebetrau, C.; Heck, M.; Gunther, A.; Wehling, M. Glucose increases endothelial-dependent superoxide formation in coronary arteries by NAD(P)H oxidase activation: attenuation by the 3-hydroxy-3-methylglutaryl coenzyme A reductase inhibitor atorvastatin. Diabetes 51:2648-2652; 2002.

[42]　Akbari, C. M.; Saouaf, R.; Barnhill, D. F.; Newman, P. A.; LoGerfo, F. W.; Veves, A. Endothelium-dependent vasodilatation is impaired in both microcirculation and macrocirculation during acute hyperglycemia. J. Vasc. Surg. 28:687-694; 1998.

[43]　Du, X.; Stocklauser-Farber, K.; Rosen, P. Generation of reactive oxygen intermediates, activation of NF-kappaB, and induction of apoptosis in human endothelial cells by glucose: role of nitric oxide synthase? Free Radic. Biol Med. 27:752-763; 1999.

[44]　Du, X. L.; Sui, G. Z.; Stockklauser-Farber, K.; Weiss, J.; Zink, S.; Schwippert, B.; Wu, Q. X.; Tschope, D.; Rosen, P. Introduction of apoptosis by high proinsulin and glucose in cultured human umbilical vein endothelial cells is mediated by reactive oxygen species. Diabetologia 41:249-256; 1998.

[45]　Du, X.; Matsumura, T.; Edelstein, D.; Rossetti, L.; Zsengeller, Z.; Szabo, C.; Brownlee, M. Inhibition of GAPDH activity by poly(ADP-ribose) polymerase activates three major pathways of hyperglycemic damage in endothelial cells. J. Clin. Invest 112:1049-1057; 2003.

[46]　Ceriello, A.; Bortolotti, N.; Crescentini, A.; Motz, E.; Lizzio, S.; Russo, A.; Ezsol, Z.; Tonutti, L.; Taboga, C. Antioxidant defences are reduced during the oral glucose tolerance test in normal and non-insulin-dependent diabetic subjects. Eur. J. Clin. Invest 28:329-333; 1998.

[47]　Ceriello, A. The emerging role of post-prandial hyperglycaemic spikes in the pathogenesis of diabetic complications. Diabet. Med. 15:188-193; 1998.

[48]　Lee, I. K.; Kim, H. S.; Bae, J. H. Endothelial dysfunction: its relationship with acute hyperglycaemia and hyperlipidemia. Int. J. Clin. Pract. Suppl 59-64; 2002.

[49]　Schinkovitz, A.; Dittrich, P.; Wascher, T. C. Effects of a high-fat meal on resistance vessel reactivity and on indicators of oxidative stress in healthy volunteers. Clin. Physiol 21:404-410; 2001.

[50]　Li, J. M.; Shah, A. M. Endothelial cell superoxide generation: regulation and relevance for cardiovascular pathophysiology. Am. J Physiol Regul. Integr. Comp Physiol 287:R1014-R1030; 2004.

[51]　Mueller, C. F.; Widder, J. D.; McNally, J. S.; McCann, L.; Jones, D. P.; Harrison, D. G. The role of the multidrug resistance protein-1 in modulation of endothelial cell oxidative stress. Circ. Res 97:637-644; 2005.

[52]　Pagano, P. J.; Ito, Y.; Tornheim, K.; Gallop, P. M.; Tauber, A. I.; Cohen, R. A. An NADPH oxidase superoxide-generating system in the rabbit aorta. Am. J Physiol 268:H2274-H2280; 1995.

[53]　Droge, W. Free radicals in the physiological control of cell function. Physiol Rev. 82:47-95; 2002.

[54]　Cadenas, E.; Davies, K. J. Mitochondrial free radical generation, oxidative stress, and aging. Free Radic. Biol. Med 29:222-230; 2000.

[55]　Finkel, T. Opinion: Radical medicine: treating ageing to cure disease. Nat. Rev. Mol. Cell Biol. 6:971-976; 2005.

[56]   Raha, S.; Robinson, B. H. Mitochondria, oxygen free radicals, disease and ageing. Trends Biochem. Sci. 25:502-508; 2000.

[57]   Venugopal, J.; Hanashiro, K.; Yang, Z. Z.; Nagamine, Y. Identification and modulation of a caveolae-dependent signal pathway that regulates plasminogen activator inhibitor-1 in insulin-resistant adipocytes. Proc. Natl. Acad. Sci. U. S. A 101:17120-17125; 2004.

[58]   Roberts, C. K.; Barnard, R. J.; Sindhu, R. K.; Jurczak, M.; Ehdaie, A.; Vaziri, N. D. Oxidative stress and dysregulation of NAD(P)H oxidase and antioxidant enzymes in diet-induced metabolic syndrome. Metabolism 55:928-934; 2006.

[59]   Bellin, C.; de Wiza, D. H.; Wiernsperger, N. F.; Rosen, P. Generation of reactive oxygen species by endothelial and smooth muscle cells: influence of hyperglycemia and metformin. Horm Metab Res 38:732-739; 2006.

[60]   Goldstein, B. J.; Mahadev, K.; Wu, X. Redox paradox: insulin action is facilitated by insulin-stimulated reactive oxygen species with multiple potential signaling targets. Diabetes 54:311-321; 2005.

[61]   Avogaro, A.; de Kreutzenberg, S. V.; Fadini, G. P. Oxidative stress and vascular disease in diabetes: is the dichotomization of insulin signaling still valid? Free Radic. Biol. Med. 44:1209-1215; 2008.

[62]   McClung, J. P.; Roneker, C. A.; Mu, W.; Lisk, D. J.; Langlais, P.; Liu, F.; Lei, X. G. Development of insulin resistance and obesity in mice overexpressing cellular glutathione peroxidase. Proc. Natl. Acad. Sci. U. S. A 101:8852-8857; 2004.

[63]   McGarry, J. D. Banting lecture 2001: dysregulation of fatty acid metabolism in the etiology of type 2 diabetes. Diabetes 51:7-18; 2002.

[64]   Boden, G. Role of fatty acids in the pathogenesis of insulin resistance and NIDDM. Diabetes 46:3-10; 1997.

[65]   Hotamisligil, G. S.; Peraldi, P.; Budavari, A.; Ellis, R.; White, M. F.; Spiegelman, B. M. IRS-1-mediated inhibition of insulin receptor tyrosine kinase activity in TNF-alpha- and obesity-induced insulin resistance. Science 271:665-668; 1996.

[66]   Cohen, B.; Novick, D.; Rubinstein, M. Modulation of insulin activities by leptin. Science 274:1185-1188; 1996.

[67]   Randle, P. J.; Kerbey, A. L.; Espinal, J. Mechanisms decreasing glucose oxidation in diabetes and starvation: role of lipid fuels and hormones. Diabetes Metab Rev. 4:623-638; 1988.

[68]   Steppan, C. M.; Bailey, S. T.; Bhat, S.; Brown, E. J.; Banerjee, R. R.; Wright, C. M.; Patel, H. R.; Ahima, R. S.; Lazar, M. A. The hormone resistin links obesity to diabetes. Nature 409:307-312; 2001.

[69]   Steinberg, H. O.; Chaker, H.; Leaming, R.; Johnson, A.; Brechtel, G.; Baron, A. D. Obesity/insulin resistance is associated with endothelial dysfunction. Implications for the syndrome of insulin resistance. J. Clin. Invest 97:2601-2610; 1996.

[70]   Laakso, M.; Edelman, S. V.; Brechtel, G.; Baron, A. D. Decreased effect of insulin to stimulate skeletal muscle blood flow in obese man. A novel mechanism for insulin resistance. J. Clin. Invest 85:1844-1852; 1990.

[71]   Ritz, P.; Berrut, G. Mitochondrial function, energy expenditure, aging and insulin resistance. Diabetes Metab 31 Spec No 2:5S67-5S73; 2005.

[72]   Frisard, M.; Ravussin, E. Energy metabolism and oxidative stress: impact on the metabolic syndrome and the aging process. Endocrine. 29:27-32; 2006.

[73]   Petersen, K. F.; Befroy, D.; Dufour, S.; Dziura, J.; Ariyan, C.; Rothman, D. L.; DiPietro, L.; Cline, G. W.; Shulman, G. I. Mitochondrial dysfunction in the elderly: possible role in insulin resistance. Science 300:1140-1142; 2003.

[74]   Inoguchi, T.; Sonta, T.; Tsubouchi, H.; Etoh, T.; Kakimoto, M.; Sonoda, N.; Sato, N.; Sekiguchi, N.; Kobayashi, K.; Sumimoto, H.; Utsumi, H.; Nawata, H. Protein kinase C-dependent increase in reactive oxygen species (ROS) production in vascular tissues of diabetes: role of vascular NAD(P)H oxidase. J Am Soc. Nephrol. 14 S227-S232; 2003.

[75]   Brownlee, M. A radical explanation for glucose-induced beta cell dysfunction. J. Clin. Invest 112:1788-1790; 2003.

[76]   Kim, J. A.; Wei, Y.; Sowers, J. R. Role of mitochondrial dysfunction in insulin resistance. Circ. Res 102:401-414; 2008.

[77]   Crimi, E.; Ignarro, L. J.; Napoli, C. Microcirculation and oxidative stress. Free Radic. Res 41:1364-1375; 2007.

[78]   Wiernsperger, N.; Nivoit, P.; De Aguiar, L. G.; Bouskela, E. Microcirculation and the metabolic syndrome. Microcirculation. 14:403-438; 2007.

[79]   Wang, Y.; Marsden, P. A. Nitric oxide synthases: biochemical and molecular regulation. Curr. Opin. Nephrol. Hypertens. 4:12-22; 1995.

[80]   Cooke, J. P.; Dzau, V. J. Nitric oxide synthase: role in the genesis of vascular disease. Annu. Rev. Med. 48:489-509; 1997.

[81]   Ignarro, L. Activation and regulation of the nitric oxide-cGMP pathway by oxidative stress. In Forman, H.; Cadenas, E. eds. Oxidative stress and signal transduction. New York: Chapmann & Hall; 1997:32-51.

[82]   Archer, S. L.; Huang, J. M.; Hampl, V.; Nelson, D. P.; Shultz, P. J.; Weir, E. K. Nitric oxide and cGMP cause vasorelaxation by activation of a charybdotoxin-sensitive K channel by cGMP-dependent protein kinase. Proc. Natl. Acad. Sci. U. S. A 91:7583-7587; 1994.

[83]   Robertson, B. E.; Schubert, R.; Hescheler, J.; Nelson, M. T. cGMP-dependent protein kinase activates Ca-activated K channels in cerebral artery smooth muscle cells. Am. J. Physiol 265:C299-C303; 1993.

[84]   Spear, N.; Estévez, A.; Radi, R.; Beckmann, J. Activation and regulation of the nitric oxide-cyclich GMP signal transduction pathway by oxidative stress. In Forman, H.; Cadenas, E. eds. Oxidative stress and signal transduction. New York: Chapmann & Hall; 1997:3-31.

[85]   Ohara, Y.; Peterson, T. E.; Harrison, D. G. Hypercholesterolemia increases endothelial superoxide anion production. J Clin. Invest 91:2546-2551; 1993.

[86]   Bouloumie, A.; Bauersachs, J.; Linz, W.; Scholkens, B. A.; Wiemer, G.; Fleming, I.; Busse, R. Endothelial dysfunction coincides with an enhanced nitric oxide synthase expression and superoxide anion production. Hypertension 30:934-941; 1997.

[87]   Zou, M. H.; Shi, C.; Cohen, R. A. Oxidation of the zinc-thiolate complex and uncoupling of endothelial nitric oxide synthase by peroxynitrite. J Clin. Invest 109:817-826; 2002.

[88]   Schmidt, T. S.; Alp, N. J. Mechanisms for the role of tetrahydrobiopterin in endothelial function and vascular disease. Clin. Sci. (Lond) 113:47-63; 2007.

[89]   Cai, S.; Khoo, J.; Mussa, S.; Alp, N. J.; Channon, K. M. Endothelial nitric oxide synthase dysfunction in diabetic mice: importance of tetrahydrobiopterin in eNOS dimerisation. Diabetologia 48:1933-1940; 2005.

[90]   Frisbee, J. C.; Delp, M. D. Vascular function in the metabolic syndrome and the effects on skeletal muscle perfusion: lessons from the obese Zucker rat. Essays Biochem. 42:145-161; 2006.

[91]   Dell'Omo, G.; Penno, G.; Pucci, L.; Mariani, M.; Del Prato, S.; Pedrinelli, R. Abnormal capillary permeability and endothelial dysfunction in hypertension with comorbid Metabolic Syndrome. Atherosclerosis 172:383-389; 2004.

[92]   Sun, Y. X.; Hu, S. J.; Zhang, X. H.; Sun, J.; Zhu, C. H.; Zhang, Z. J. [Plasma levels of vWF and NO in patients with metabolic syndrome and their relationship with metabolic disorders]. Zhejiang. Da. Xue. Xue. Bao. Yi. Xue. Ban. 35:315-318; 2006.

[93]   Hsueh, W. A.; Quinones, M. J. Role of endothelial dysfunction in insulin resistance. Am. J. Cardiol. 92:10J-17J; 2003.

[94]   Laakso, M.; Sarlund, H.; Mykkanen, L. Insulin resistance is associated with lipid and lipoprotein abnormalities in subjects with varying degrees of glucose tolerance. Arteriosclerosis 10:223-231; 1990.

[95]   Murdie, P. Link between insulin resistance, ethnicity and endothelial dysfunction. Nat Clin Pract Cardiovasc Med 2, 498. 2005.

[96]   Anastasiou, E.; Lekakis, J. P.; Alevizaki, M.; Papamichael, C. M.; Megas, J.; Souvatzoglou, A.; Stamatelopoulos, S. F. Impaired endothelium-dependent vasodilatation in women with previous gestational diabetes. Diabetes Care 21:2111-2115; 1998.

[97]   Tooke, J. E.; Goh, K. L. Endotheliopathy precedes type 2 diabetes. Diabetes Care 21:2047-2049; 1998.

[98]   Balletshofer, B. M.; Rittig, K.; Enderle, M. D.; Volk, A.; Maerker, E.; Jacob, S.; Matthaei, S.; Rett, K.; Haring, H. U. Endothelial dysfunction is detectable in young normotensive first-degree relatives of subjects with type 2 diabetes in association with insulin resistance. Circulation 101:1780-1784; 2000.

[99]   Caballero, A. E. Metabolic and vascular abnormalities in subjects at risk for type 2 diabetes: the early start of a dangerous situation. Arch. Med Res 36:241-249; 2005.

[100]   Caballero, A. E. Endothelial dysfunction, inflammation, and insulin resistance: a focus on subjects at risk for type 2 diabetes. Curr. Diab. Rep. 4:237-246; 2004.

[101]   Caballero, A. E.; Arora, S.; Saouaf, R.; Lim, S. C.; Smakowski, P.; Park, J. Y.; King, G. L.; LoGerfo, F. W.; Horton, E. S.; Veves, A. Microvascular and macrovascular reactivity is reduced in subjects at risk for type 2 diabetes. Diabetes 48:1856-1862; 1999.

[102]   Freeman, D. J.; Norrie, J.; Caslake, M. J.; Gaw, A.; Ford, I.; Lowe, G. D.; O'Reilly, D. S.; Packard, C. J.; Sattar, N. C-reactive protein is an independent predictor of risk for the development of diabetes in the West of Scotland Coronary Prevention Study. Diabetes 51:1596-1600; 2002.

[103]   Festa, A.; D'Agostino, R., Jr.; Tracy, R. P.; Haffner, S. M. Elevated levels of acute-phase proteins and plasminogen activator inhibitor-1 predict the development of type 2 diabetes: the insulin resistance atherosclerosis study. Diabetes 51:1131-1137; 2002.

[104]   Enderle, M. D.; Benda, N.; Schmuelling, R. M.; Haering, H. U.; Pfohl, M. Preserved endothelial function in IDDM patients, but not in NIDDM patients, compared with healthy subjects. Diabetes Care 21:271-277; 1998.

[105]   Houben, A. J.; Schaper, N. C.; de Haan, C. H.; Huvers, F. C.; Slaaf, D. W.; de Leeuw, P. W.; Nieuwenhuijzen Kruseman, A. C. The effects of 7-hour local hyperglycaemia on forearm macro and microcirculatory blood flow and vascular reactivity in healthy man. Diabetologia 37:750-756; 1994.

[106]   Clarkson, P.; Celermajer, D. S.; Donald, A. E.; Sampson, M.; Sorensen, K. E.; Adams, M.; Yue, D. K.; Betteridge, D. J.; Deanfield, J. E. Impaired vascular reactivity in insulin-dependent diabetes mellitus is related to disease duration and low density lipoprotein cholesterol levels. J. Am. Coll. Cardiol. 28:573-579; 1996.

[107]   Arcaro, G.; Zenere, B. M.; Saggiani, F.; Zenti, M. G.; Monauni, T.; Lechi, A.; Muggeo, M.; Bonadonna, R. C. ACE inhibitors improve endothelial function in type 1 diabetic patients with normal arterial pressure and microalbuminuria. Diabetes Care 22:1536-1542; 1999.

[108]   Schalkwijk, C. G.; Stehouwer, C. D. Vascular complications in diabetes mellitus: the role of endothelial dysfunction. Clin. Sci. (Lond) 109:143-159; 2005.

[109]   Clark, M. G.; Wallis, M. G.; Barrett, E. J.; Vincent, M. A.; Richards, S. M.; Clerk, L. H.; Rattigan, S. Blood flow and muscle metabolism: a focus on insulin action. Am. J Physiol Endocrinol. Metab 284:E241-E258; 2003.

[110]   Assumpcao, C.; Brunini, T.; Matsuura, C.; Resende, A.; Mendes-Ribeiro, A. Impact of the L-arginine-nitric oxide pathway and oxidative stress on the pathogenesis ogf the metabolic syndrome. The Open Biochem J 2:108-115; 2008.

[111]   Zeng, G.; Nystrom, F. H.; Ravichandran, L. V.; Cong, L. N.; Kirby, M.; Mostowski, H.; Quon, M. J. Roles for insulin receptor, PI3-kinase, and Akt in insulin-signaling pathways related to production of nitric oxide in human vascular endothelial cells. Circulation 101:1539-1545; 2000.

[112]   He, Z.; Opland, D. M.; Way, K. J.; Ueki, K.; Bodyak, N.; Kang, P. M.; Izumo, S.; Kulkarni, R. N.; Wang, B.; Liao, R.; Kahn, C. R.; King, G. L. Regulation of vascular endothelial growth factor expression and vascularization in the myocardium by insulin receptor and PI3K/Akt pathways in insulin resistance and ischemia. Arterioscler. Thromb. Vasc. Biol. 26:787-793; 2006.

[113]   Forman, H. J.; Cadenas, E. Oxidative stress and signal transduction: New York Chapman & Hall; 1997.

[114]   Schulze-Osthoff, K.; Bauer, M.; Wesselborg, S.; Baeuerle, P. Reactive oxygen species as primary signals and second messenger in the activation of transcription factors. In Forman, H.; Cadenas, E. eds. Oxidative stress and signal transduction. New York: Chapmann & Hall; 1997:239-259.

[115]   Simon, A.; Fanburg, B.; Cochran, B. STAT activation by oxidative stress. In Forman, H.; Cadenas, E. eds. Oxidative stress and signal transduction. New York: Chapmann & Hall; 1997:260-271.

[116]   Lenardo, M. J.; Baltimore, D. NF-kappa B: a pleiotropic mediator of inducible and tissue-specific gene control. Cell 58:227-229; 1989.

[117]   Xie, Q. W.; Kashiwabara, Y.; Nathan, C. Role of transcription factor NF-kappa B/Rel in induction of nitric oxide synthase. J Biol. Chem. 269:4705-4708; 1994.

[118]   He, Z.; King, G. L. Microvascular complications of diabetes. Endocrinol. Metab Clin North Am. 33:215-xii; 2004.

[119]   King, G. L.; Ishii, H.; Koya, D. Diabetic vascular dysfunctions: a model of excessive activation of protein kinase C. Kidney Int. Suppl 60:S77-S85; 1997.

CHAPTER 7

Microalbuminuria and Insulin Resistance

Börje Haraldsson

Institute of Medicine, Department of molecular and clinical medicine - Nephrology, University of Gothenburg, Gothenburg, Sweden

Abstract: The glomerular barrier is highly selective and an only minute amount reaches the urine. Normally, the daily loss of albumin in urine is less than 30 mg and microalbuminuria denotes losses between 30-300 mg per day. Overt proteinuria means daily losses between 300- 3000 mg, whereas larger albumin losses are in the nephrotic range. There are a wide variety of conditions that cause microalbuminuria or proteinuria, but recently our understanding of these phenomena has improved considerably. Microalbuminuria is one of the first signs of diabetic nephropathy where it reflects endothelial dysfunction and increased risk of microvascular complications. Microalbuminuria is also an independent predictor of cardiovascular disease in non-diabetic individuals. Insulin resistance is an interesting condition that precedes the development of type II diabetes. Patients with severe kidney disease have insulin resistance without developing diabetes. Insulin resistance is also associated to microalbuminuria, hypertension and obesity. Finally, there is an association between all these conditions and certain inflammatory vascular reactions. In this chapter, I will try to review our current understanding of microalbuminuria and how it is related to insulin resistance.

Keywords: Albumin, diabetes, endothelium, glomerular, glycocalyx, kidney, podocytes.

1. INTRODUCTION

Microalbuminuria is seen in several conditions such as diabetes and hypertension. The term depicts the presence of slightly more albumin than normal in urine. Diabetes is a common cause of microalbuminuria, but it may also occur due to hypertension, obesity, metabolic syndrome, or a variety of other disorders. In 1995, Agewall et al showed that microalbuminuria was associated with insulin resistance, but obesity was a confounding factor [1]. More recently, Lin et al found that insulin resistance is the main determinant for microalbuminuria [2]. Others question the notion that microalbuminuria is a marker of metabolic disorder [3, 4], and consider it mainly to reflect glomerular endothelial dysfunction [3]. Mogensen et al showed that albuminuria occurred after acute infusions of insulin in a dose-dependent manner under conditions of normoglucemia [5]. Today, it seems clear that there is a strong association between microalbuminuria and cardiovascular disease [6, 7].

In patients with insulin resistance, normal insulin concentration does not produce an adequate response in the target organs. As a result, the patient develops hyperinsulinemia to ensure a normal turnover of glucose. In the kidneys, there seems to be a strong relationship between microalbuminuria, insulin resistance and endothelial dysfunction [3]. Recently, there has been a renewed interest since the glomerular epithelial cells, the podocytes express several glucose transporters (GLUT1-5 and GLUT8) [8], and seem to be highly sensitive to insulin.

2. THE GLOMERULAR BARRIER

A normal day, the entire human plasma volume is filtered 50 to 60 times across the glomerular barrier to form 180 litres of primary urine [9]. Fortunately, 99 % of the fluid is reabsorbed in the proximal tubules, thereby ensuring homeostasis and continuing life. Approximately 1-2 litres is left as final urine containing minute amounts of sodium, potassium, glucose, amino acids, vitamins and protein. If the glomerular capillary properties were similar to those of skeletal muscle, 5-10 % of the proteins would cross the glomerular barrier.

Nicolas Wiernsperger (Ed.)

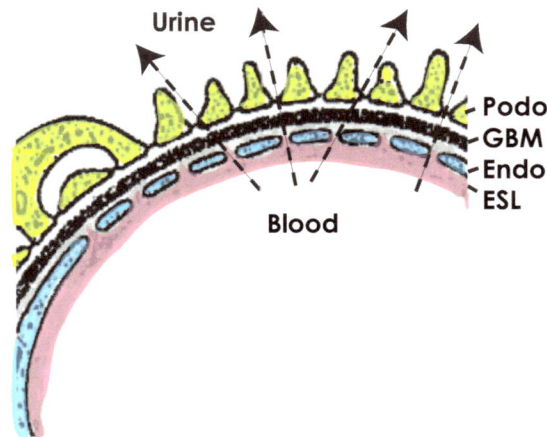

Figure 1: Illustrates the four principle components of the glomerular barrier. From blood to urine, the glomerular filtrate fluid and solutes cross the endothelial surface layer (ESL), the fenestrated endothelial cells (Endo), the glomerular basement membrane (GBM) and the glomerular epithelial cells, the podocytes (Podo).

With an albumin concentration of 40 g/l that would mean more than 360 g/day, i.e. more than three times the total intravascular content of albumin. Naturally, such losses are incompatible with life, unless there is rapid uptake of intact albumin from the proximal tubules [10]. However, recent data on the tubular uptake of albumin have shown that it is mediated by the megalin-cubulin-complex and obligatory destruction of the protein in lyzosomes [11]. Indeed, most precise measurements on glomerular selectivity indicates that 0.01 to 0.1 % of the plasma albumin crosses the normal glomerular barrier [9], i.e. less than 1g/day. The glomerular barrier discriminate solutes depending on their size, charge and shape. Thus, there is high degree of size- and charge selectivity [9].

2.1. The Podocytes

Current data show that the podocytes is of utmost importance for an intact barrier and to prevent albumin to reach urine, other than in minute quantities. Thus, several hereditary conditions causing nephritic syndrome have been shown to be due to defects in the production in certain podocytes-specific proteins such as nephrin [12], podocin [13], CD2AP [14], alpha-actinin-4 [15], and others [16].

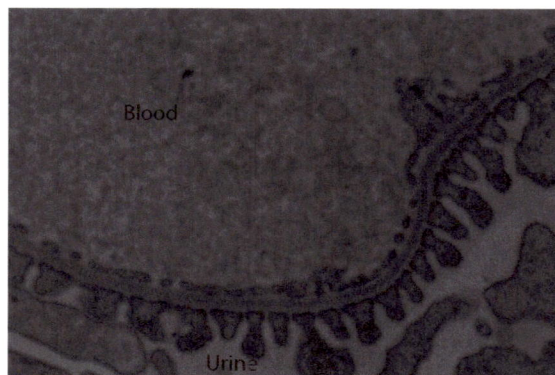

Figure 2: In the normal glomerulus, slender podocyte foot processes connected by a thin slit membrane cover the GBM on the urine side. Here a picture from a mouse glomerulus.

2.2. The Glomerular Basement Membrane, GBM

Previously, the GBM was considered to be the most important component of the glomerular barrier. Today, it is clear that certain genetic disorders in the GBM cause proteinuria. Thus, laminin seems to be essential for an intact barrier in mice and men [17-19]. However, it does not seem to contribute to glomerular charge selectivity since neither defect agrin nor perlecan seem to induce proteinuria [20, 21].

2.3. Glomerular Endothelium

The endothelium has hitherto been a neglected part of the glomerular barrier since it is highly fenestrated. In recent years, the structure has attracted more interest, since it affects glomerular permselectivity and prevents proteinuria by at least three mechanisms. Firstly, the endothelium seems to be an important part of the glomerular barrier per se, due to the presence of a thick (0.3 um) endothelial surface layer (ESL or glycocalyx) as illustrated below. The endothelial cells produce components of the surrounding matrix. Secondly, the endothelium communicates with the podocytes causing proteinuria. Thirdly, the endothelium may affect the mesangial cell matrix production by similar, but so far not studied, signaling mechanisms. Eremina et al recently showed that inhibition of vascular endothelial growth factor, VEGF, cause damage to the glomerular endothelium resulting in proteinuria [22]. Since VEGF is produced by the podocytes, those cells seem to control the entire glomerular barrier.

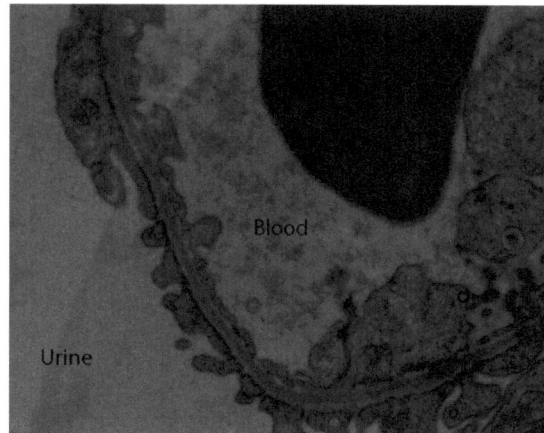

Figure 3: In practically all cases of heavy proteinuria, the podocytes become flattened and there is effacement. Note also, that in this mouse glomerulus, the endothelium seems to be affected as well.

2.4. Endothelial Surface Layer, ESL

All cells are surrounded by a more or less developed glycocalyx composed of cell-bound proteoglycans. A thick surface layer constituting a fiber matrix or a gel also covers the endothelial cells. This gel restricts the passage of larger solutes, such as albumin and prevents proteinuria [23]. The production has been studied of these proteoglycans by glomerular endothelial cells [24], by podocytes [25] and the changes induced by long-term diabetes in mice [26]. Earlier this year, the thickness of ESL was found to be markedly reduced in certain experimental conditions of nephrotic syndrome such as adriamycin-induced proteinuria in mice [27].

2.5. Cross-talk between glomerular cells

There is accumulating evidence of an intense crosstalk between the endothelial and the epithelial cells of the barrier [28]. One important factor produced by the endothelium is endothelin, which may cause proteinuria [29]. This has mainly been studied in eclampsia, where patient serum contains large amounts of endothelin that cause nephrin shedding of podocyte due to release of endothelin from the endothelial cells [29, 30]. Also, the release of VEGF by the podocytes modifies the properties of the glomerular endothelium [22]. Thus, VEGF rapidly diffuses against the convective flow and reaches high concentrations at the endothelium due to the short distance. In fact the Peclet number estimated in the barrier suggest diffusion-dominated transport for molecules the size of VEGF [9]. Less is known about endothelial and podocyte crosstalk in diabetes, apart from the renin angiotensin system [31]. Far less is known about mesangial and endothelial cell crosstalk [32] in general and the effects of diabetes needs to be investigated.

3. REASONS FOR PROTEINURIA

Just like fever can be caused by viral or bacterial infections, or malignancies, albuminuria can be due to several conditions. From a theoretical point of view, proteinuria can be the result of defects in the glomerular filter causing more protein to enter into Bowman's space. In addition, the urine may contain more protein if the uptake of proximal tubular cells is defect for some reason. Indeed, in Fanconi, or Dent's syndrome the megalin-cubulin-complex is mutated and as a result the patients loose protein in their urine. Such conditions only induce milder forms of proteinuria and it requires a glomerular defect to obtain a nephritic syndrome.

According to the integrative view of glomerular selectivity, proteinuria can be caused by defects in any of the four components of the barrier, i.e. the podocytes, GBM, endothelium or ESL.

3.1. Classification of Proteinuria

The amount of protein can be determined, but measurements of albumin are more precise. Several clinics request that their patients collect urine during 24 hours. Approximately 50% of patients will bring true collections of all urine, but others will bring a fraction of the total urine. This can be avoided by calculating the albumin to creatinine concentration ratio. Hereby, corrections are made for diluted or concentrated urine and any spot urine can be used. Below is the classification of proteinuria most often used:

Table 1: The degree of proteinuria can be classified from normal minute quantities to nephrotic range proteinuria.

Degree of Proteinuria	Urinary Albumin Excretion Rate (ug/min)	Daily Albumin Excretion in Urine (mg)	Albumin – Creatinine Concentration Ratio (mg/umol)
Normal	<20	< 30	<3
Microalbuminuria	20-200	30-300	3-30
Proteinuria	200-2000	300-3000	30-300
Nephrotic range	>2000	> 3000	>300

3.2. Podocytes and Insulin Resistance

As cited above, podocytes express several glucose transporters. Coward et al demonstrated that human immortalized podocytes in culture double their glucose uptake in response to insulin [33] mainly through GLUT1 (and 4). Insulin affects the actin cytoskeleton of the podocyte and may thereby affect selectivity and proteinuria. In contrast, they found no effect on immortalize human glomerular endothelium [33].

The mesangial cell is another important player in the glomerulus and these cells express GLUT1, and respond to insulin stimulation [34]. Indeed, the mesangial cells seems to produce substances such as VEGF and IL-6.

During insulin resistance there may be increased turnover by podocytes, which Hakamura et al showed to be improved by pioglitazone [35]. Hyperinsulinemia and insulin resistance is associated by podocyte injury and albuminuria [5, 36]. However, the glomerular endothelium seems to have a crucial pathogenetic role for the development of diabetic micro- and macrovascular complications as revealed by studied on eNOS knockout mice [37]. VEGF seems to control the expression of eNOS in glomerular endothelium. Also, inflammation has a role in diabetic nephropathy [38].

3.3. Microalbuminuria and Cardiovascular Risks

It is known that any degree of albuminuria is a risk factor for cardiovascular events in diabetic and non-diabetic individuals with a history of cardiovascular events [7]. However, the same is true for non-diabetic normotensive middle-aged persons in the general population. Thus, albuminuria even below the threshold for microalbuminuria was found to be associated with an increased risk of cardiovascular events [6].

4. CONCLUSIONS

Albuminuria is a hallmark of kidney disease and microalbuminuria can be seen as a foreboding of things to come. The strong association between microalbuminuria and cardiovascular events is useful but does not provide insight into the underlying molecular mechanisms. There does however seem to be a connection between insulin resistance and microalbuminuria and further studies on glomerular cells are required. Our knowledge has advanced dramatically in recent years regarding the components of the glomerular barrier and their communication. The glomerular endothelium with its surface layer (ESL or glycocalyx) has a key role, but may be controlled by actions in the podocytes and/or the mesangial cells. It is also true that the endothelium can modify the properties of the podocytes. With further understanding of these intricate processes we will hopefully be able to prevent some of the complications to diabetes and cardiovascular disease in general.

5. ACKNOWLEDGEMENTS

The author is grateful for the support by the Swedish Research Council 9898.

6. REFERENCES

[1]　Agewall S, Fagerberg B, Attvall S, Ljungman S, Urbanavicius V, Tengborn L, et al. Microalbuminuria, insulin sensitivity and haemostatic factors in non-diabetic treated hypertensive men. Risk Factor Intervention Study Group. J Intern Med. 1995 Feb;237(2):195-203.

[2]　Lin CY, Chen MF, Lin LY, Liau CS, Lee YT, Su TC. Insulin resistance is the major determinant for microalbuminuria in severe hypertriglyceridemia: implication for high-risk stratification. Intern Med. 2008;47(12):1091-7.

[3]　Solbu MD, Jenssen TG, Eriksen BO, Toft I. Changes in insulin sensitivity, renal function, and markers of endothelial dysfunction in hypertension--the impact of microalbuminuria: a 13-year follow-up study. Metabolism. 2009 Mar;58(3):408-15.

[4]　Kronborg J, Jenssen T, Njolstad I, Toft I, Eriksen BO. Metabolic risk factors associated with serum creatinine in a non-diabetic population. Eur J Epidemiol. 2007;22(10):707-13.

[5]　Mogensen CE, Christensen NJ, Gundersen HJ. The acute effect of insulin on heart rate, blood pressure, plasma noradrenaline and urinary albumin excretion. The role of changes in blood glucose. Diabetologia. 1980 Jun;18(6):453-7.

[6]　Arnlov J, Evans JC, Meigs JB, Wang TJ, Fox CS, Levy D, et al. Low-grade albuminuria and incidence of cardiovascular disease events in nonhypertensive and nondiabetic individuals: the Framingham Heart Study. Circulation. 2005 Aug 16;112(7):969-75.

[7]　Gerstein HC, Mann JF, Yi Q, Zinman B, Dinneen SF, Hoogwerf B, et al. Albuminuria and risk of cardiovascular events, death, and heart failure in diabetic and nondiabetic individuals. JAMA. 2001 Jul 25;286(4):421-6.

[8]　Schiffer M, Susztak K, Ranalletta M, Raff AC, Bottinger EP, Charron MJ. Localization of the GLUT8 glucose transporter in murine kidney and regulation in vivo in nondiabetic and diabetic conditions. Am J Physiol Renal Physiol. 2005 Jul;289(1):F186-93.

[9]　Haraldsson B, Nyström J, Deen WM. Properties of the glomerular barrier and mechanisms of proteinuria. Physiol Rev. 2008 Apr;88(2):451-87.

[10]　Russo LM, Sandoval RM, Campos SB, Molitoris BA, Comper WD, Brown D. Impaired tubular uptake explains albuminuria in early diabetic nephropathy. J Am Soc Nephrol. 2009 Mar;20(3):489-94.

[11]　Christensen EI, Birn H, Rippe B, Maunsbach AB. Controversies in nephrology: renal albumin handling, facts, and artifacts! Kidney Int. 2007 Nov;72(10):1192-4.

[12]　Kestila M, Lenkkeri U, Mannikko M, Lamerdin J, McCready P, Putaala H, et al. Positionally cloned gene for a novel glomerular protein--nephrin--is mutated in congenital nephrotic syndrome. Molecular cell. 1998 Mar;1(4):575-82.

[13]　Boute N, Gribouval O, Roselli S, Benessy F, Lee H, Fuchshuber A, et al. NPHS2, encoding the glomerular protein podocin, is mutated in autosomal recessive steroid-resistant nephrotic syndrome. Nature genetics. 2000 Apr;24(4):349-54.

[14]　Shih NY, Li J, Karpitskii V, Nguyen A, Dustin ML, Kanagawa O, et al. Congenital nephrotic syndrome in mice lacking CD2-associated protein. Science. 1999 Oct 8;286(5438):312-5.

[15]　Kaplan JM, Kim SH, North KN, Rennke H, Correia LA, Tong HQ, et al. Mutations in ACTN4, encoding alpha-actinin-4, cause familial focal segmental glomerulosclerosis. Nature genetics. 2000 Mar;24(3):251-6.

[16]　Tryggvason K, Patrakka J, Wartiovaara J. Hereditary proteinuria syndromes and mechanisms of proteinuria. N Engl J Med. 2006 Mar 30;354(13):1387-401.

[17]　Jarad G, Cunningham J, Shaw AS, Miner JH. Proteinuria precedes podocyte abnormalities inLamb2-/- mice, implicating the glomerular basement membrane as an albumin barrier. J Clin Invest. 2006 Aug;116(8):2272-9.

[18]　Miner JH, Morello R, Andrews KL, Li C, Antignac C, Shaw AS, et al. Transcriptional induction of slit diaphragm genes by Lmx1b is required in podocyte differentiation. J Clin Invest. 2002 Apr;109(8):1065-72.

[19]　Zenker M, Aigner T, Wendler O, Tralau T, Muntefering H, Fenski R, et al. Human laminin beta2 deficiency causes congenital nephrosis with mesangial sclerosis and distinct eye abnormalities. Human molecular genetics. 2004 Nov 1;13(21):2625-32.

[20]　Harvey SJ, Jarad G, Cunningham J, Rops AL, van der Vlag J, Berden JH, et al. Disruption of glomerular basement membrane charge through podocyte-specific mutation of agrin does not alter glomerular permselectivity. Am J Pathol. 2007 Jul;171(1):139-52.

[21]　Rossi M, Morita H, Sormunen R, Airenne S, Kreivi M, Wang L, et al. Heparan sulfate chains of perlecan are indispensable in the lens capsule but not in the kidney. The EMBO journal. 2003 Jan 15;22(2):236-45.

[22]　Eremina V, Jefferson JA, Kowalewska J, Hochster H, Haas M, Weisstuch J, et al. VEGF inhibition and renal thrombotic microangiopathy. The New England journal of medicine. 2008 Mar 13;358(11):1129-36.

[23]　Haraldsson B, Nystrom J, Deen WM. Properties of the glomerular barrier and mechanisms of proteinuria. Physiol Rev. 2008 Apr;88(2):451-87.

[24]   Björnson A, Moses J, Ingemansson A, Haraldsson B, Sörensson J. Primary human glomerular endothelial cells produce proteoglycans, and puromycin affects their posttranslational modification. Am J Physiol Renal Physiol. 2005 Apr;288(4):F748-56.

[25]   Björnson Granqvist A, Ebefors K, Saleem MA, Mathieson PW, Haraldsson B, Sörensson Nyström J. Podocyte proteoglycan synthesis is involved in the development of nephrotic syndrome. Am J Physiol Renal Physiol. 2006 Apr 18.

[26]   Jeansson M, Granqvist AB, Nyström JS, Haraldsson B. Functional and molecular alterations of the glomerular barrier in long-term diabetes in mice. Diabetologia. 2006 Sep;49(9):2200-9.

[27]   Jeansson M, Björck K, Tenstad O, Haraldsson B. Adriamycin Alters Glomerular Endothelium to Induce Proteinuria. J Am Soc Nephrol. 2009 Dec 10;20(1):114-22.

[28]   Eremina V, Baelde HJ, Quaggin SE. Role of the VEGF--a signaling pathway in the glomerulus: evidence for crosstalk between components of the glomerular filtration barrier. Nephron Physiol. 2007;106(2):p32-7.

[29]   Hauser PV, Collino F, Bussolati B, Camussi G. Nephrin and endothelial injury. Curr Opin Nephrol Hypertens. 2009 Jan;18(1):3-8.

[30]   Collino F, Bussclati B, Gerbaudo E, Marozio L, Pelissetto S, Benedetto C, et al. Preeclamptic sera induce nephrin shedding from podocytes through endothelin-1 release by endothelial glomerular cells. Am J Physiol Renal Physiol. 2008 May;294(5):F1185-94.

[31]   Gross ML, El-Shakmak A, Szabo A, Koch A, Kuhlmann A, Munter K, et al. ACE-inhibitors but not endothelin receptor blockers prevent podocyte loss in early diabetic nephropathy. Diabetologia. 2003 Jun;46(6):856-68.

[32]   Lopez-Ongil S, Diez-Marques ML, Griera M, Rodriguez-Puyol M, Rodriguez-Puyol D. Crosstalk between mesangial and endothelial cells: angiotensin II down-regulates endothelin-converting enzyme 1. Cell Physiol Biochem. 2005;15(1-4):135-44.

[33]   Coward RJ, Welsh GI, Yang J, Tasman C, Lennon R, Koziell A, et al. The human glomerular podocyte is a novel target for insulin action. Diabetes. 2005 Nov;54(11):3095-102.

[34]   Pfafflin A, Brodbeck K, Heilig CW, Haring HU, Schleicher ED, Weigert C. Increased glucose uptake and metabolism in mesangial cells overexpressing glucose transporter 1 increases interleukin-6 and vascular endothelial growth factor production: role of AP-1 and HIF-1alpha. Cell Physiol Biochem. 2006;18(4-5):199-210.

[35]   Nakamura T, Ushiyama C, Osada S, Hara M, Shimada N, Koide H. Pioglitazone reduces urinary podocyte excretion in type 2 diabetes patients with microalbuminuria. Metabolism. 2001 Oct;50(10):1193-6.

[36]   Whaley-Connell A, DeMarco VG, Lastra G, Manrique C, Nistala R, Cooper SA, et al. Insulin resistance, oxidative stress, and podocyte injury: role of rosuvastatin modulation of filtration barrier injury. Am J Nephrol. 2008;28(1):67-75.

[37]   Mohan S, Reddick RL, Musi N, Horn DA, Yan B, Prihoda TJ, et al. Diabetic eNOS knockout mice develop distinct macro- and microvascular complications. Lab Invest. 2008 May;88(5):515-28.

[38]   Fornoni A, Ijaz A, Tejada T, Lenz O. Role of inflammation in diabetic nephropathy. Curr Diabetes Rev. 2008 Feb;4(1):10-7.

CHAPTER 8

Importance of Microparticles in Microcirculation and Diseases

Maria Carmen Martínez and Ramaroson Andriantsitohaina

INSERM, U771; CNRS UMR 6214; Université d'Angers, Angers (France)
Address correspondence to: R. Andriantsitohaina, INSERM U771-CNRS UMR 6214, Faculté de Médecine, Université d'Angers, Rue haute de reculée; F-49045 Angers cedex (France). Tel: +33 2 41 73 58 29; Fax: +33 2 41 73 58 95; e-mail: ramaroson.andriantsitohaina@univ-angers.fr

Abstract: Although generation of microparticles from stimulated cells is a universal event of the cell life, little is known about the mechanisms regulating this process. Only in the last ten years, microparticles are considered as vectors of biological information between cells. Levels of circulating microparticles are enhanced in a large number of cardiovascular pathologies including changes in the microcirculation associated with insulino-resistance and this has been associated with deleterious effects on cells from vascular wall, mainly, endothelial cells. However, under several conditions, microparticles released from different vascular cells can induce beneficial effects, such as repair of injured tissue favoring angiogenesis, release of nitric oxide from injured endothelium, for instance. This review emphasizes the increasing significance of microparticles in major cardiovascular pathological situations, as well as, the recent progress in the identification of other biological functions for microparticles, mainly, considering microparticles as potential therapeutic tools.

1. INTRODUCTION

During cell stimulation, intracellular events, such as the increase of the intracellular calcium concentration, can induce modifications at the surface of cell through mechanisms not completely elucidated up to now. In particular, changes in plasma membrane phospholipid repartition between internal and external leaflets lead to membrane blebbing and release of small size fragments of the plasma membrane. These vesicles, called microvesicles or microparticles, are very heterogeneous in size and in protein composition. Indeed, molecular profiling approaches using proteomic techniques, performed in order to determine the protein composition of microparticles, have shown that not only protein composition depends on cell type, but also on the conditions of cell stimulation [10, 26, 39]. Although in the past, microparticles have been considered as cell dust, during the last years, a large number of studies have illustrated the «novel» role of microparticles: they can either be used as biomarkers or act as vectors of biological information playing diverse roles in intercellular communication [9, 21, 23, 42, 43]. Levels of microparticles are easily measurable in plasma from blood samples using different techniques such as protein concentration, flow cytometry, or ELISA assays associated with their procoagulant activity. Using the two latter approaches, it is possible to quantify the total circulating level of microparticles, as well as, their origin through specific determination of their surface antigens. Circulating level of microparticles is increased in numerous cardiovascular pathologies linked to inflammatory and/or procoagulant states, and in other diseases such as cancer, sepsis and HIV, for instance [22]. Concerning the pathologies associated with cardiovascular complications, microparticles from platelets are the major subpopulation of circulating microparticles, and in general, their levels are enhanced in cardiovascular diseases. However, other subpopulations such as microparticles from endothelial and red cells or leukocytes can also be increased as described in metabolic syndrome [2], acute coronary syndrome [7], severe hypertension [36] and type 2 diabetes [33]. All these pathologies are associated with endothelial dysfunction and microcirculation disturbances suggesting that microparticles may, at least in part, play a key role in the pathogenesis of these diseases. In this review, we focus on the underestimated evidence for the potential role of microparticles in the development and/or the maintenance of several cardiovascular pathologies.

2. Formation and characterization of microparticles

Although it is largely accepted that all cells are able to release microparticles, the mechanisms leading to microparticle formation are not completely elucidated. During cell stimulation, and after the increase of intracellular calcium concentration, the phospholipid asymmetry of the plasma membrane is disrupted and aminophospholipids, which are sequestered in the internal leaflet of the membrane bilayer in rest cells, are exposed at the external surface of cells. The negative surcharge at the external leaflet of the membrane, mainly due to phosphatidylserine externalization, and the concomitant proteolysis of the cytoskeletal proteins result in the blebbing of the plasma membrane and then, vesiculation [15]. For this, it is has been shown that a sustained, but not transient, increase in intracellular calcium concentration is necessary for phospholipid externalization. In non-excitable cells such as erythroleukemia HEL cells and platelets, it has been proposed that both calcium entry through store-operated calcium channels and cytoskeleton architectural organization are implicated in the regulation of phosphatidylserine transbilayer migration [6, 19]. Little is known concerning the molecular targets linked to the increase of intracellular calcium concentration. Among the proposed pathways, extracellular signal-regulated kinase (ERK) [19], small GTPase Rho A [18], myosin light chain and ROCKI [37] have been shown as candidates to regulate phosphatidylserine externalization and release of microparticles.

In the last years, the research field of microparticles is focused on the identification of the profile of proteins harbored by these vesicles. Indeed, the content of microparticles and their biological function depend on the cell of origin and the stimulation used for their generation. Current proteomic technology is able to detect and identify proteins carried by microparticles even if they are not abundant [40]. Proteins from endothelial microparticles are mainly metabolic enzymes, proteins involved in adhesion and fusion processes, and cytoskeleton-associated proteins [5], whereas proteins from platelet microparticles are surface glycoproteins or chemokines [14]. Concerning the effects of the stimulation on the protein composition of microparticles, it has been reported that more proteins are recovered in samples from microparticles generated from human apoptotic T lymphocytes those than generated from human activated T lymphocytes [26]. Although near to 70% of proteins are represented in both conditions, differences are observed concerning mainly ribosomal proteins and nuclear histones that were only identified in apoptotic microparticles [26]. Peterson *et al.* [34] have compared the protein profile of microparticles from non-treated endothelial cells versus those obtained from plasminogen activator inhibitor type 1 (PAI-1) - or tumor necrosis factor-alpha (TNFα)-treated endothelial cells. Interestingly, ~22, 10 and 7% of the proteins identified are unique to the control, PAI-1, and TNFα group of endothelial microparticles, respectively. Proteins from the cellular membrane compartment are enriched in control endothelial microparticles, whereas in microparticles generated with PAI-1 and TNFα stimulation, enrichment in proteins from the proteasome complex is described. These differences suggest that each microparticle population may display functional differences.

Differential lipid composition of microparticles, regarding the cell type from which they originate and the stimulation used for their generation, has not yet been studied. However, several reports have shown that the lipid environment could modify the activity of certain proteins carried by microparticles. For instance, cholesterol enrichment of human monocytes induces the generation of highly procoagulant active microparticles [20]. Taken together, one can advanced the hypothesis that microparticles from patients with metabolic pathologies, for instance, may have different lipid composition, which may account for different functional effects. Future lipidomic studies should be addressed to evaluate the role of lipid environment of microparticle effects.

Very recently, it has been reported that some cells including glioblastoma tumour cells release microparticles containing mRNA and miRNA in addition to angiogenic proteins [38]. These microvesicles can be taken up by normal host cells, such as brain microvascular endothelial cells. By incorporating an mRNA for a reporter protein into these microvesicles, the authors demonstrate that messages delivered by microvesicles are translated by recipient cells. Thus, tumour-derived microparticles, therefore, serve as a means of delivering genetic information and proteins to recipient cells in the tumour environment.

3. Effects of microparticles on vascular vessel

One of the main targets of microparticles is the endothelium, the key component of the microcirculation contributing to the local balance between relaxing and constrictor mediators, and regulating hemostasis and vascular permeability. Whereas normal shear stress controls homeostasis of endothelium monolayer, alterations in shear stress induce the unbalance of endothelial-derived factor release leading to endothelial dysfunction. Among these alterations, a decrease of nitric oxide (NO) release and bioavailability, an increase of vasoconstrictor factors, and an enhanced oxidative stress favor a disturbance of the vascular reactivity, induce vascular inflammation and remodeling through the upregulation of gene expression. Theoretically, all of these vascular events can be mediated by microparticles.

3.1. Microparticles and Endothelial Function

3.1.1. Effects of Microparticles on NO Pathway

It has been described that total circulating microparticles, as well as, each subpopulation of them, can affect NO pathway, but the mechanisms involved can vary. Thus, circulating microparticles, rich in endothelial and platelet surface markers, from patients with acute myocardial infarction cause severe endothelial dysfunction in rat aorta by affecting the endothelial NO transduction pathway but not endothelial NO synthase expression [7]. By contrast, circulating microparticles from type 2 diabetic patients, also mainly from endothelial cells and platelets, are able to decrease NO release from endothelial cells by decreasing endothelial NO synthase expression [21]. Also, apoptotic T lymphocyte-derived microparticles, at concentrations that can be reached in circulating blood under immunological dysfunction (e.g., HIV), impair endothelium-dependent relaxation in both conductance and small resistance arteries in response to agonists and shear stress, respectively [21]. Interestingly, microparticle treatment affects NO- and prostacyclin- but not endothelium-derived hyperpolarizing factor-mediated dilatation Fig. (**1**). These effects are linked to the decrease in expression of endothelial NO synthase, and the increased caveolin-1 expression that probably impairs of translocation of endothelial NO synthase into the cytosol and its activation by Ca^{2+}/calmodulin [21]. Recently, we have shown that the same type of microparticles (from apoptotic T lymphocytes) is able to increase reactive oxygen species production that may reduce the bioavailability of NO [28].

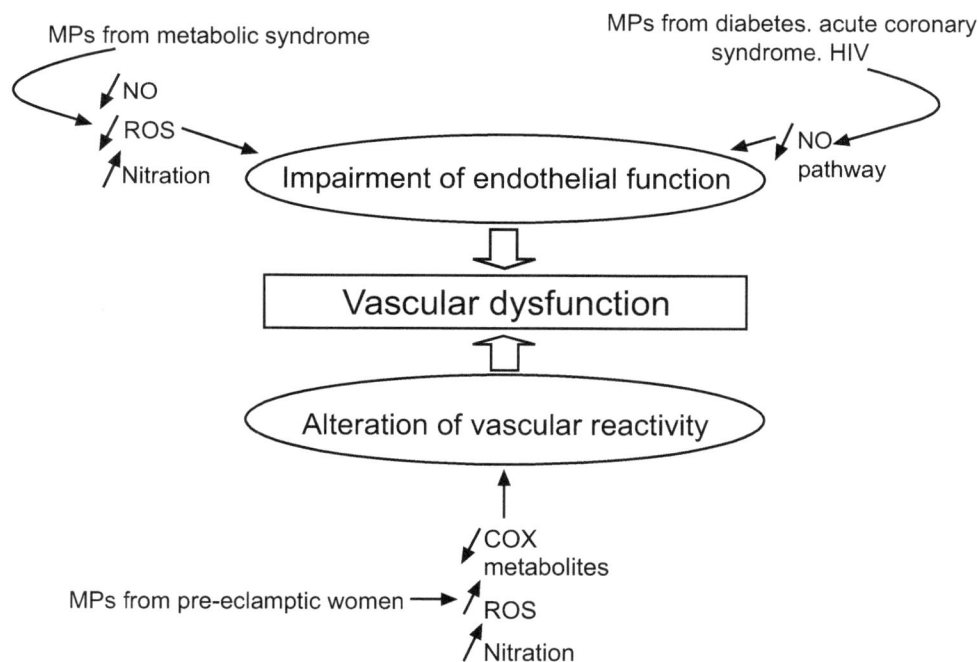

Figure 1

In metabolic syndrome, it has been reported an increase of total circulating microparticles, as well as, microparticles from platelets, endothelial and red cells without modifications in levels of microparticles from leukocytes [2]. Regarding the effects of microparticles from syndrome metabolic patients on endothelial function, a decrease of NO, being these effects associated with enhanced phosphorylation of endothelial NO synthase at the site of inhibition, and reactive oxygen species generation is described, and this results in the reduction of the endothelium-dependent relaxation in mice aorta. These data suggest that microparticles from metabolic syndrome cause endothelial dysfunction [2] Fig. (**1**). In addition, the separation of the different subpopulation of microparticles, using the magnetic beads coupled to specific antibodies, has shown that the decrease in NO production was triggered by non-platelet-derived microparticles [2].

On the other hand, endothelial microparticles can aggravate endothelial dysfunction being thus implicated in the generation and in the maintenance of endothelial disturbances. Indeed, microparticles generated from endothelial cells impair endothelium-dependent relaxation and NO production in the rat aorta [9]. It has also been shown that the effect induced by endothelial microparticles is related to an increase in superoxide anion production [9], which might reduce the bioavailability of NO. Also, endothelial microparticles generated *in vitro* are able to attenuate of endothelium-mediated vasodilation through a reduction of NO production [11]. Indeed, endothelial microparticles decrease endothelial NO synthase phosphorylation at the activator site of this enzyme and also, they are able to increase capillary permeability in mice, suggesting that endothelial microparticles may induce endothelial injury. Also, the same group reports that endothelial micropaticles inhibit proliferation and migration of human valve endothelial cells suggesting that endothelial microparticles may be responsible of valvular leaflet injury by affecting growth and repair of the valve endothelium [17]. In addition, in several pathologies, a correlation between the circulating levels of endothelial microparticles and endothelial dysfunction has been described [4]. *In vitro*, microparticles from patients with end-stage renal failure impair endothelium-dependent relaxation and cyclic guanosine monophosphate generation, whereas microparticles from healthy subjects have no effects on the endothelium. Moreover, *in vitro* endothelial dysfunction, assayed in mice aorta, correlates with endothelial-derived microparticle concentrations [4], suggesting that circulating microparticles of endothelial origin are tightly associated with endothelial dysfunction end-stage renal failure. In patients with coronary artery disease, endothelial apoptotic microparticle levels are positively correlated with coronary endothelial dysfunction, suggesting that endothelial cell apoptosis *in vivo* may participate in the development of endothelial dysfunction in coronary diseases [44].

Few studies have determined the effects of microparticles from smooth muscle cells on endothelial function. Essayagh *et al.* [12] have shown that microparticles from smooth muscle cells reduce the endothelium-dependent vasodilatory response to acetylcholine in mouse aorta by a mechanism sensitive to beta3-integrin antagonists and by inhibition of NO production. These data indicate that microparticles from cells of the wall vessels, in addition of endothelial microparticles, may impair vascular perfusion and beta3-integrin antagonists may improve deleterious effects induced by microparticles generated from injured smooth muscle cells.

3.1.2. Effects of Microparticles on Oxidative Stress

In metabolic syndrome, microparticles induce a reduction of superoxide anion production, which is associated with both decreased expression of p47 phox subunit of NADPH oxidase and overexpression of extracellular superoxide dismutase [2]. In addition, these authors have shown that nitration of proteins, as result of the increase of nitrosative stress, is most important in the presence of microparticles from metabolic syndrome patients than those from healthy subjects, although they reduce both NO and superoxide anions productions under the experimental conditions used.

Using microparticles from apoptotic T lymphocytes, Mostefai *et al.* [28] have shown that the mechanism involved in the increase of reactive oxygen species production is sensitive to xanthine oxidase and phospho-IkappaB inhibitors. Also, phosphoinositide 3-kinase (PI3-kinase) inhibition enhance the effects of microparticles on superoxide anion production suggesting that microparticles from apoptotic T lymphocytes lead to an increase of oxidative stress that may account for the deleterious effects of these microparticles on endothelial function.

3.1.3. Effects of Microparticles on Endothelial Thrombogenicity and Apoptosis

In patients with type 2 diabetes, elevated levels of circulating microparticles have been described [33]. In particular, both platelet- and monocyte-derived microparticles are increased, being higher in diabetic patients with complications such as hypertension, nephropathy, retinopathy or neuropathy [30, 33]. In addition, monocyte-derived microparticle levels correlate with platelet activation markers. Treatment of these patients with lipid-lowering or anti-hypertensive agents decrease the level of platelet- and monocyte-derived microparticles suggesting that hypercholesterolemia and/or hypertension induce platelet and monocyte activation and the subsequent membrane vesiculation [31, 32]. Monocyte-derived microparticles are of particular interest, because in addition to procoagulant phospholipids they expose at their surface active tissue factor [3], a key element in physiological and pathophysiological hemostasis. Microparticles from monocytes are able to increase cell surface thrombogenicity of endothelial cells through the enhancement of endothelial tissue factor expression. This is associated with an increase of endothelial apoptosis and membrane blebbing. Essayagh *et al.* [13] have shown that up-regulation of tissue factor by endothelial cells induced by monocyte-derived microparticles are regulated by reactive oxygen species and the phosphorylation of p38 mitogen-activated protein kinase. Altogether, these results suggest that endothelial integrity may be comprised in pathologies with elevated levels of monocyte-derived microparticles.

3.2. Microparticles and Vascular Reactivity

In addition to the direct effects of microparticles on the endothelium, they can act on smooth muscle cells and modify the vascular reactivity. The direct evidence that microparticles can reach smooth muscle cells has been provided by Tesse *et al.* [43]. In this study, it has been found increased human CD4 labeling, specific for human leukocytes, in the media layer of aortas from mice treated with microparticles from human T lymphocytes, suggesting that microparticles can affect directly the function of smooth muscle cells. Furthermore, both microparticles from human T lymphocytes or from plasma of diabetic patients with vascular complications induced vascular hyporeactivity in response to vasoconstrictor agents in mouse aorta. Hyporeactivity was reversed by NO synthase plus cyclooxygenase-2 (COX-2) inhibitors, and associated with an increased production of vasodilatory products such as NO and prostacyclin. Microparticles induced an upregulation of proinflammatory protein expressions, inducible NO-synthase and COX-2, mainly in the medial layer of the vessels as evidenced by immunochemical staining. In addition, microparticles evoke nuclear factor-kappaB activation probably through the interaction with the Fas/Fas Ligand pathway. These data provide a rationale to explain the paracrine role of microparticles as vectors of transcellular exchange of message in promoting vascular dysfunction during inflammatory diseases.

In accordance with the above data, it has been shown that microparticles from patients with other pathologies can also alter vascular smooth muscle contraction. Microparticles from preeclamptic women induce *ex vivo* vascular hyporeactivity to serotonin in human omental arteries and mouse aortas [25]. Microparticle-induced hyporeactivity is associated with increased NO production through the up-regulation of inducible NO synthase. Also, hyporeactivity evoked by preeclamptic microparticles is associated with increased 8-isoprostane production and COX-2 expression, nuclear factor-kappaB activation, and enhanced oxidative and nitrosative stresses Fig. (**1**). Interestingly, the authors show that microparticles originating most probably from leukocytes are responsible for the COX-2 vasoconstrictor component of preeclamptic microparticles, whereas those of platelet origin are mainly involved in NO release.

On the contrary, microparticles from septic patients enhance sensitivity of serotonin-evoked contraction of aortae from non-treated and lipopolysaccharide-treated mice [27]. Indeed, these authors provide evidence of the physiological relevance of septic microparticles in the regulation of vascular contraction. Surprisingly, septic microparticles enhance, but do not reduce, the sensitivity of contraction in response to serotonin without affecting endothelium-dependent vasodilation. Interestingly, septic microparticles enhance the contraction of aortas from endotoxin-treated mice, and this effect is linked neither to increased calcium entry nor to Rho kinase inhibitor–sensitive mechanisms. In addition, the effect of septic microparticles is not modified in the presence either of NO synthase inhibitor or COX-2 inhibitor, and is not associated with changes in NO or superoxide anions productions. By contrast, the nonselective COX inhibitor, indomethacin, either reduces or abolishes contraction to serotonin in aorta from mice treated with nonseptic and septic microparticles, respectively. Interestingly, the effect of septic microparticles is not linked to changes in COX-1 and COX-2 expression, but is associated both with a mechanism sensitive to the thromboxane A2 receptor antagonist, SQ-29548, and increased thromboxane A2 production. Thus, septic microparticles may, rather, be protective in counteracting the drop in peripheral resistance and progressive hypotension during severe sepsis under the experimental conditions used in this study [27]. These results may also explain the fact that increased levels of microparticles may predict a more favorable outcome in severe sepsis in terms of mortality rate and organ dysfunction [41]. Whereas the protective effects of septic micropaticles are displayed mainly by non-platelet microparticles, Pfister [35] has shown that platelet microparticles enhanced contractions in rabbit aorta and pulmonary arteries through the production of thromboxane A2.

4. MICROPARTICLES AND THE GENERATION OF NEW VESSEL NETWORKS

Another interesting aspect of microparticles is their ability to control the new creation of a network of capillaries. Several works have shown that microparticles depending on their origin and/or their concentration can favor or reduce angiogenesis (for review: [29]). For instance, microparticles generated from platelets are able to favor angiogenesis acting at the different steps that regulate this phenomenon. Thus, platelet-derived microparticles increase proliferation, migration and capillary-like structures formation in endothelial cells [16]. Regarding the mechanisms involved, these authors have shown that microparticles from platelets have pro-angiogenic effects through the activation of PI-3kinase and extracellular signal-regulated kinase (ERK) pathways. Most interestingly, Brill *et al.* [8] have reported that, in rat chronic ischemic heart, injection of platelet-derived microparticles into the myocardium increase the number of functioning capillaries, suggesting that, at least in this pathological state, microparticles from platelets may control the formation of microcirculatory vessels.

Another type of microparticles, those generated from apoptotic T lymphocytes, suppress microvessel sprouting due to a down-regulation of the VEGF receptor type 2 and an increase of the activity of NADPH oxidase and the subsequent production of reactive oxygen species [45]. As commented above, microparticles from apoptotic T lymphocytes activate pathways related to NO and reactive oxygen productions [28] suggesting that, in addition to key role of NO in angiogenesis, induction of oxidative stress by this type of microparticles may also be involved in angiogenesis impairment. In this respect, it has been shown that endothelial microparticles affect angiogenesis through the increase of superoxide anion production [24]. Indeed, endothelial microparticles, at the concentration of 10^5 microparticles/ml, decrease the formation of capillary-like structures by a mechanism sensitive to a cell-permeable superoxide dismutase mimetic, suggesting that oxidative stress play an important role in the effects of microparticles on angiogenesis independently of the type of microparticles. By contrast, at lower concentration, endothelial microparticles, through the metalloproteinase activity that they carry, promote matrix degradation and favor new vessel network formation resulting in a pro-angiogenic effect [42].

5. A NOVEL ASPECT OF MICROPARTICLES: THERAPEUTIC TOOLS

Our group has described that engineered microparticles from apoptotic/stimulated human T lymphocytes are able to improve endothelial function of conductance and small resistance vessels as well as human cultured endothelial cells [1]. These microparticles have the particularity to carry at their surface the morphogen Sonic Hedgehog [23]. Due to Sonic Hedgehog morphogen, these microparticles are able to stimulate NO production from endothelial cells by direct activation of the Sonic Hedgehog receptor and PI3-kinase pathway [1]. Most interestingly, these microparticles reverse endothelial dysfunction after myocardial ischemia/reperfusion. Studies performed using these microparticles show that they favor angiogenesis of endothelial cells, via the capillary-like formation through the activation of adhesion proteins and up-regulation of pro-angiogenic genes even if they are able to inhibit endothelial cell migration and proliferation (unpublished results). Taken together, these data suggest that microparticles harboring Sonic Hedgehog may represent a new therapeutic approach against endothelial dysfunction during acute endothelial injury. Accordingly, we suggest that engineering microparticles may be considered a new therapeutic tool in the same order that cell or gene therapies.

6. REFERENCES

[1]   Agouni A, Mostefai HA, Porro C, *et al.* Sonic hedgehog carried by microparticles corrects endothelial injury through nitric oxide release. FASEB J 2007; 21: 2735-41.

[2]   Agouni A, Lagrue-Lak-Hal AH, Ducluzeau PH, *et al.* Endothelial dysfunction caused by circulating microparticles from patients with metabolic syndrome. Am J Pathol 2008; 173: 1210-9.

[3]   Aharon A, Tamari T, Brenner B. Monocyte-derived microparticles and exosomes induce procoagulant and apoptotic effects on endothelial cells. Thromb Haemost 2008; 100: 878-85.

[4]   Amabile N, Guérin AP, Leroyer A, *et al.* Circulating endothelial microparticles are associated with vascular dysfunction in patients with end-stage renal failure. J Am Soc Nephrol 2005; 16: 3381-8.

[5]   Banfi C, Brioschi M, Wait R, *et al.* Proteome of endothelial cell-derived procoagulant microparticles. Proteomics 2005; 5: 4443-55.

[6]   Bergmeier W, Oh-Hora M, McCarl CA, Roden RC, Bray PF, Feske S. R93W mutation in Orail causes impaired calcium influx in platelets. Blood 2008. doi: blood-2008-08-174516v1.

[7]   Boulanger CM, Scoazec A, Ebrahimian T, *et al.* Circulating microparticles from patients with myocardial infarction cause endothelial dysfunction. Circulation 2001; 104: 2649-52.

[8]   Brill A, Dashevsky O, Rivo J, Gozal Y, Varon D. Platelet-derived microparticles induce angiogenesis and stimulate post-ischemic revascularization. Cardiovasc Res 2005; 67: 30-8.

[9]   Brodsky SV, Zhang F, Nasjletti A, Goligorsky MS. Endothelium-derived microparticles impair endothelial function in vitro. Am J Physiol Heart Circ Physiol 2004; 286: H1910-5.

[10]   Choi DS, Lee JM, Park GW, *et al.* Proteomic analysis of microvesicles derived from human colorectal cancer cells. J Proteome Res 2007; 6: 4646-55.

[11]   Densmore JC, Signorino PR, Ou J, *et al.* Endothelium-derived microparticles induce endothelial dysfunction and acute lung injury. Shock 2006; 26: 464-71.

[12]   Essayagh S, Brisset AC, Terrisse AD, *et al.* Microparticles from apoptotic vascular smooth muscle cells induce endothelial dysfunction, a phenomenon prevented by beta3-integrin antagonists. Trhomb Haemost 2005; 94: 853-8.

[13]   Essayagh S, Xuereb JM, Terrisse AD, Tellier-Cirioni L, Pipy B, Sié P. Microparticles from apoptotic monocytes induce transient platelet recruitment and tissue factor expression by cultured human vascular endothelial cells via a redox-sensitive mechanism. Thomb Haemost 2007; 98: 831-7.

[14]   Garcia BA, Smalley DM, Cho H, Shabanowitz J, Ley K, Hunt DF. The platelet microparticle proteome. J Proteome Res 2005; 4: 1516-21.

[15]   Hugel B, Martinez MC, Kunzelmann C, Freyssinet JM. Membrane microparticles: two sides of the coin. Physiology, 2005; 20: 22-7.

[16]   Kim HK, Song KS, Chung JH, Lee KR, Lee SN. Platelet microparticles induce angiogenesis in vitro. Br J Haematol 2004; 124: 376-84.

[17]   Klinkner DB, Densmore JC, Kaul S, *et al.* Endothelium-derived microparticles inhibit human cardiac valve endothelial cell function. Shock 2006; 25: 575-80.

[18]   Kunzelmann C, Freyssinet JM, Martínez MC. Rho A participates in the regulation of phosphatidylserine-dependent procoagulant activity at the surface of megakaryocytic cells. J Thromb Haemost 2004; 2: 644-50.

[19]   Kunzelmann-Marche C, Freyssinet JM, Martínez MC. Regulation of phosphatidylserine transbilayer redistribution by store-operated Ca2+ entry: role of actin cytoskeleton. J Biol Chem 2001; 276: 5134-9.

[20]   Liu ML, Reilly MP, Casasanto P, McKenzie SE, Williams KJ. Cholesterol enrichment of human monocyte/macrophages induces surface exposure of phosphatidylserine and the release of biologically active tissue factor-positive microvesicles. Arterioscler Thromb Vasc Biol 2007; 27: 430-5.

[21]   Martin S, Tesse A, Hugel B, *et al.* Shed membrane particles from T lymphocytes impair endothelial function and regulate endothelial protein expression. Circulation 2004; 109: 1653-9.

[22]   Martinez MC, Tesse A, Zobairi F, Andriantsitohaina R. Shed membrane microparticles from circulating and vascular cells in regulating vascular function. Am J Physiol Herat Circ Physiol 2005; 288: H1004-9.

[23]   Martinez MC, Larbret F, Zobairi F, *et al.* Transfer of differentiation signal by membrane microvesicles harboring hedgehog morphogens. Blood 2006; 108: 3012-20.

[24]   Mezentsev A, Merks RM, O'Riordan E, *et al.* Endothelial microparticles affect angiogenesis in vitro: role of oxidative stress. Am J Physiol Heart Circ Physiol 2005; 289: H1106-14.

[25]   Meziani F, Tesse A, David E, *et al.* Shed membrane particles from preeclamptic women generate vascular wall inflammation and blunt vascular contractility. Am J Pathol 2006; 169: 1473-83.

[26]   Miguet L, Pacaud K, Felden C, *et al.* Proteomic analysis of malignant lymphocyte membrane microparticles using double ionization coverage optimization. Proteomics 2006; 6: 153-71.

[27]   Mostefai HA, Meziani F, Mastronardi ML, *et al.* Circulating microparticles from patients with septic shock exert protective role in vascular function. Am J Respir Crit Care Med 2008; 178: 1148-55.

[28]   Mostefai HA, Agouni A, Carusio N, *et al.* Phosphatidylinositol 3-kinase and xanthine oxidase regulate nitric oxide and reactive oxygen species productions by apoptotic lymphocyte microparticles in endothelial cells. J Immunol 2008; 180: 5028-35.

[29]   Mostefai HA, Andriantsitohaina R, Martinez MC. Plasma membrane microparticles in angiogenesis: role in ischemic disease and in cancer. Physiol Res 2008; 57: 311-20.

[30]   Nomura S, Kanazawa S, Fukuhara S. Effects of efonidipine on platelet and monocyte activation markers in hypertension patients with and without type 2 diabetes mellitus. J Hum Hypertens 2002; 16: 539-47.

[31]   Nomura S, Shouzu A, Omoto S, Nishikawa M, Iwasaka T. Effects of losartan and simvastatin on monocyte-derived microparticles in hypertensive patients with and without type 2 diabetes mellitus. Clin Appl Thromb Hemost 2004; 10: 133-41.

[32]   Nomura S, Shouzu A, Omoto S, Nishikawa M, Iwasaka T. Long-term treatment with nifedipine modulates procoagulant marcker and C-C chemokine in hypertensive patients with type 2 diabetes mellitus. Thromb Res 2005; 115: 277-85.

[33]   Omoto S, Nomura S, Shouzu A, Nishikawa M, Fukuhara S, Iwasaka T. Detection of monocyte-derived microparticles in patients with type II diabetes mellitus. Diabetologia 2002; 45: 550-5.

[34]   Peterson DB, Sander T, Kaul S, *et al.* Comparative proteomic analysis of PAI-1 and TNF-alpha-derived endothelial microparticles. Proteomics 2008; 8: 2430-46.

[35]   Pfister SL. Role of platelet microparticles in the production of thromboxane by rabbit pulmonary artery. Hypertension 2004; 43: 428-33.

[36]   Preston RA, Jy W, Jimenez JJ, *et al.* Effects of severe hypertension on endothelial and platelet microparticles. Hypertension 2003; 41: 211-7.

[37]   Sebbagh M. Renvoizé C, Hamelin J, Riché N, Bertoglio J, Bréard J. Caspase-3-mediated cleavage of ROCK I induces MLC phosphorylation and apoptotic membrane blebbing. Nat Cell Biol 2001; 3: 346-52.

[38]   Skog J, Würdinger T, van Rijn S, *et al.* Glioblastoma microvesicles transport RNA and proteins that promote tumour growth and provide diagnostic biomarkers. Nat Cell Biol 2008; 10: 1470-6.

[39]   Smalley DM, Root KE, Cho H, Ross MM, Ley K. Proteomic discovery of 21 proteins expressed in human plasma-derived but not platelet-derived microparticles. Thromb Haemost 2007; 97: 67-80.

[40]   Smalley DM, Ley K. Plasma-derived microparticles for biomarker discovery. Clin Lab 2008; 54: 67-79.

[41]   Soriano AO, Wenche J, Chirinos JA, *et al.* Levels of endothelial and platelet microparticles and their interactions with leukocytes negatively correlate with organ dysfunction and predict mortality in severe sepsis. Crit Care Med 2005; 33: 2540-6.

[42]   Taraboletti G, D'Ascenzo S, Borsotti P. Giavazzi R, Pavan A, Dolo V. Shedding of the matrix metalloproteinases MMP-2, MMP-9, and MT1-MMP as membrane vesicle-associated components by endothelial cells. Am J Pathol 2002; 160: 673-80.

[43]   Tesse A, Martinez MC, Hugel B, *et al.* Upregulation of pro-inflammatory proteins through NF-kappaB pathway by shed membrane microparticles results in vascular hyporeactivity. Arterioscler Thromb Vasc Biol 2005; 25: 2522-7.

[44]   Werner N, Wassmann S, Ahlers P, Kosiol S, Nickenig G. Circulating CD31+/Annexin V+ apoptotic microparticles correlate with coronary endothelial function in patients with coronary artery disease. Arterioscler Thromb Vasc Biol 2006; 26: 112-6.

[45]   Yang C, Mwaikambo BR, Zhu T, *et al.* Lymphocytic microparticles inhibit angiogenesis by stimulating oxidative stress and negatively regulating VEGF-induced pathways. Am J Physiol Regul Integr Comp Physiol 2008; 294: R467-76.

CHAPTER 9

Hemorheology in Insulin Resistance

Jean-Frédéric Brun[1][*], Emmanuelle Varlet-Marie[1, 2], Ikram Aloulou[1], Mathieu Sardinoux[1], Eric Raynaud de Mauverger [1], and Jacques Mercier[1]

[1]*INSERM ERI 25 Muscle et Pathologies, Service Central de Physiologie Clinique, Centre 'Exploration et de Réadaptation des Anomalies du Métabolisme Musculaire (CERAMM), CHU Lapeyronie, 34295 Montpellier cédex 5, France email: drjfbrun@dixinet.com;*

[2]*Laboratoire de Biophysique & Bio-Analyses, Faculté de Pharmacie, Université Montpellier I, France*

Abstract: The insulin resistance syndrome is associated with hemorheologic abnormalities whose understanding is complex, since rheological properties of plasma and blood cells are to a large extent determined by the surrounding milieu: physicochemical factors, metabolism and hormones. It is thus difficult to delineate the specific role of adiposity, endothelial dysfunction, and the hormonal disturbance by its own in this complex picture. Nevertheless, low insulin sensitivity which is associated with both increased body fat and increased circulating lipids, together with impaired fibrinolysis, is characterized by a mild hyperviscosity syndrome. Those rheological alterations are more closely related to insulin resistance than to the clinical scoring of the metabolic syndrome. Low insulin sensitivity is associated with increased erythrocyte aggregability. When low insulin sensitivity is associated with hyperinsulinemia there is an increase in plasma viscosity. Among those factors, plasma viscosity appears, in multivariate analysis, to be "independently" related to insulin resistance. Moreover, plasma hyperviscosity is corrected by insulin-sensitizing procedures (such as exercise training) and is thus to some extent a marker of this disease.

1. INTRODUCTION

Biorheology is the branch of biological sciences that studies flow and deformation of biological material under the influence of the constraints which are applied to it. The branch of biorheology focusing more specifically on blood is termed hemorheology. Its purpose is therefore to study the flow of blood, in interaction with its surrounding environment, in both macro and microcirculation. One of the historical fathers of biorheology, AL Copley, used to say that hemorheology was the "missing link" among biological science, since rheological properties of blood where modified in many physiological and pathological situations, and were also likely to play a role in most body functions.

Recent physiological and pathophysiological studies have emphasized the importance of blood rheology in microcirculatory and venous hemodynamics, while large evidence emerges for an involvement of factors of blood viscosity as vascular risk factors [1, 2].

Not surprisingly, metabolic disorders are associated with hemorheologic alterations [3], so that blood reheology has been said to represent a mirror of metabolic status [3].

2. SOME FUNDAMENTAL CONCEPTS IN HEMORHEOLOGY

When blood circulates through vessels, its flow is driven by a pressure gradient between heart and periphery, and results in a force of friction over the surface of endothelium. This force results in a shear stress τ applied on the vessel wall. Due to forces of cohesion between the wall and blood and within blood itself, the velocity of blood flow is lower in the vicinity of the endothelial surface than in the middle of the vessel, thus defining the *shear rate* $\dot{\gamma}$. This difference in velocity reflects an intrinsic resistance to flow which is termed *apparent blood viscosity* $\eta = \tau / \dot{\gamma}$.

Blood viscosity η is well described by a classical robust model, Quemada's equation [4].

$$\eta = \eta_P (1 - 1/2 \, \mathbf{k} \, \phi)^{-2}$$

where ϕ is hematocrit, η_p is plasma viscosity, and $k(\dot\gamma)$ is a shear-dependent parameter quantifying the contribution of erythrocyte rheological properties to whole blood viscosity. At high shear rate $k(\dot\gamma)$ is representative of red cell rigidity (ie, the lower $k(\dot\gamma)$, the higher is erythrocyte deformability), while at low shear rate $k(\dot\gamma)$ which tends to a maximum k_0 that is proportional to the ability to form erythrocyte aggregates (red cell aggregability).

It is beyond the scope of this review to describe the physiology of these different parameters, but the important point for our purpose is that Quemada's equation states that blood viscosity actually relies on 3 factors:
- plasma viscosity η_p, explained by plasma content in proteins;
- hematocrit ϕ, which may rapidly vary according to the area of the circulation and the physiological condition,
- red cell deformability and aggregability, which, as mentioned above, are influenced by metabolism and hormones [3] have also a marked circulatory influence in the microcirculatory bed that is beyond its physical effects on whole blood viscosity [5-6].

Therefore, our review will focus on individual factors of viscosity (η_p, , ϕ, red cell deformability and aggregability) considered separately rather than η alone.

In fact, the traditional picture of circulatory physiology provided by Hagen-Poiseuille's law involves blood viscosity as a factor of peripheral resistance that might hamper blood flow if it were not easily overcome by vasomodilation. This equation can be written as follows :

$$Q = (\pi \cdot R^4 \cdot \Delta P) / (8 \cdot \eta_e \cdot L)$$

Where Q is the suspension volumetric flow rate through a tube of radius R under a pressure difference ΔP over the vessel length L; η_e is an effective viscosity - i.e. the ratio of shear stress to shear rate with shear stress corresponding to the force that moves the fluid layers or laminae and shear rate corresponding to the velocity gradient in the fluid. As discussed below, terms of this equation can be re-arranged in order to describe a theoretical effect of viscosity on O_2 supply to tissues. Actually, this simplistic picture of circulation is not relevant to in vivo reality, and modern investigators like Holger Schmid-Schönbein have proposed more complex models in which the effect of blood viscosity is markedly more important, as developed below [7].

3. CORRELATIONS BETWEEN INSULIN SENSITIVITY AND HEMORHEOLOGY

Relationship between insulin sensitivity (SI) and rheology have been reported since 1994, by our team [8-9] and others [10]. Moan [10] performed a stepwise regression analysis in 21 young men (mean age = 21) and found two explanatory variables related to the glucose disposal rate: body mass index (even within a normal range), and whole blood viscosity. In this study only whole-blood viscosity and body mass index were independent explanatory variables of the glucose disposal rate. Together they accounted for 63% of the variability in the glucose disposal rate in the study subjects, suggesting that hemorheologic, and therefore indirectly hemodynamic, factors were correlates to insulin sensitivity.

In 22 nondiabetic women (20-54 years) presenting a wide range of body mass index (from 20 to 48 kg/m²), we assessed insulin sensitivity with the minimal model procedure, over a 180 min intravenous glucose tolerance test with frequent sampling. The insulin sensitivity index SI (i.e. the slope of the dose-response relationship between insulin increased above baseline and glucose disposal) ranges between 0.1 and 20.1 x 10(-4) min-1/microU/ml) i.e all the range of insulin sensitivity. SI was negatively correlated with blood viscosity (r = -0.530 p < 0.02), body mass index (r = 0.563 p < 0.01) and baseline insulinemia (r = 0.489 p < 0.05). These correlations were independent of each other and were not explained by relationships between insulin sensitivity and fibrinogen or blood lipids. Thus, we concluded that blood fluidity was correlated with insulin sensitivity when it is measured with an accurate technique, suggesting that blood hyperviscosity is a symptom of insulin resistance that might be involved in the cardiovascular risk of this syndrome.

Further works by Høieggen [11-12] confirmed these earlier findings. These authors measured whole blood viscosity in 105 healthy blood donors and found that it correlated with systolic blood pressure, cholesterol, cholesterol/HDL cholesterol ratio, triglycerides, body mass index and waist-hip ratio.

Interestingly, subjects with systolic blood pressure > 130 mmHg had higher whole blood viscosity than those with lower blood pressure [11].

In another study in healthy young men they performed a hyperinsulinemic isoglycemic glucose clamp, and found statistically significant negative correlations between glucose disposal rate and whole-blood viscosity. Both insulin sensitivity and blood viscosity exhibited strong correlations with lipid parameters (serum triglyceride, total cholesterol, cholesterol subfractions.

All these studies provide consistent results and demonstrate that insulin sensitivity, measured with the two better recognized procedures, is negatively correlated to whole blood viscosity, so that the more a patient is insulin resistant, the higher is his viscosity.

However, whole blood viscosity is an in vitro measurement that is not by itself relevant to in vivo hemodynamics. It should be analyzed as indicated above in terms of hematocrit, plasma viscosity, red cell deformability and red cell aggregation. These correlations cannot demonstrate any pathophysiological relationship, and have the only interest to point out an overall tendency to worsen blood rheology when insulin sensitivity decreases.

4. WHICH FACTOR OF VISCOSITY?

The next step in these investigations was thus to determine which factor of blood viscosity is mostly impaired in insulin resistant subjects. For this purpose we investigated 108 nondiabetic subjects the relationships between insulin sensitivity measured with the minimal model and factors of blood viscosity: hematocrit, plasma viscosity, red cell deformability and red cell aggregation [13]. Across quartiles of insulin sensitivity (defined after log transformation since distribution of insulin sensitivity was not normal), hematocrit and red cell rigidity remained stable, while aggregability and plasma viscosity (η_p) increased in the lowest quartile. insulin sensitivity appeared to be correlated to only two rheological parameters: η_p and Myrenne index of red cell aggregability M1. Among SI, fasting insulin, age and BMI multivariate analysis selected only BMI as a determinant of either whole blood viscosity, and erythrocyte disaggregation threshold, only fasting insulin as determinant of M1, and a combination of BMI (p=0.009) and insulin sensitivity (p=0.007) for η_p .

Thus, although age and obesity are factors of hyperviscosity, the hemorheological disturbances found in insulin resistance are not fully statistically "explained" by those two factors. While hyperaggregability (measured with M1) is rather related to hyperinsulinism, η_p is influenced by SI.

Therefore η_p was the hemorheological parameter that in a population of nondiabetic subjects was the more closely related to insulin-resistance, although other viscosity factors may also be modified in patients exhibiting low values of insulin sensitivity [13].

On the basis of this finding we suggested that η_p may be a simple marker for the follow up of insulin-resistant states [13].

5. INSULIN RESISTANCE OR METABOLIC SYNDROME?

What makes a little confusing the issue of "Metabolic syndrome", "Insulin resistance syndrome" and "Syndrome X", is that there are three possibilities to define it: on the basis of a measurement of insulin sensitivity, on the basis of a surrogate of insulin sensitivity, or on the basis of a purely clinical classification that does no longer take into account the insulin and insulin sensitivity status. Clearly, these three approaches do not select the same patients [14]. Initially, G. Reaven [15] defined an "insulin resistance syndrome" as a cluster of abnormalities responsible of higher cardiovascular risk. However, further definition of the 'Metabolic Syndrome', although they aimed at refer to the same clinical entity, did no longer mention insulin resistance in the criteria [16, 17] and it became rapidly obvious that this later approach did not select only insulin resistant patients, while some insulin resistant patients were not classified as suffering from the metabolic syndrome. Despite the simplicity of use of the new definition, some leading authors still insisted on the fact that insulin resistance is really the core of a cluster of deleterious abnormalities. A defect in insulin action associated with a compensatory increase in insulin secretion, and therefore hyperinsulinemia, results in impaired glucose tolerance or type 2 diabetes, obesity, dyslipidemia, coronary artery disease and hypertension [18, 19]. Therefore, insulin resistance and metabolic syndrome are two distinct, although closely related, concepts.

We tried to delineate the combined effects of obesity, insulin resistance, and hyperinsulinemia in 157 nondiabetic subjects divided in 6 groups according to BMI (cut-off point 25 kg/m²) and insulin sensitivity measured with the minimal model and divided into quartiles (lowest quartile, highest quartile, and the two middle quartiles put together). Thus, we investigated the effect of varying levels of insulin sensitivity with or without obesity. Results showed that both obesity and insulin resistance impair blood rheology by inducing alterations in on red cell rigidity and plasma viscosity. Whole blood viscosity at high shear rate reflects rather obesity than insulin resistance. In this sample erythrocyte aggregation seemed to be rather a marker of hyperinsulinemia [20].

In another study, we classified a sample of 90 subjects into 4 subgroups according to the clinical score "NCEP-ATPIII" of metabolic syndrome. Results show no significant changes of blood rheology across classes of NCEP score despite a borderline rank correlation between erythrocyte aggregability and the score. This study thus suggested that the hyperviscosity syndrome of the metabolic syndrome is not proportional to its clinical scoring. By contrast we found the classical correlations between blood viscosity and blood lipid profile, suggesting that the individual items of the syndrome are better correlates of blood rheology than its clinical scoring [21]. This applies at least to the NCEP-ATPIII definition [16], since we are not aware of a similar study using the IDF definition [17]. Some degree of discrepancy exists between these two definitions, so that this needs to be studied also with the IDF definition.

At this stage of the investigation, it thus appeared that the factors of blood viscosity are correlated to insulin resistance but not to the score of the metabolic syndrome, consistent with the discrepancy between the two concepts that was pointed out by several authors [14, 18]. All this can be summarized by the statement that **blood rheology is likely to be a marker of insulin resistance rather than a marker of the metabolic syndrome.** Obviously, lipid abnormalities that directly influence erythrocyte rheology [3] play a major role in this story, as does obesity.

6. INSULIN RESISTANCE OR HYPERINSULINEMIA?

Even more, there is another confusing issue due to the fact that insulin resistance is associated with a compensatory increase in insulin secretion, and thus hyperinsulinemia, due to the physiological feedback loop between insulin sensitivity and insulin secretion pointed out by the team of RN Bergman [22-23]. This physiological relationship underlies the validity of 'surrogates of insulin sensitivity' that have been developed in order to easily measure insulin resistance without performing a dynamic test [24]. Actually indices based on fasting insulin have been demonstrated to correctly fit with insulin sensitivity measurements in some situations like polycystic ovary syndrome or nondiabetic obesity, suggesting that they really could help to evaluate insulin sensitivity over a wide range of clinical situations. However, there are clearly situations of complete discrepancy between insulin sensitivity and indices based on insulin, such as trained athletes, reactive hypoglycemia, and diabetes, so that the general use of insulin as a mirror of insulin sensitivity should not be recommended outside of conditions where its validity has been well demonstrated [25]. However, although hyperinsulinemia and insulin resistance are reciprocally related to one another, the association is not constant [26]. Therefore, some studies showing relationships between insulin resistance and other parameters, when they use these surrogates rather than a dynamic measurement of insulin sensitivity, actually reflect a relationship of these parameters with hyperinsulinemia.

Recently, Ferrannini and Balkau [26] investigated the issue of the separate effect of insulin sensitivity and insulinemia on the database of the European Group for the study of Insulin Resistance (EGIR). Using clamp-derived insulin sensitivity and fasting plasma insulin concentrations available in 1308 non-diabetic subjects with a wide range of age and body mass index, they were able to define three situations. In this cohort, 40% of the whole population had insulin resistance and/or hyperinsulinemia. In this subgroup 60% of subjects had the two abnormalities, but there were subjects with insulin resistance but without hyperinsulinemia and others with hyperinsulinemia but without insulin resistance. Their clinical phenotypes were slightly different. Subjects with 'pure' insulin resistance had a more central fat distribution and presented evidence of excessive lipolysis and endogenous glucose production. Subjects with 'pure' hyperinsulinemia had suppressed lipolysis, endogenous glucose production and insulin clearance, higher values of systolic blood pressure and lower values of serum HDL-cholesterol concentrations. The only abnormality common to both phenotypes was the presence of raised serum triglycerides concentrations. This study supported the idea of three different subgroups of individuals in a non-diabetic population, and suggested that hyperinsulinemia and insulin resistance carry distinct pathogenic potential in terms of the components of the insulin resistance syndrome [26].

Actually, this classification of patients can be criticized and considered rather as a sequence of steps than separate phenotypes (RN Bergman, personal communication). According to Bergman's 'portal hypothesis' of insulin resistance [27-28], the natural history of this syndrome can involve a first stage of purely hepatic insulin resistance with compensatory hyperinsulinism (ie the phenotype of 'pure' hyperinsulinemia), followed by a generalized insulin resistance with compensatory hyperinsulinism (the phenotype of insulin resistance plus hyperinsulinemia), and then due to beta-cell progressive failure, a situation of 'pure' insulin resistance, in which insulin resistance is no longer compensated by hyperinsulinemia.

Notwithstanding, this leaded us to investigate the same issue for blood rheology, ie, are they different pictures according to the insulin status ('pure' hyperinsulinemia, 'pure' insulin resistance, insulin resistance plus hyperinsulinemia) [29]. In this study we aimed at defining the specific hemorheologic profile of insulin resistance and hyperinsulinemia by separating a sample of 81 subjects into 4 subgroups according to quartiles of insulin sensitivity (SI) (measured with the minimal model) and baseline insulin. Results show that (1) values of insulin sensitivity within the upper quartile are associated with low blood viscosity and plasma viscosity; (2) that low insulin sensitivity regardless insulinemia is associated with increased erythrocyte aggregation indexes; (3) that when low insulin sensitivity is associated with hyperinsulinemia (insulin the upper quartile and insulin sensitivity in the lower) there is a further increase in blood viscosity due to an increase in plasma viscosity. Interestingly, hematocrit was not related to insulin sensitivity or insulinemia.

This study, consistent with the classification proposed by Ferranini and Balkau, shows thus that hyperinsulinemia and insulin resistance induce hyperviscosity syndromes which are somewhat different, although they are associated most of the time. Low insulin sensitivity increased red cell aggregation while hyperinsulinemia increases plasma viscosity.

It should be emphasized that this picture [29] was somewhat different from our first findings where plasma viscosity appeared to be the factor of blood viscosity that was the most specifically related to insulin resistance [13]. The reason for this discrepancy in studies performed on similar samples performed with the same methods of measurement of insulin, insulin sensitivity and blood rheology is unclear.

7. FIBRINOGEN AND INSULIN SENSITIVITY

Since fibrinogen is a major determinant of blood theology, we also studied the relationships between insulin sensitivity and plasma fibrinogen. We found that there was a fair negative correlation between insulin sensitivity and plasma fibrinogen. Using partial correlation analysis, the negative relation between insulin sensitivity and fibrinogen was maintained independently from the body mass index [30-32].

8. IMPROVING INSULIN SENSITIVITY AND BLOOD RHEOLOGY

Since exercise is one of the key treatments of the metabolic syndrome [33] and is a major insulin sensitizer [34], and in addition is one of the stronger available tools for improving blood rheology [35-37] we studied the specific effect of endurance training on the hemorheological aspects of the metabolic syndrome [38-39].

The training procedure employed in this work requires some comments. It was based on Brooks and Mercier's "crossover concept" [40] and thus on the notion of a power intensity that elicits a maximal rate of lipid oxidation (LIPOXmax) that can be determined with graded exercise calorimetry [41]. Exercise is targeted at this level, resulting in a selective improvement in the ability to oxidize fats at exercise [42]. Interestingly, the ability to oxidize lipids at exercise seems to be associated with lower blood viscosity and thus a favorable hemorheologic profile [43]. Correlations found between erythrocyte deformability and the ability to oxidize at exercise more lipids may be due to effects of endurance training on lipid oxidation which may in turn modify both lipid metabolism and free radical generation, thus influencing erythrocyte rheology [43].

A first study was performed on thirty-two obese insulin resistant subjects that were tested before and after 2 months. Twenty-one of them were trained (3x45 min/wk) at the LIPOXmax and eleven served as controls. Blood rheology was unchanged in the control group while training markedly improved plasma viscosity whose mean values decrease from 1.43 mPa.s down to 1.35 mPa.s. There was no change in either hematocrit red cell rigidity or red cell aggregation. Besides, training improved body composition with a mean weight loss of 2.5 kg that was totally explained by a loss in fat mass (-2.7 kg) while fat free mass remained unchanged, and the balance of substrates oxidation shifted towards a higher use of lipids.

Relationship among these variuos exercise-induced alterations were investigated in a second study that employed the same training protocol in 24 patients, all submitted to training [39]. This study showed that variations of whole blood viscosity at high shear rate were explained by two statistically independent determirants: hematocrit and red cell rigidity. Whole blood viscosity decreased in 16 subjects, but increased in 8, due to a rise in hematocrit. Changes in erythrocyte rigidity appeared to reflect weight loss and decrease in LDL cholesterol. Plasma viscosity was related to cholesterol and its training-induced changes are related to those of the maximal aerobic capacity $VO_{2\ max}$, but not to lipid oxidation. Red cell aggregability reflected both the circulating lipids (Cholesterol and its fractions HDL and LDL) and the ability to oxidize lipids at exercise. Factors associated to a post-training decrease in erythrocyte aggregab:lity were weight loss and more precisely decrease in fat mass, improvement in lipid oxidation, rise in HDL-Cholesterol, and decrease in fibrinogen. On the whole the major determinant of hemorheologic improvement was an increase in cardiorespiratory fitness ($VO_{2\ max}$), correlated with a decrease in plasma viscosity, rather than an improvement in lipid metabolism, although erythrocyte aggregability and deformability exhibited clear relationships with lipid metabolism. For wh:ch reason hematocrit increased in 30% of the patients during this kind of training remains unclear at present.

These two studies show that, consistent with observations in athletes, the metabolic and ergometric improvements induced by training reduces plasma viscosity in sedentary, insulin resistant patients, i.e. the parameter that appeared in our first studies to be more related to insulin resistance itself. Plasma viscosity appears to mirror metabolic disturbances, since it is correlated to cholesterol levels. Its training-induced changes are related to those of the maximal aerobic capacity $VO_{2\ max}$, but not to lipid oxidation. Lipid ox:dation seems to be rather related to erythrocyte rheology. Besides, at those low levels training the response in hematocrit that reflects a beneficial phenomenon of "autohemodilution" [35-37] is not evidenced. Probably a longer period or a stronger training intensity is required to observe these classical hematocrit changes.

Another approach of the impact of therapeutic of insulin resistance on blood rheology is shown by Aksnes [43] who compared the effect of vasodilating agents on levels whole blood viscosity in the same 21 hypertensive patients with cardiovascular risk factors. Patients were randomized double-blindly to additional treatment with amlodipine 5 mg or losartan 100 mg and after 8 weeks of treatment, all patients were crossed over to the opposite treatment regimen for another 8 weeks. Although no significant differences in whole blood viscosity and blood pressure were observed between the 2 treatment regimens, a consistent trend toward lower viscosity was found at all shear rates as vasodilatory treatment was intensified (baseline to amlodipine 5 mg to amlodipine 10 mg to losartan 100 mg + amlodipine 5 mg). The author hypothesized that whole blood viscosity changes could explain improved insulin sensitivity seen on AT1-receptor blockade.

9. CONCLUSIONS: EGG OR CHICKEN?

At present there is no information to discuss whether hemorheology is by itself a factor governing insulin sensitivity, due to vascular effects, according to A. Baron's findings that insulin is an important muscular vasodilator [44] and that a decrease in its action in the vascular bed accounts for a significant part of glucose disposal impairment in insulin resistance. Such a mechanism has been hypothesized [43] and cannot be ruled out. However, the bulk of studies presented here shows that metabolic alterations found in the metabolic syndrome and more or less associated with insulin resistance are potent modifyers of blood rheology, while the correlations between insulin resistance itself are less elusive. Since the lipid discrders typically associated with the metabolic syndrome are unequivocally able to impair by their own blood rheology, we believe that the most obvious conclusions that can be drawn from these studies is that the metabolc disturbances associated to lowered insulin sensitivity and/or hyperinsulinemia result in hemorheologic disturbances. Whether those hemorheologic disturbances are in turn able to impair insulin sensitivity via vascular effects is an attractive hypothesis but, as far as we know, poorly supported until now by the literature.

10. REFERENCES

[1]   Tzoulaki I, Murray GD, Lee AJ, Rumley A, Lowe GD, Fowkes FG. Inflammatory, haemostatic, and rheological markers for incident peripheral arterial disease: Edinburgh Artery Study. Eur Heart J. 2007;28(3): 354-62.

[2]   Lowe GD. Virchow's triad revisited: abnormal flow. Pathophysiol Haemost Thromb. 2003; 33(5-6): 455-7.

[3]   Brun JF. Hormones, metabolism and body composition as major determinants of blood rheology: potential pathophysiological meaning. Clin Hemorheol Microcirc. 2002; 26(2):63-79.

[4]   Quemada D. Rheology of concentrated disperse systems. II. A model of non newtonian shear viscosity in steady flows. Rheol Acta 1978; 17 : 632-642

[5]   Baskurt OK, Meiselman HJ.Blood rheology and hemodynamics. Semin Thromb Hemost. 2003; 29(5): 435-50.

[6]   Baskurt OK.In vivo correlates of altered blood rheology. Biorheology. 2008;45(6):629-38.

[7]   Gaudard A, Varlet-Marie E, Bressolle F, Mercier J, Brun JF. Hemorheological correlates of fitness and unfitness in athletes: moving beyond the apparent "paradox of hematocrit"? Clin Hemorheol Microcirc. 2003;28(3):161-73.

[8]   Brun JF Brun, C Dupuy-Fons, JF Monnier, JP Micallef, D Bouix, C Peyreigne and A Orsetti. Blood viscosity is negatively correlated to insulin sensitivity. Biorheology 32 (1995), 387-388

[9]   Brun JF, Monnier JF, Kabbaj H, Orsetti A. La viscosité sanguine est corrélée à l'insulino-résistance. J Mal Vasc (Paris) 21 (1996), 171-174.

[10]   Moan, G. Nordby, I. Os, K.I. Birkeland and S.E. Kjeldsen, Relationship between hemorrheologic factors and insulin sensitivity in healthy young men, Metabolism 1994; 43: 423-427.

[11]   Fossum E, Høieggen A, Moan A, Nordby G, Velund TL, Kjeldsen SE. Whole blood viscosity, blood pressure and cardiovascular risk factors in healthy blood donors. Blood Press. 1997 ; 6(3): 161-5.

[12]   Høieggen A, Fossum E, Moan A, Enger E, Kjeldsen SE. Whole-blood viscosity and the insulin-resistance syndrome. J Hypertens. 1998; 16(2):203-10.

[13]   Perez-Martin A, Dumortier M, Pierrisnard E, Raynaud E, Mercier J, Brun JF. Multivariate analysis of relationships between insulin sensitivity and blood rheology: is plasma viscosity a marker of insulin resistance? Clin Hemorheol Microcirc. 2001;25(3-4): 91-103.

[14]   Reaven G. The metabolic syndrome or the insulin resistance syndrome? Different names, different concepts, and different goals. Endocrinol Metab Clin North Am. 2004; 33(2):283-303

[15]   Reaven GM. Banting lecture 1988. Role of insulin resistance in human disease. Diabetes. 1988; 37(12): 1595-607.

[16]   Executive summary of the third report of the National Cholesterol Education Program (NCEP) Expert Panel on Detection, Evaluation, And Treatment of High Blood Cholesterol in Adults (Adult Treatment Panel III). JAMA 2001; 285:2486-2497.

[17]   Alberti, KG, Zimmet P, Shaw J. The metabolic syndrome—a new worldwide definition, Lancet 366 (9491) (2005), pp. 1059–1062

[18]   Reaven G. Why a cluster is truly a cluster: insulin resistance and cardiovascular disease. Clin Chem. 2008; 54(5): 785-7

[19]   Kashyap SR, Defronzo RA.The insulin resistance syndrome: physiological considerations. Diab Vasc Dis Res. 2007; 4(1): 13-9.

[20]   Brun JF, Aloulou I, Varlet-Marie E. Hemorheological aspects of the metabolic syndrome: markers of insulin resistance, obesity or hyperinsulinemia? Clin Hemorheol Microcirc. 2004;30(3-4):203-9

[21]   Aloulou I, Varlet-Marie E, Mercier J, Brun JF. Hemorheological disturbances correlate with the lipid profile but not with the NCEP-ATPIII score of the metabolic syndrome. Clin Hemorheol Microcirc. 2006;35(1-2):207-12.

[22]   Kahn SE, Prigeon RL, McCulloch DK, Boyko EJ, Bergman RN, Schwartz MW, Neifing JL, Ward WK, Beard JC, Palmer JP, et al.Quantification of the relationship between insulin sensitivity and beta-cell function in human subjects. Evidence for a hyperbolic function.Diabetes. 1993; 42(11):1663-72.

[23]   Bergman RN. Pathogenesis and prediction of diabetes mellitus: lessons from integrative physiology. Mt Sinai J Med. 2002; 69(5):280-90.

[24]   Wallace TM, Levy JC, Matthews DR.Use and abuse of HOMA modeling. Diabetes Care. 2004; 27(6): 1487-95

[25]   Brun JF, Raynaud E, Mercier J. Homeostasis model assessment and related simplified evaluations of insulin sensitivity from fasting insulin and glucose. Diabetes Care. 2000; 23(7):1037-8

[26]   Ferrannini E, Balkau B. Insulin: in search of a syndrome. Diabet Med. 2002;19(9):724-9.

[27]   Bergman RN and Ader M. Free fatty acids and pathogenesis of type 2 diabetes mellitus. Trends Endocrinol Metab 11: 351–356, 2000

[28]   Kabir M, Catalano KJ, Ananthnarayan S, Kim SP, Van Citters GW, Dea MK, Bergman RN. Molecular evidence supporting the portal theory: a causative link between visceral adiposity and hepatic insulin resistance. Am J Physiol Endocrinol Metab. 2005; 288(2):E454-61.

[29]   Aloulou I, Varlet-Marie E, Mercier J, Brun JF. The hemorheological aspects of the metabolic syndrome are a combination of separate effects of insulin resistance, hyperinsulinemia and adiposity. Clin Hemorheol Microcirc. 2006; 35(1-2):113-9.

[30]   Worth H. Comparison of hydrofluoroalkane-beclomethasone dipropionate autohaler with budesonide Turbuhaler in asthma con-trol. Respiration 2001; 68: 517-26.

[31]   Raynaud E, Brun JF, Perez-Martin A, Orsetti A, Solère M. Negative correlation between plasma fibrinogen and insulin sensitivity measured with the minimal model technique. Clin Hemorheol Microcirc. 1998 ; 18(4): 323-30.

[32]   Raynaud E, Brun JF, Perez-Martin A, Mercier J. Association between fibrinogen levels and insulin resistance. Diabetes Care. 1998; 21(11): 2040-1

[33] Raynaud E, Pérez-Martin A, Brun JF, Aissa Benhaddad A, Fédou C, Mercier J. Relationships between fibrinogen and insulin resistance. Atherosclerosis 2000; 150 (2): 365-370

[34] Dumortier M, Brandou F, Perez-Martin A, Fedou C, Mercier J, Brun JF. Low intensity endurance exercise targeted for lipid oxidation improves body composition and insulin sensitivity in patients with the metabolic syndrome. Diabetes Metab. 2003; 29(5):509-18.

[35] Manetta J, Brun JF, Maimoun L, Callis A, Préfaut C, Mercier J. Effect of training on the GH/IGF-I axis during exercise in middle-aged men: relationship to glucose homeostasis. Am J Physiol Endocrinol Metab. 2002; 283(5):E929-36.

[36] Brun JF, Khaled S, Raynaud E, Bouix D, Micallef JP, Orsetti A.The triphasic effects of exercise on blood rheology: which relevance to physiology and pathophysiology? Clin Hemorheol Microcirc. 1998; 19: 89-104

[37] Brun JF. Exercise hemorheology as a three acts play with metabolic actors: is it of clinical relevance? Clin Hemorheol Microcirc. 2002;26(3):155-74.

[38] Brun JF, Bouchahda C, Chaze D, Benhaddad AA, Micallef JP, Mercier J. The paradox of hematocrit in exercise physiology: which is the "normal" range from an hemorheologist's viewpoint? Clin Hemorheol Microcirc. 2000; 22(4):287-303.

[39] Dumortier M, Pérez-Martin A, Pierrisnard E, Mercier J, Brun JF. Regular exercise (3x45 min/wk) decreases plasma viscosity in sedentary obese, insulin resistant patients parallel to an improvement in fitness and a shift in substrate oxidation balance. Clin Hemorheol Microcirc. 2002;26(4):219-29.

[40] Aloulou I, Varlet-Marie E, Mercier J, Brun JF.Hemorheologic effects of low intensity endurance training in sedentary patients suffering from the metabolic syndrome. Clin Hemorheol Microcirc. 2006; 35(1-2):333-9.

[41] Brooks GA, Mercier J. Balance of carbohydrate and lipid utilization during exercise: the "crossover" concept. J Appl Physiol. 1994; 76(6): 2253-61

[42] Brun JF, Jean E, Ghanassia E, Flavier S, Mercier J.Metabolic training: new paradigms of exercise training for metabolic diseases with exercise calorimetry targeting individuals. Ann Readapt Med Phys. 2007; 50(6): 528-34

[43] Brun JF, Varlet-Marie E, Cassan D, Manetta J, Mercier J. Blood fluidity is related to the ability to oxidize lipids at exercise. Clin Hemorheol Microcirc. 2004; 30(3-4): 339-43.

[44] Aksnes TA, Seljeflot I, Torjesen PA, Höieggen A, Moan A, Kjeldsen SE. Improved insulin sensitivity by the angiotensin II-receptor blocker losartan is not explained by adipokines, inflammatory markers, or whole blood viscosity. Metabolism. 2007; 56(11): 1470-7.

[45] Baron AD. Hemodynamic actions of insulin. Am J Physiol. 1994 ; 267(2 Pt 1): E187-202.

Microcirculation and Insulin Resistance, 2009, 107-118

Post-Myocardial Infarction Insulin Resistance: A Sentinel Role for the Muscle Microcirculation

David C. Poole and Timothy I. Musch

Departments of Kinesiology, Anatomy and Physiology Kansas State University, Manhattan, Kansas 66506

Address correspondence to: David C. Poole; Department of Anatomy and Physiology, Kansas State University, Manhattan, Kansas 66506; E-mail: poole@vet.ksu.edu

Abstract: Patients who have suffered a myocardial infarction (MI) and live with chronic heart failure (CHF) exhibit a substantial reduction in peripheral insulin sensitivity and increase their risk for developing diabetes by several-fold. To establish the putative role for post-myocardial infarction (MI) microcirculatory dysfunction in insulin resistance several questions must be addressed. Paramount amongst these are: 1. What are the microcirculatory hemodynamic characteristics in healthy resting muscle? 2. How are these impacted in post-infarction CHF? 3. Can current models of blood-tissue substrate delivery/exchange support a role for CHF-induced functional alterations in insulin resistance? This brief review considers that skeletal muscle, in part because of its great mass, prodigious capillarity and metabolic plasticity, constitutes a primary organ in body glucose homeostasis. The myriad changes in arteriolar vasoregulation post-MI, whilst certainly important with respect to the control of bulk muscle blood flow and its distribution, will not be addressed in depth herein. Rather, the questions posed above will be focussed within the context of recent novel observations at the capillary level i.e., at the primary site of blood-muscle exchange. These observations challenge the dogma that, in resting muscle, most capillaries are not recruited at rest which, if correct, would restrict their participation in glucose uptake and homeostasis. This is a crucial issue because direct observations suggest that, in healthy muscle, most capillaries do support continuous red blood cell (RBC) flux. In contrast, in post-MI CHF, a substantial proportion of skeletal muscle capillaries cease to support RBC flux both at rest and during contractions and it is likely that this constitutes a sentinel event in insulin resistance. Development and optimization of treatment strategies designed to ameliorate insulin resistance and halt or reverse the progression towards overt diabetes in CHF patients are dependent upon resolving these issues.

1. INTRODUCTION

In humans skeletal muscle constitutes 30-40% of body mass and is estimated to contain some nine to ten billion capillaries. These capillaries form a dense, tortuous, interconnected network possessing a total length of 10,000 kilometers and a surface area approaching two hundred square meters. Access of substrates such as oxygen and blood glucose as well as insulin to muscle tissue and individual muscle fibers depends on the blood flow and the distribution of that flow within and among the capillaries. Textbook values for total skeletal muscle blood flow at rest approximate 1 L/min (20% cardiac outputs) which can increase up to 80-90% of a cardiac output of 30 L/min during maximal exercise [e.g., 1].

Given that, at rest, skeletal muscle has access essentially to the entire blood volume every 5 min or so (and every 10 s during intense exercise) it is ideally placed to play a major role in regulating blood glucose homeostasis. Moreover, because blood glucose and muscle glycogen constitute important energy sources at rest and particularly during intense exercise, there is the opportunity for skeletal muscle to correct deficits of glucose regulation caused by, for example, pancreatic dysfunction. By the same token, if the normal access of glucose and insulin to exchange vessels is compromised, for example by the cessation of blood flow in a substantial portion of the post-MI muscle capillary bed, it is possible that this causes or contributes to the increased insulin resistance and incidence of diabetes in CHF patients [2,3 rev. 4].

Unfortunately, our knowledge of skeletal muscle capillary function has been hampered by the challenges of observing capillary hemodynamics *in vivo* and a rigid adherence to possibly erroneous

Nicolas Wiernsperger (Ed.)

models and principles first conceived nearly a hundred years ago [rev. 5]. This paper argues strongly for examining the compelling weight of evidence which supports that most capillaries in healthy skeletal muscle can, and do, support RBC and plasma flow at rest and thus blood glucose has access to the prodigious capillary surface area, and thus exchange capacity, of skeletal muscle. Against this backdrop, pathophysiological sequelae to MI - such as a reduction in total capillary numbers and importantly the proportion of these capillaries supporting RBC and plasma flow [6, 7] – are examined with respect to their putative link to insulin resistance.

2. MICROCIRCULATORY HEMODYNAMIC CHARACTERISTICS OF HEALTHY MUSCLE

2.1 The 'Classical View'

In the early 20th Century the extraordinary physiologist and Nobel laureate August Krogh performed high-pressure India ink infusions of the microvasculature in resting and contracted skeletal muscles [8]. Based on the absence of India ink in many capillaries at rest and its presence in many more capillaries following contractions, he concluded that the majority of capillaries were not flowing at rest and that these capillaries were then recruited (i.e., initiated perfusion) during contractions. These observations were central to the development of Krogh's theoretical O_2 diffusion model which presupposed that the partial pressure of O_2 (PO_2) within muscle fell systematically with increasing distance from the capillary. This notion predicted that those mitochondria furthest from a RBC-flowing capillary would see the lowest PO_2 and be most prone to anoxia under conditions of lowered muscle O_2 delivery or increased metabolic rate. It is pertinent that, in the last two decades, analyses of contracting intramyocyte PO_2 by cryomicrospectrophotometry in canine muscle [9] and magnetic resonance spectroscopy in human muscle [10] have not found evidence for intramyocyte O_2 gradients. Rather, the low and uniform intramyocyte PO_2 suggests that intramyocyte O_2 transport is not limited by diffusion distances *per se* which brings into question the necessity for reducing such distances – via capillary 'recruitment' - as metabolic rate increases during contractions.

Krogh himself recognized that his India ink perfusion technique had major flaws. Specifically, the India ink particles clumped together which was more likely to prevent complete perfusion of the capillary bed at rest than during exercise. This would give the erroneous conclusion that more capillaries are flowing during/following muscle contractions. Moreover, the perfusions themselves were made at very high pressure likely to cause substantial tissue edema and structural damage. One wonders whether these latter considerations were responsible for Krogh, on occasion, calculating O_2 diffusion distances in resting muscle based on the presumption that all capillaries supported RBC flux. Despite Krogh's misgivings regarding his techniques and subsequent technological advances that enable demonstration of RBC flux in the majority of capillaries in resting muscle (see *"An Alternative Contemporary Perspective"* below), Krogh's studies are still cited as state-of-the art by researchers invoking capillary 'recruitment' as an explanation for their findings [rev. 5,11].

In the contemporary literature a plethora of publications, most of which have not observed capillaries *in vivo*, consider that in resting muscle most, or at least, many, capillaries do not support RBC and plasma flux [rev. 5,11,12]. Each particular study which invokes the capillary 'recruitment' hypothesis deserves consideration on its own merit. When this is done it is possible to explain the findings, of many capillaries at rest that do not support RBC flux, by one of the following: 1. Resting muscle PO_2 is quite low (<20 mmHg [13]) and raising this to non-physiological levels will cause arteriolar vasoconstriction and stop flow in many capillaries [14]. 2. Anesthesia may induce hypovolemia and reduce mean arterial blood pressure resulting in a reflex arteriolar vasoconstriction. This effect is particularly pronounced in resting muscle. 3 Capillaries themselves are extremely delicate structures which can easily be damaged by inadvertent tissue stretching or other trauma induced during surgery. 4. Histological examination of muscle reveals more RBCs in the capillary lumens after contractions than at rest [e.g., 15]. Whereas this has been interpreted as *de novo* RBC flow in previously non-flowing capillaries it likely resulted from the increased capillary hematocrit (i.e., more RBCs per unit length of capillaries) that occurs with hyperemic conditions [16]. The contractions-induced elevation of capillary hematocrit raises the statistical probability that an RBC will be present in capillary cross-sections examined histologically *ex-vivo* and does not provide any evidence that RBC flux is, or is not, present in a given capillary.

One troubling consequence of accepting the capillary 'recruitment' concept is that it has reinforced a black box approach to interpreting blood-muscle exchange and metabolism data. Specifically, rather than appreciating the enormous heterogeneity of RBC (and presumably plasma) flux across capillaries the presumption has been made that each capillary has a unitary exchange capacity and blood-muscle flux is increased during exercise or with insulin, for example, by simple addition (i.e., recruitment) of capillaries [e.g., 17-19].

Today capillary 'recruitment' during exercise is accepted by many to explain important physiological phenomena including: 1. Increased blood-muscle delivery of O_2, free fatty acids and glucose, and 2. Decreased capillary-to-mitochondrial diffusion distances [rev. 5]. However, as considered in *"An Alternative Contemporary Perspective"* below, there is a substantial body of literature, much of which is based on intravital microscopic observations of capillary hemodynamics, made in muscle *in vivo*, which suggests that most capillaries support RBC and plasma flux at rest. The importance of this issue to understanding microcirculatory function cannot be overstated and forces a radical rethinking of the control of blood-myocyte substrate flux within the capillary bed that is particularly germane to understanding the mechanistic bases for the predations of CHF on microcirculatory function.

2.2. An Alternative Contemporary Perspective

Direct observation of the capillary bed *in vivo* in a range of healthy resting skeletal muscles reveals that over 80% of capillaries support RBC flux e.g., rat spinotrapezius [12,20,21], rat diaphragm [22], hamster cremaster and sartorius [23], cat sartorius [24], cat tenuissimus [25], and rabbit tenuissimus [26]. Within these RBC-flowing capillaries there is a substantial heterogeneity of RBC fluxes suggesting that some capillaries are much more important for O_2 (as well as glucose and free fatty acid, FFA) delivery than others. However, notwithstanding this heterogeneity the majority of capillary endothelial surface area will be available for blood-tissue exchange at some level.

This view of a muscle microcirculation, in which most capillaries flow continuously, presents a paradigm shift for adherents of the capillary 'recruitment' hypothesis. Consequently, it is important that these data are viewed within the context of the technical limitations inherent with intravital microscopy and also that the conclusions can be corroborated by independent techniques.

2.3. Technical Limitations

One paramount limitation for these intravital microscopy observations of exteriorized muscles is the necessity for anesthesia which raises the concern that either the anesthetic used or the surgical procedures themselves may alter the blood flow to the muscle or the matching between O_2 delivery and O_2 utilization ($\dot{V}O_2$). Bailey and colleagues [27] reasoned that, if the presence of RBC flux in most capillaries was an artifact of anesthesia and/or surgical manipulation this would be reflected by an increased bulk blood flow and therefore O_2 delivery which could be detected using radioactive microspheres and also microvascular PO_2 (a sensitive measure of O_2 delivery-to-$\dot{V}O_2$ matching). Their results demonstrated that neither anesthesia nor the exteriorization procedure impacted blood flow or microvascular PO_2. Importantly, the dynamic matching of O_2 delivery and $\dot{V}O_2$ present at the onset of contractions *in situ* was maintained intact in the exteriorized muscle. Given these results, it is difficult to conceive that the anesthesia regimen and/or surgical manipulation used in those investigations impacted arteriolar smooth muscle function at rest (to produce a falsely high % RBC-perfused capillaries) whilst conserving the ability to regulate its blood flow-to-$\dot{V}O_2$ ratio at ~6:1 which is precisely that seen in intact voluntary exercising animals and humans [28,29].

2.4. Corroborating Evidence of Flow in Most Capillaries Obtained Using Different Techniques.

A. In both anesthetized and conscious rats Snyder and colleagues [30] infused FITC-albumin into the central circulation and arrested blood flow at discrete intervals thereafter. They demonstrated the presence of flow in essentially all capillaries within several seconds (i.e., < 1 circulation time) in each muscle examined (e.g. vastus lateralis, soleus). As with the intravital microscopy observations their data suggested that there was a great range of flow rates among individual capillaries consistent with some being more important for substrate delivery than others. Moreover, that flow was demonstrated in all capillaries, even in resting muscle (vastus lateralis), was inconsistent with the ability to 'recruit' additional capillaries during contractions or other hyperemic conditions. B. When one follows the logic that, if most muscle capillaries don't flow at rest and that these are subsequently recruited during exercise, it would be anticipated that muscle hemoglobin concentration ([Hb]) might be expected to increase many-fold at exercise onset. For instance, if it were assumed that 20% of capillaries sustained RBC flux at rest and this increased to 90% during exercise and also that within RBC-flowing capillaries the hematocrit increased from a resting of ~20% towards systemic (45%) [16] then a greater than 9-fold increase in [Hb] would be expected. However, near infrared spectroscopy (NIRS) measurements reveal that, from rest to exercise in the human quadriceps, [Hb] increases less than 1-fold [31]. This more modest increase in [Hb] can be explained solely on the basis of increased capillary hematocrit and leaves little room for recruitment of previously non-RBC containing/flowing capillaries.

In conclusion, the compelling weight of evidence indicates that most skeletal muscle capillaries support flow at rest albeit with a broad range of flow rates such that the potential for participation in blood-myocyte flux differs widely among capillaries. This scenario leaves little room for recruitment of previously non-flowing capillaries to initiate flow following the onset of muscle contractions/exercise. Pertinent to the consideration of blood glucose homeostasis this means that most of the capillary surface area in resting skeletal muscle is available for glucose removal from the blood. It is from this understanding that the impact of CHF on capillary function must be considered.

2.5. Effects of Post-MI CHF on Microcirculatory Hemodynamics

Chronic heart failure (CHF) secondary to MI is now recognized as a syndrome comprised of central hemodynamic and skeletal muscle dysfunction. Thus, impaired exercise tolerance and increased fatigability are associated with compromised skeletal muscle function which emanates, in part, from disturbed vascular control and metabolic alterations, such as a reduction in oxidative enzyme capacity within myocytes, as well as a shift to proportionally more fast-twitch fibers. The rat model of CHF has been invaluable for studying these processes in the absence of confounding effects of medications and altered or poorly-controlled activity levels [32, 33].

At rest and during exercise increased vasoconstriction is pathognomonic to CHF and results from an upregulation of the adrenergic and renin-angiotension systems as well as increased endothelin levels combined with a reduced bioavailability of, and sensitivity to, vasodilators such as nitric oxide (NO) [rev. 34-36]. In addition, the presence of venous congestion, microvascular rarefaction and altered mechanical characteristics of the blood vessels themselves all are likely to affect the ability to increase blood flow rapidly and to a level appropriate to the (changing) metabolic demand [rev. 7, 37, 38].

In healthy skeletal muscle there appears to be a superb regulation of blood flow with respect to metabolic demand (expressed as $\dot{V}O_2$). Thus, although fast twitch muscle(s) and muscle fibers may have a lower blood flow-to- $\dot{V}O_2$ ratio (and hence microvascular PO_2, [39,40]) at rest, during the exercising steady-state blood flow to both slow- and fast-twitch muscles increases with a proportionality of ~6:1 [28].

Although these steady-state responses can be insightful, it is the dynamic responsiveness to altered metabolic demands that may be most sensitive to pathologically altered regulation of blood flow (O_2 delivery) with respect to $\dot{V}O_2$. In this regard, Diederich *et al.* [37] and Behnke *et al.* [38] have used phosphorescence quenching measurements of microvascular PO_2 to resolve the effects of CHF on the dynamic relationship between O_2 delivery and $\dot{V}O_2$. As demonstrated in Fig. (**1**), in healthy animals following the onset of contractions muscle microvascular PO_2 displays a distinct and characteristic profile with a delay where microvascular PO_2 remains at resting levels for several seconds (reflecting O_2 delivery and $\dot{V}O_2$ increasing at the same rate) followed by an exponential fall to the new contracting steady-state as fractional O_2 extraction increases. The corresponding profile for CHF animals is very different and depends crucially on the severity of CHF and the age of the animals. Notice, in Fig (**1**) that for the soleus muscle in a rat with severe CHF, microvascular PO_2 at rest (time 0) is much reduced and falls, with little delay, to extremely low steady-state values. This is significant functionally because it means that the driving pressure for blood-myocyte O_2 flux is severely reduced. The overarching conclusion from these studies is that CHF impairs the normal exquisite matching of blood flow-to- $\dot{V}O_2$ present immediately following the onset of contractions and also in the steady-state impairing conditions for appropriate blood-myocyte O_2 flux and likely other substrates such as glucose.

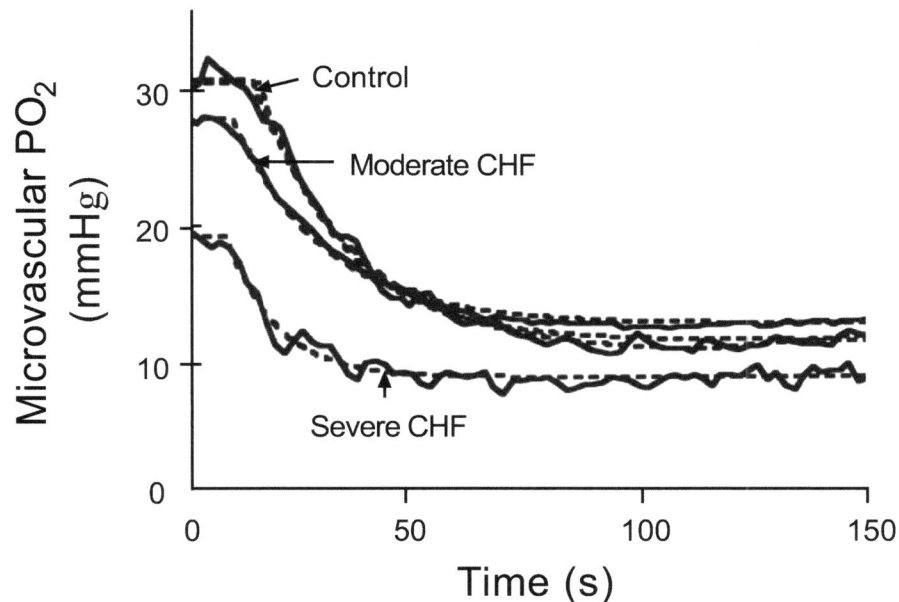

Figure 1: Profile of microvascular O_2 partial pressure (PO_2) in the soleus muscle following the onset of 1 Hz twitch contractions in control (healthy) rats and rats with ~7 weeks of moderate (left ventricular end-diatolic pressure, LVEDP >control< 20 mmHg) and severe (LVEDP> 20 mmHg) chronic heart failure (CHF). CHF was induced by myocardial infarction caused by ligation of the left coronary artery. Notice the lowered microvascular PO_2 at rest and during contractions particularly in the severe CHF muscle suggestive of a lowered resting capillary RBC flux and an impaired response to contractions. Redrawn from Behnke *et al.* [38].

Because of the difficulty of visualizing microcirculatory function in intact muscle our understanding, historically, of the effects of CHF on muscle vascular control has emphasized alternative approaches such as: 1. Assessment of integrated organ dysfunction from pulmonary O_2 measurements (i.e., maximal $\dot{V}O_2$ and $\dot{V}O_2$ kinetics at the onset of exercise) [e.g., 41-45]. 2. Description of structural vascular and fiber adaptations *ex-vivo* [6, 46-52]. 3. Bulk blood flow alterations at rest and during exercise. [32, 53-58] 4. Determination of altered vasomotor control [59-64] and endothelial function [65]. 5. Intravital microscopic evaluation of single vessel (arteriolar) function [66, 67].

In toto these investigations have provided evidence for CHF reducing maximal $\dot{V}O_2$ and slowing $\dot{V}O_2$ kinetics as well as decreasing and redistributing exercising muscle blood flow. In CHF a mild degree of capillary involution may be present in oxidative muscles which decrease the maximal capillary surface area available for blood-muscle substrate flux. In addition severe CHF reduces muscle oxidative enzyme capacity and induces a shift towards a more fast-twitch fiber population accompanied by a mild fiber atrophy. Importantly, within single arterioles there may be a down-regulation of vasodilatory function and an up-regulation of vasoconstrictor tone; the net effect of which may be to retard vasodilation and reduce the blood flow increase to a given level of muscle contractile activity. The present review will not dissect these findings or the underlying mechanisms further, but, rather, will examine the consequences of these events as they impact muscle capillary hemodynamics at rest and following the onset of contractions. This approach is directly germane to establishing a connection between the microcirculatory functional sequellae to CHF and putative mechanistic bases for the development of insulin resistance.

Intravital Microscopy studies in the Rat Spinotrapezius Muscle. Based upon muscle fiber type and oxidative capacity the rat spinotrapezius muscle is an excellent analog of the human quadriceps [c.f., 68,69] and, crucially, possesses optical properties amenable to intravital microscopy. Using this preparation Kindig and colleagues [6] determined that CHF has a profound impact on microcirculatory hemodynamics in resting muscle. Specifically, rats with an average infarction size of 33% (range 13-45%) of the left ventricular endocardial circumference demonstrated a reduction in the percentage of capillaries supporting continuous RBC flux from 87 to 66%. Moreover there was a significant correlation between infarction size and RBC-flowing capillaries indicating that the perfused capillary surface area available for blood-muscle substrate delivery was substantially reduced Fig. (**2**).

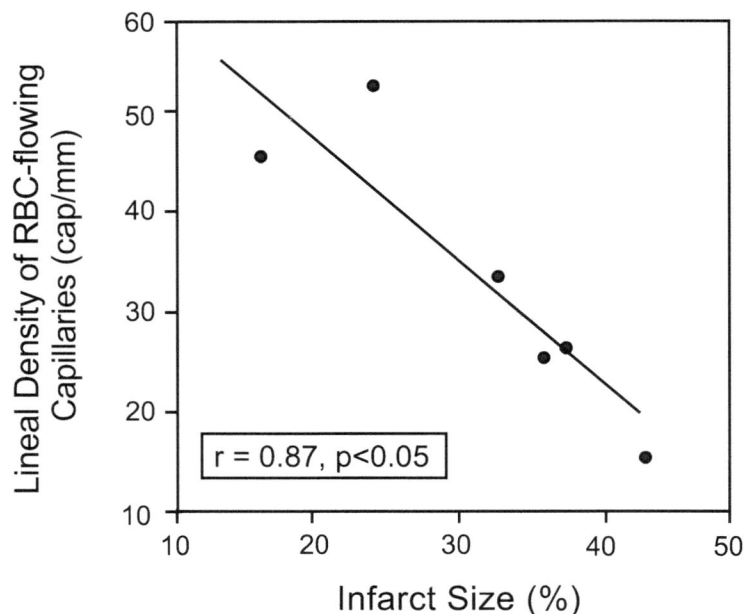

Figure 2: Relationship between the lineal density of red blood cell-perfused capillaries in the spinotrapezius muscle and infarction size in rats with chronic heart failure (CHF) (from Kindig *et al.* [6], with permission).

Within the RBC-flowing capillaries RBC velocity and flux were reduced in synchrony; severely compromising substrate delivery and presumably increasing the number of capillaries in which RBC and plasma flow is so low that they become functionally insignificant for substrate delivery. Notice that, when this is expressed as RBC flux per unit of muscle (i.e., lineal capillary density x capillary RBC flux) there was ~50% decrease in O_2 delivery in CHF Fig. (**3**). Germane to microcirculatory glucose and insulin delivery this presumably indicates that plasma flux is also halved in CHF.

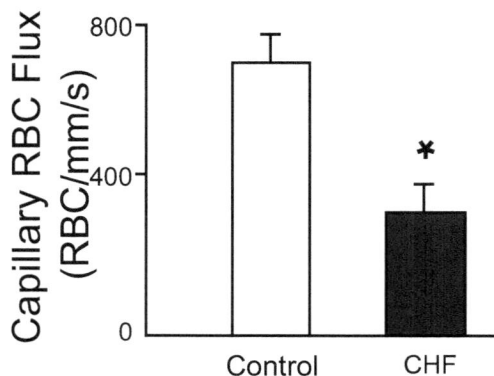

Figure 3: Reduction in spinotrapezius capillary RBC flux (lineal density of flowing capillaries x RBC flux) in chronic heart failure rats ~ 7 weeks following myocardial infarction induced by left coronary artery ligation (from Kindig *et al.* [6], with permission). *P<0.05 compared with control.

One of the key questions that arose from the Kindig *et al.* [6] study was to what extent muscle contractions could modify the capillary hemodynamics in CHF. Of particular interest was whether or not those capillaries not supporting RBC flux at rest would initiate flow during contractions. To this end, Richardson and colleagues [7] compared the muscle capillary hemodynamic response to contractions in healthy vs CHF rats Fig (**4**). They observed that, in muscles of CHF rats, those capillaries not supporting RBC flux at rest did not initiate flow during contractions. Moreover, although RBC flux did increase with contractions the dynamic profile was blunted. Specifically, in *healthy* muscle RBC flux evinces a rapid and biphasic increase rising 50-60% within 1-2 s and subsequently achieving its new elevated steady-state after about 20-30 s (i.e., with a half-time (T_{50}) for the response of ~11 s, Fig. (**4**). In marked contrast, capillaries supporting RBC flux at rest in muscles from CHF rats demonstrated no rapid increase of RBC flux or velocity, rather, both increased sluggishly from the onset of contractions such that by the end of the 180 s contraction bout, they were still increasing - but at levels far below those present in their healthy counterparts [7].

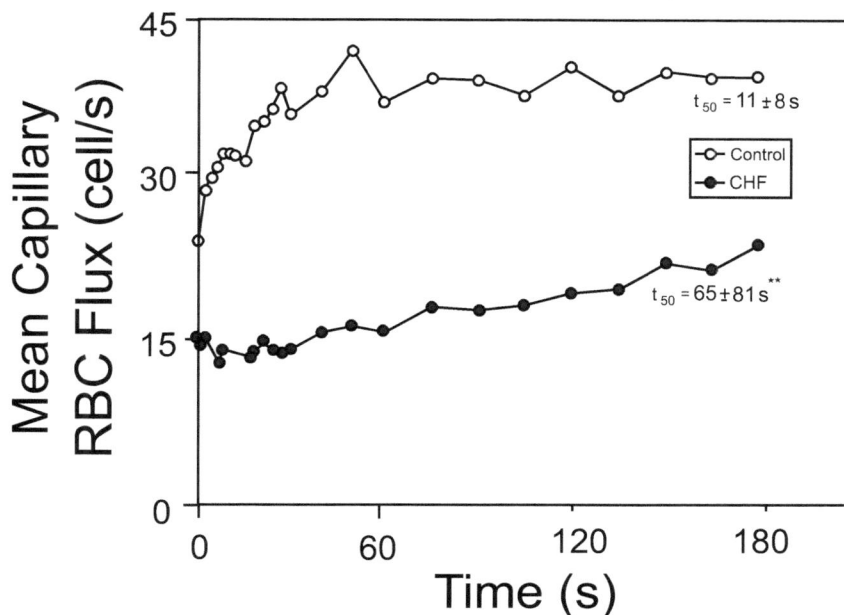

Figure 4: Capillary RBC flux in 20 spinotrapezius capillaries from control rats and chronic heart failure (CHF) rats. Standard error bars are omitted for clarity. Notice the rapid increase in RBC flux witin the first contraction cycle in control rats which is completely absent in the CHF rats. The overall very sluggish nature of the increase in RBC flux in CHF is exemplified by the half-times (t_{50}) of the responses presented which were nearly 6-fold longer (slower) in CHF. **P<0.05 vs control. Redrawn from Richardson *et al.* [7].

The profile for RBC flux and therefore capillary O_2 delivery seen in Fig. (**4**) is close to that predicted from the microvascular PO_2 profile for CHF presented in Fig. (**1**). Collectively, these findings demonstrate that CHF impairs microvascular O_2 delivery to a proportionally greater extent than $\dot{V}O_2$. One consequence of this disparity is that microvascular PO_2 falls to very low, and likely limiting, levels at the same time that blood-myocyte O_2 flux is increasing (or trying to) at its greatest rate. Because the capillary-to-subsarcolemmal PO_2 differential is decreased and it is this differential that provides the sole motive force for transmembrane O_2 flux the blood-muscle O_2 flux will be compromised and hence $\dot{V}O_2$ kinetics slowed. As mentioned above, slowed $\dot{V}O_2$ kinetics at the onset of exercise constitute a hallmark of CHF in human patients which causes greater muscle phosphocreatine depletion and compromises exercise tolerance [70, 71]. Whereas the focus of this review is on glucose homeostasis the capillary hemodynamic dysfunction that impairs O_2 flux will also apply to glucose transport and delivery to muscle. In addition, the $\dot{V}O_2$ kinetics in-and-of themselves will result in greater intracellular perturbations that are known to limit exercise tolerance. Hence, the CHF patients' ability, and often willingness, to use exercise as a therapeutic intervention to manage their reduced insulin sensitivity is compromised.

The mechanisms responsible for the CHF-induced deficits in capillary hemodynamic function at rest and during exercise are complex and, as discussed above, likely involve vasoregulatory dysfunction at multiple levels. In CHF inflammatory mediators such as the cytokines C-reactive protein [72], interleukin 1β [73] and TNFα [74] are elevated. There is reduction of bioavailable NO [75] and redox status is perturbed [76]. All of these features may contribute to the microvascular dysfunction described above. Delineation of exactly how each vasodilatory mechanism may be impacted by CHF remains to be determined and presents a valuable arena for future research. However, at present we do have some important clues regarding the participation of CHF-induced dysregulation at several levels. For instance: A. the rapid increase in RBC flux occurring within the first contraction-relaxation cycle in healthy but not CHF individuals [7] can be restored, in part, by removing the venous congestion present in CHF [77]. B. The recent recognition that capillary endothelial cell caveoli (small plasma membrane invaginations) form microdomains of vascular control that include eNOS, endothelium-derived hyperpolarizing factor (EDHF), large capacity calcium (BK) channels, and insulin receptor signaling might provide a control locus that helps link vascular control directly to the metabolic requirements of the muscle and, as such, constitute a putative site for CHF-induced dysregulation and mediating insulin resistance [rev. 4]. C. In addition to ablating the almost instantaneous increase in capillary hemodynamics following the onset of contractions CHF constrains the subsequent less rapid increase that has been attributed, in part, to shear stress, sympatholysis (i.e., both NO-related mechanisms), ascending vasodilation and metabolic feedback from the contracting fibers [7]. Despite the complexity of candidate control mechanisms involved in the precise matching of O_2 delivery to VO_2 (and thus microvascular PO_2 regulation), in our laboratory, Ferreira *et al.* [35,36] recently demonstrated that muscle superfusion with the NO-donor sodium nitroprusside (SNP) restored the CHF muscle microvascular PO_2 profile close to that seen in healthy animals Fig. (**5**). Whereas it would be convenient to interpret these results as NO exerting an overarching control over the entire capillary hemodynamic response this conclusion must be tempered by an important caveat. Elevations in microvascular PO_2 may result from either increased O_2 delivery or decreased $\dot{V}O_2$. NO impairs mitochondrial function [35,36,78] and thus the elevation of microvascular PO_2 seen with SNP was likely due, at least in part, to decreased muscle $\dot{V}O_2$. Thus, it remains to be determined exactly how much of the restoration of microvascular PO_2 seen in Fig. (**5**) was due to improved microvascular function *per se*.

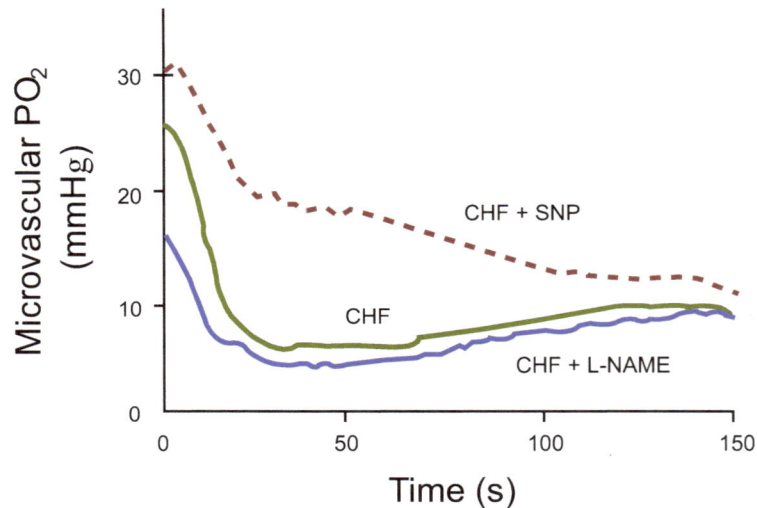

Figure 5: Profile of microvascular O_2 partial pressure (PO_2) in the spinotrapezius muscle following the onset of 1 Hz twitch contractions in rats in chronic heart failure (CHF) ~7 weeks after myocardial infarction induced by ligation of the left coronary artery. Notice that the depressed microvascular PO_2 characteristic of CHF appears to be completely restored by increased availability of nitric oxide (NO) supplied by sodium nitroprusside (SNP) superfusion. In contrast blockade of NO synthase with L-NAME has little effect on the control CHF profile suggesting that, in CHF muscles, NO plays only a limited role in increasing O2 delivery to match O_2 demands during contractions. Please see text for additional details. Redrawn from Ferreira *et al.* [36].

3. MECHANISTIC CONNECTION BETWEEN POST-MI MICROCIRCU-LATORY DYSFUNCTION AND INSULIN RESISTANCE.

For many years the observation that the arterial-to-venous O_2 difference was maintained or even increased in CHF lead to the erroneous conclusion that muscle microcirculatory function was preserved post-MI. However, following elegant theoretical and empirical investigations [79, 80] it is now appreciated that fractional O_2 extraction is determined by the ratio of diffusing capacity for O_2 (DO_2) to blood flow (Q and therefore, O_2 delivery, QO_2) according to:

$$\text{Fractional } O_2 \text{ extraction} = QO_2 \left(1 - e^{-DO2/\beta Q}\right)$$

Where β is the slope of the O_2 dissociation curve in the physiologically relevant range. Thus, in pathologically low-Q conditions such as CHF, as long as Q falls proportionally more than DO_2, fractional O_2 extraction (i.e., arterial-venous O_2 difference) will increase even in the face of a reduced total O_2 flux [81]. It is now appreciated that CHF leads to profound microcirculatory flow abnormalities which will act to reduce muscle DO_2 and that fractional O_2 extraction is only preserved because the low

Q condition reduces capillary RBC velocity thereby increasing capillary RBC transit time which increases the opportunity for O_2 extraction from each RBC.

O_2 transport and flux should not be used as direct surrogates for glucose transport and flux for many reasons including the most obvious that the overwhelming majority of O_2 is carried in the RBC whereas the plasma is more important for glucose transport. However, even accepting the fact that RBCs and plasma behave differently (e.g., travel at different speeds) in the microcirculation, the observed behavior of RBCs in the capillary bed in CHF may provide important clues for the role of skeletal muscle in CHF-induced insulin resistance. For instance, it is difficult to envision that capillaries which do not support RBC flux at rest or during contractions can provide important avenues for plasma flow. Additionally, within RBC-flowing capillaries, where RBC flux and velocity are reduced in CHF, the unchanged hematocrit suggests that plasma flux is decreased in proportion to that of RBCs. What this means is that, irrespective of any regulatory effect of CHF on insulin receptors *per se*, the access of glucose and insulin to a substantial portion of the skeletal muscle capillary bed is impaired in CHF. Not only is this effect present at rest but also in contracting muscles; experimental evidence suggesting that capillaries which do not supporting flow at rest do not initiate flow and therefore glucose and insulin access to this endothelial surface area is denied. It is also pertinent that the cessation of fluid flow within capillaries leads to the formation of endothelial projections into the capillary lumen which may constitute a critical event leading to involution of those capillaries [82]. Thus, with increased CHF duration, and absence of capillary flux, these vessels may be resorbed and the muscle capillary bed undergoes rarefaction [49].

4. CONCLUSIONS

Post-MI CHF induces profound capillary hemodynamic dysfunction within skeletal muscle such that the ability to match blood flow to the tissue metabolic requirements impaired. This process involves stoppage of RBC and plasma flow in many capillaries and reduces flux in those capillaries that do sustain flow. Recognition of these abnormalities is dependent entirely on the acknowledgement that, in healthy skeletal muscle, the vast majority of capillaries support RBC and plasma flow. Such recognition is a necessary first-step to investigating the mechanistic bases for this phenomenon. The scenario described above for skeletal muscle in CHF, which resembles closely that for type II diabetes [82, 83], will restrict the access of glucose and insulin to a substantial portion of the capillary bed and, importantly, is not alleviated during an acute bout of muscle contractions. Whether repeated bouts of exercise that induce capillary neogenesis, elevated muscle oxidative capacity and improved endothelial function can restore flow in non-flowing capillaries is uncertain. However, what is certain is that therapeutic reversal of post-MI skeletal muscle capillary flow stoppage presents a putative avenue for enhancing glucose delivery to, and uptake by, skeletal muscle.

5. REFERENCES

[1]   Rowell LB. *Human cardiovascular control.* Oxford University Press, Inc., Oxford, 1993.
[2]   Pajunen P, Koukkunen H, Ketonen M *et al.* Five-year risk of developing clinical diabetes after first myocardial infarction: the FINAMI study. Diabet Med 2005; 22: 1334-7.
[3]   Swan JW, Ealton C, Godsland IF, Clark AL, Coats AJ, Oliver MF. Insulin resistance in chronic heart failure. Eur Heart J 1994; 15: 1528-32.
[4]   Wiernsperger N, Nivoit P, Kraemer De Aguiar LG, Bouskela E. Microcirculation and the metabolic syndrome. Microcirculation 2007; 14: 403-38.
[5]   Poole, DC, Brown MD, Hudlicka O. Point-Counterpoint: There is not capillary recruitment in skeletal muscle during exercise. J Appl Physiol 2008: 104: 891-3.
[6]   Kindig, C.A., T.I. Musch, R. Basaraba, and D.C. Poole. Impaired capillary hemodynamics in skeletal muscle of rats in chronic heart failure. J Appl Physiol 1999; 87: 652-60.
[7]   Richardson, T.S., C.A. Kindig, T.I. Musch, and D.C. Poole. Effects of chronic heart failure on skeletal muscle capillary hemodynamics at rest and during contractions. J Appl Physiol 2003; 95: 1055-62.
[8]   Krogh A. The number and distribution of capillaries in muscles with calculations of the oxygen pressure head necessary for supplying the tissue. J Physiol Lond 1919; 52: 409-15.
[9]   Voter WA, Gayeski TE. Determination of myoglobin saturation of frozen specimens using a reflecting cryospectrophotometer. Am J Physiol 1995; 269: H1328-41.
[10]   Richardson, R.S., E.A. Noyszewski, K.F. Kendrick, J.S. Leigh, and P.D. Wagner. Myoglobin O_2 desaturation during exercise: Evidence of limited O_2 transport. J Clin Invest 1995; 96: 1916-26.
[11]   Clark MG, Rattigan S, Barrett EJ, Vincent MA. There is capillary recruitment in active skeletal muscle during exercise. J Appl Physiol 2008; 104: 889-91.

[12]   Kindig CA, Richardson TE, Poole DC. Skeletal muscle capillary hemodynamics from rest to contractions: implications for oxygen transfer. J Appl Physiol 2002; 92: 2513-20.

[13]   Whalen WJ,Buerk D, Kanoy BE, Duran WN. Tissue PO_2, $\dot{V}O_2$, venous PO_2 and perfusion pressure in resting dog gracilis muscle perfused at constant flow. Adv Exp Med Biol 1976; 75: 639-55.

[14]   Parthasarathi K, Lipowsky HH. Capillary recruitment in response to tissue hypoxia and its dependence on red blood cell deformability. *Am* J Physiol Heart Circ Physiol 1999; 277:H2145-57.

[15]   Honig CR, Odoroff CL, Frierson JL. Capillary recruitment in exercise: rate, extent, uniformity, and relation to blood flow. Am J Physiol Heart Circ Physiol. 1980; 238:H31-42.

[16]   Klitzman B, Duling BR. Microvascular hematocrit and red cell flow in resting and contracting striated muscle. Am J Physiol 1979; 237:H481-90.

[17]   Baron AD, Tarshoby M, Hook G, Lazaridis EN, Cronin J, Johnson A, Steinberg HO. Interaction between insulin sensitivity and muscle perfusion on glucose uptake in human skeletal muscle: Evidence for capillary recruitment. Diabetes 2000; 49: 768-74.

[18]   Clark ADH, Barrett EJ, Rattigan S, Wallis MG, Clark MG. Insulin stimulates laser Doppler signal by rat muscle which is consistent with nutritive flow recruitment. Clin Science 2001; 100: 283-90.

[19]   Wheatley CM, Rattigan S, Richards SM, Barrett EJ, Clark MG. Skeletal muscle contraction stimulates capillary recruitment and glucose uptake in insulin-resistant obese Zucker rats. Am J Physiol Endocrinol Metab 2004; 287:E804-9.

[20]   Hudlicka O, Zweifach BW, Tyler KR. Capillary recruitment and flow velocity in skeletal muscle after contractions. Microvasc Res 1982; 23: 201-13.

[21]   Poole DC, Musch TI, Kindig CA. In vivo microvascular structural and functional consequences of muscle length changes. Am J Physiol 1997; 272: H2107-14.

[22]   Kindig CA, Poole DC. A comparison of the microcirculation in the rat spinotrapezius and diaphragm muscles. Microvasc Res 1998; 55: 249-59.

[23]   Damon DH, Duling BR. Distribution of capillary blood flow in the microcirculation of the hamster: An in vivo study using epifluorescent microscopy. Microvasc Res. 1984; 27: 81-95.

[24]   Burton KS, Johnson PC. Reactive hyperemia in individual capillaries of skeletal muscle. Am J Physiol. 1972; 223:517-24.

[25]   Erickson E, Myrhage R. Microvascular dimensions and blood flow in skeletal muscle. Acta Physiol Scand 1972; 86; 211-22.

[26]   Vrielink HH, Slaaf DW, Tangelder GJ, Reneman RS. Does capillary recruitment exist in young rabbit skeletal muscle? Int J Microcirc Clin Exp 1987; 6:321-32.

[27]   Bailey JK, Kindig CA, Behnke BJ, Musch TI, Schmid-Schoenbein GW, Poole DC. Spinotrapezius muscle microcirculatory function: effects of surgical exteriorization. Am. J. Physiol 2000; 279: H1331-7.

[28]   Ferreira LF, McDonough P, Behnke BJ, Musch TI, Poole DC. Blood flow and O_2 extraction as a function of O_2 uptake in muscles composed of different fiber type. Respir Physiol Neurobiol 2006; 153: 237-49.

[29]   Poole DC. Influence of exercise training on skeletal muscle oxygen delivery and utilization. In: *The Lung:Scientific Foundations.* Eds: R.G. Crystal, J.B. West, E.R. Weibel, P.J. Barnes, Raven Press, New York, 1997, pp. 1957-67.

[30]   Snyder GK, Farrelly C, Coelho JR. Capillary perfusion in skeletal muscle. Am J Physiol Heart Circ Physiol 1992; 262:H828-32.

[31]   Ferreira LF, Lutjemeier BJ, Townsend DK, Barstow TJ. Effects of pedal frequency on estimated muscle microvascular O_2 extraction. Eur J Appl Physiol 2006; 96:558-63.

[32]   Musch TI, Terrell JA. Skeletal muscle blood flow abnormalities in rats with a chronic myocardial infarction: rest and exercise. Am J Physiol Heart Circ Physiol 1992; 262: H411-9. .

[33]   Simonini A, Long CS, Dudley GA, Yue P, McElhinney J, Massie BM. Heart failure in rats causes changes in skeletal muscle morphology and gene expression that are not explained by reduced activity. Circ Res 1996; 79: 128-36.

[34]   Ventura-Clapier R, De Sousa E, Veksler V. Metabolic myopathy in heart failure. News Physiol Sci 2002; 17: 191-6.

[35]   Ferreira LF, Padilla DJ, Williams J, Hageman KS, Musch TI, Poole DC. Effects of altered nitric oxide availability on rat muscle microvascular oxygenation during contractions. Acta Physiol. (Oxf.) 2006; 186: 223-32.

[36]   Ferreira LF, Padilla DJ, Williams J, Hageman KS, Poole DC, Musch TI. Muscle microvascular oxygenation in chronic heart failure: role of nitric oxide availability. Acta Physiol (Oxf.) 2006; 188:3-13.

[37]   Diederich ER, Behnke BJ, McDonough P, Kindig CA, Barstow TJ, Poole DC, Musch TI. Effects of chronic heart failure on microvascular PO_2 dynamics in contracting muscle. Cardiovasc Res 2002; 56: 479-86.

[38]   Behnke BJ, Delp MD, McDonough P, Spier SA, Poole DC, Musch TI. Effects of chronic heart failure on microvascular oxygen exchange dynamics in muscles of contrasting fiber type. Cradiovasc Res 2004; 61: 325-32.

[39]   Behnke BJ, McDonough P, Padilla DJ, Musch TI, Poole DC. Oxygen exchange profile in muscles of contrasting fibre types. J. Physiol. (Lond.) 2003; 549:597-605.

[40]   McDonough P, Behnke BJ, Padilla DJ, Musch TI, Poole DC. Control of microvascular oxygen pressures in muscles comprised of different fibre types. J Physiol 2005; 563: 903-13.

[41]   Meakins J, Long CNH. Oxygen consumption, oxygen debt and lactic acid in circulatory failure. *J* Clin Invest 1927; 4: 273-93.

[42]   Weber KT, Janicki JS. Cardiopulmonary exercise testing for evaluation of chronic heart failure. Am J Cardiol 1985; 55: 22-31.

[43]   Ceretelli P, Grassi B, Colombini A, Caru B, Marconi C. Gas exchange and metabolic transients in heart transplant recipients. Respir Physiol 1988; 74: 355-71.

[44]   Grassi B, Marconi C, Meyer M, Rieu M, Cerretelli P. Gas exchange and cardiovascular kinetics with different exercise protocols in heart transplant recipients. J Appl Physiol 1997; 82: 1952-62.

[45]   Hepple RT, Liu PP, Plyley MJ, Goodman JM. Oxygen uptake kinetics during exercise in chronic heart failure influence of peripheral vascular reserve. Clin Sci (Lond) 1999; 97: 569-77.

[46]   Ralston MA, Merola AJ, Leier CV. Depressed aerobic enzyme activity of skeletal muscle in severe chronic heart failure. J Lab Clin Med 1991; 117: 370-2.

[47]   Drexler H, Riede R, Munzel T, Konig H, Funke E, Just H. Alterations of skeletal muscle in chronic heart failure. Circulation 1992; 85: 1751-9.

[48]   Schaufelberger M, Eriksson BO, Grimby G, Held P, Swedberg K. Skeletal muscle fiber composition and capillarization in patients with chronic heart failure: relation to exercise capacity and central hemodynamics. J. Card Fail 1995; 1: 267-72.

[49]   Xu L, Poole DC, Musch TI. Effect of heart failure on muscle capillary geometry: implications for O_2 exchange. Med Sci Sports Exerc 1998; 30: 1230-7.

[50]   Delp MD, Duan C, Mattson JP, Musch TI. Changes in skeletal muscle biochemistry and histology relative to fiber type in rats with heart failure. J Appl Physiol 1997; 83: 1291-99.

[51]   Degens H, Anderson RK, Always SE. Capillarization in skeletal muscle of rats with cardiac hypertrophy. Med Sci Sports Exerc 2002; 34: 258-66.

[52]   Nusz DJ, White DC, Dai Q *et al.* Vascular rarefaction in peripheral skeletal muscle after experimental heart failure. Am J Physiol Heart Circ Physiol 2003; 285: H1554-62.

[53]   Zelis R, Longhurst J, Capone RJ, Mason DT. A comparison of regional blood flow and oxygen utilization during dynamic forearm exercise in normal subjects and patients with congestive heart failure. Circulation 1974; 50: 137-43.

[54]   Wilson JR, Martin JL, Schwartz D, Ferraro N. Exercise intolerance in patients with chronic heart failure: role of impaired nutritive flow to skeletal muscle. Circulation 1984; 69: 1079-87.

[55]   Drexler H, Toggart EJ, Glick MR, Heald J, Flaim SF, Zelis R. Regional vascular adjustments during recovery from myocardial infarction in rats. J Am Coll Cardiol 1986; 8: 134-42.

[56]   Sullivan MJ, Knight JD, Higginbotham MB, Cobb FR. Relation between central and peripheral hemodynamics during exercise in patients with chronic heart failure. Circulation 1989; 80: 769-81.

[57]   Hirai T, Zelis R, Musch TI. Effects of nitric oxide synthase inhibition on the muscle blood flow response to exercise in rats with heart failure. Cardiovasc Res 1995; 30: 469-76.

[58]   Shoemaker JK, Naylor HL, Hogeman CS Sinoway LI. Blood flow dynamics in heart failure. Circulation 1999; 99: 3002-8.

[59]   Zelis R, Flaim SF. Alterations in vasomotor tone in congestive heart failure. Prog Cardiovasc Dis 1982; 24: 437-59.

[60]   Zelis R, Davis D. The sympathetic nervous system in congestive heart failure. Heart Fail 1986; 2: 21-32.

[61]   Zelis R, Sinoway LI, Musch TI, Davis D. Vasoconstrictor mechanisms in congestive heart failure, Part 1. Mod Concepts Cardiovasc Dis 1989; 58: 7-12.

[62]   Margulies KB, Hildebrand FL, Lerman A, Perrella MA, Burnett JC. Increased endothelin in experimental heart failure. Circulation 1990; 82: 2226-30.

[63]   Musch TI, Zelis R. Norepinephrine response to exercise of rats with a chronic myocardial infarction. Med Sci Sports Exerc 1991; 23: 569-77.

[64]   Thomas GD, Zhang W, Victor RG. Impaired modulation of sympathetic vasoconstriction in contracting skeletal muscle of rats with chronic myocardial infarctions. Circ Res 2001; 88: 816-23, 2001.

[65]   Kubo SH, Thomas SR, Bank AJ, Williams RE, Heifetz SM. Endothelium-dependent vasodilation is attenuated in patients with heart failure. Circulation 1991; 84: 1589-96.

[66]   Didion SP, Carmines PK, Ikenaga H, Mayhan WG. Enhanced constrictor responses of skeletal muscle arterioles during chronic myocardial infarction. Am J Physiol Heart Circ Physiol 1997; 273: H1502-8.

[67]   Didion SP, Mayhan WG. Effect of chronic myocardial infarction on *in vivo* reactivity of skeletal muscle arterioles. Am J Physiol Heart Circ Physiol 1997; 272: H2403-8.

[68]   Delp MD, Duan C. Composition and size of type I, IIA, IID/X and IIB fibers and citrate synthase activity of rat muscle. J Appl Physiol 1996; 80: 261-70.

[69]   Leek BT, Mudaliar SR, Henry R, Mathieu-Costello O, Richardson RS. Effect of acute exercise on citrate synthase activity in untrained and trained human skeletal muscle. Am J Physiol Regul Integr Comp Physiol 2001; 280: R441-7.

[70]   Massie BM, Conway M, Yonge R *et al.* 31P nuclear magnetic resonance evidence of abnormal skeletal muscle metabolism in patients with congestive heart failure. Am J Cardiol 1987; 60: 309-15.

[71]   Arnolda L, Brosnan J, Rajagopalan B, Radda GK. Skeletal muscle metabolism in heart failure rats. Am J Physiol Heart Circ Physiol 1991; 261: H4342.

[72]   Celik T, Ivisoy A, Celik M, Yuksel UC, Kardesoglu E. C-reactive protein in chronic heart failure: A new predictor of survival. Int J Cardiol 2008 In press.

[73]   Adams V, Nehrhoff B, Spate U *et al.* Induction of iNOS expression in skeletal muscle by IL-1β and NFkappaB activation: an *in vitro* and *in vivo* study. Cardiovasc Res 2002; 54: 95-104.

[74]   Berthonneche C, Sulpice T, Boucher F *et al.* New insights into the pathological role of TNFα in early cardiac dysfunction and subsequent heart failure after infarction in rats. Am J Physiol Heart Circ Physiol 2004; 287: H340-50.

[75]   Rush JW, Green HJ, Maclean DA, Code LM. Oxidative stress and nitric oxide synthase in skeletal muscles of rats with post-infarction, compensated chronic heart failure. Acta Physiol Scand 2005; 185: 211-8.

[76]   Sharma R, Davidoff MN. Oxidative stress and endothelial dysfunction in heart failure. Congest Heart Fail 2002; 8: 165-72.

[77]   Shiotani I, Sato H, Sato H *et al.* Muscle pump-dependent self-perfusion mechanism in legs in normal subjects and patients with heart failure. J Appl Physiol. 2002; 92: 1647-54.

[78]   Brown GC. Regulation of mitochondrial respiration by nitric oxide inhibition of cytochrome c oxidase. Biochim Biophys Acta 2001; 1504: 46-57.

[79]   Piiper J, Scheid P. Model for capillary-alveolar equilibration with special reference to O_2 uptake in hypoxia. Respir Physiol 1981; 46: 193-208.

[80]   Roca J, Agusti AG, Alonso A *et al.* Effects of training on muscle O_2 transport at $\dot{V}O_2$max. J Appl Physiol 1992; 73: 1067-76.

[81]   Katz SD, Maskin C, Jondeau G, Cocke T, Berkowitz R, LeJemtel T. Near-maximal fractional oxygen extraction by active skeletal muscle in patients with chronic heart failure. J Appl Physiol 2000; 88:2138-42.

[82]   Hueck IS, Rossiter K, Artmann GM, Schmid-Schonbein. Fluid shear attenuates endothelial pseudopodia formation into the capillary lumen. Microcirculation 2008; 15: 531-42.

[83]   Padilla DJ, McDonough P, Behnke BJ, Kano Y, Hageman KS, Musch TI, Poole DC. Effects of Type II diabetes on capillary hemodynamics in skeletal muscle. Am J Physiol Heart Circ 2006; 291: H2439-44.

[84]   Padilla DJ, McDonough P, Behnke BJ, Kano Y, Hageman KS, Musch TI, Poole DC. Effects of Type II diabetes on muscle microvascular oxygen pressures. Resp Physiol Neurobiol 2007; 156: 187-95.

Is Defective Microcirculation Responsible for Insulin Resistance?

PART 1: Microvascular Dysfunction and Insulin Resistance are Linked: Evidences from Clinical Observations

Nicolas Wiernsperger[1, 2]

[1]INSERM U870, INSA Lyon, Bat.L. Pasteur, 11 avenue J.Capelle, F-69621 Villeurbanne Cedex (France)

[2]Laboratorio de Pesquisas em Microcirculaçao, Centro Medico, Universidade do Estado do Rio de Janeiro, Pav. R. Haroldo Lisboa da Cunha, Rua Sao Francisco Xavier 524, 20550-013 Rio de Janeiro (Brazil)
E Mail: <u>nicolas.wiernsperger@free.fr</u>

Abstract: This chapter describes the arguments supporting our concept that microcirculatory defects may underlie insulin resistance (IR). Vascular (patho) physiology and metabolism are vast areas subjected to many confounding factors detailed here, which are cardinal to sort the many existing contradictory reports. A thorough analysis of the epidemiological and clinical literature clearly establishes that microvascular dysfunction and IR are linked and observable very early in life, well before metabolic syndrome and cardiometabolic diseases develop. In part 2 the thermodynamic, particularly microvascular effects of insulin itself are detailed and analyzed in terms of their physiological pertinence. Part 3 deals with underlying mechanisms, based on selected clinical situations. These reveal puzzling commonalities: together with cell physiology, they suggest that primary (inherited, early acquired) or secondary defects in sensing exaggerated physical forces of blood flow by the microvascular endothelial surface may be responsible. Glycocalyx and mainly caveolae, which are linked to vasomotor reactions and to insulin signalling and transport, are tentatively designed as the culprit.

Keywords: Endothelial dysfunction, insulin resistance, metabolic syndrome, microcirculation.

1. INTRODUCTION

According to a recent estimation the lifetime risk of developing non insulin dependent diabetes (NIDDM) for individuals born in 2000 is about 33% in males and 38% in females [1]. Metabolic syndrome (MS) is largely responsible for this scenario [2].

The last 20 years have generated a plethora of epidemiological and clinical data which, as a whole, have revealed that the prevalence of cardiovascular diseases (CVDs) is as high in prediabetic subjects as in established diabetes. While microangiopathy, as manifested by retinopathy, nephropathy and neuropathy in diabetics, remains a specificity of frank diabetes secondarily to the deleterious effects of hyperglycemia, large vessel diseases and other factors in the microvasculature are involved in glucose intolerance and even in normoglycemia in subjects being considered "at risk" of NIDDM. Thus the risk for subjects with MS to develop NIDDM and/or CVD is similarly high. The Framingham Offspring Study demonstrated that the presence of insulin resistance (IR) increased the risk for diabetes and CVD as strongly as did MS [3]. This led to terms such as cardiometabolic diseases or diabesity based on the concept of a "common soil" which would lead to one or both complications [4, 5].

However the multiplication of such studies has also highlighted the limitations in their their interpretation because a long list of technical and clinical confounding factors [6, 7]. As a consequence, the nature of the common soil has not been unravelled. More so, official organizations have finally rejected MS as a clinical indication [8].

2. CONFOUNDING FACTORS AND LIMITATIONS IN DATA INTERPRETATION

At first sight it may look disappointing to start with enumerating some of the many confounding factors or even artefacts characterizing this vast area but because the determinations of most vascular and metabolic parameters are essentially indirect and because the physiology of the microcirculation has many very specificities (cf E.Bouskela, this book), we feel it is absolutely necessary to make the reader aware of what he will confronted with; this should in fact help him to travel through this little 'jungle' with open eyes and provide him the necessary caution to discriminate between findings which look frequently very paradoxical.

2.1. Prediabetic Subject Populations

Prediabetic subjects differ in many aspects, making it difficult to compare different studies and introducing the need for numerous adjustments and corrections in the calculation of correlations. Some relevant illustrating examples are given below.

Race, ethnicity and geography represent a major independent factor for studies on epidemiology of NIDDM and CVD. The following few examples illustrate this aspect. Asian Indians have a high risk for both diseases and exhibit insulin resistance, dyslipidemia, increased PAI-1 levels and reduced insulin-induced vasodilatation despite being apparently healthy [9]. Vascular reactivity is very different among various populations [10, 11]. African Americans have less MS but more CVD, but a subgroup of offsprings of diabetic patients has higher prevalence of MS [12]. The arginine metabolite ADMA, considered to play a role in deficient vascular reactivity,, exhibits similar plasma levels in caucasian and african women from South Africa but is linked to MS only in the Caucasians [13]. In Colombian men, however, no involvement of ADMA could be found [14].

Patient's clinical profiles can widely differ: thus, 37% of obese subjects have no MS, while 7% of normal weight subjects have it [15]. Moreover, almost a third of obese patients have no metabolic abnormalities [16]. A cross sectional study in a Turkish population revealed that while about 34% had both IR and MS (overlapping), another 43% had MS without IR, the remaining 23% being IR without MS [17]. Interestingly the risk for CVD was more than doubled in the latter subgroup, while the group with MS and no IR had very little risk.

Gender was shown to play a major role [18] which, moreover, impacts differently according to the age of the patients. Thus while men present more MS [19, 20], more women have MS and slight NIDDM [19]. The prevalence of IR and MS increases also just in parallel to ageing of a population [21, 22].

These few examples illustrate how difficult and hazardous comparisons within and between epidemiological or clinical studies can be, just because of the difficulty linked to recruiting comparable and homogeneous subject groups.

2.2. Techniques for Evaluating Vascular Reactivity or Insulin Resistance

2.2.1. Measuring Vascular Reactivity

Endothelial dysfunction (ED) has become the easiest way to evaluate the integrity of vascular reactivity in humans. More sophisticated techniques have regularly been developed as well as more local tests. However ED is also a heterogeneous, generic term covering differing techniques and protocols which have different meanings. While some are strictly relevant for large or for small vessels, others [most] give mixed informations on the reactivity of both vessel types [Kraemer, this book]. Contrary to initial expectations, the comparison of techniques used in humans reveal significant differences and, as such, deliver different informations [E.Bouskela, this book][23-26]. Vascular reactivity is also different in upper and lower limbs, arms showing usually higher vasodilatory reponses while legs show greater constriction [27,28].The absence of standardization of protocols [29] and differences between animals species and strains in preclinical studies [30] are further confounding factors. Finally, the very limited accessibility of the microcirculation in humans (mainly the skin) limits the strength of conclusions about data if one reminds that skin has a particular physiology and that skeletal muscle is the main tissue of interest for studies on insulin resistance.

2.2.2. Measuring Insulin Resistance

IR, on the other hand, is estimated by the HOMA-index (the simplest way) or by using sophisticated (eu- or hyperglycaemic) clamp techniques. Both parameters have serious limitations, however: 1) HOMA is calculated from fasting glucose and insulin levels and does not, therefore, reflect the dynamic changes of these factors over the day [ex: glucose intolerance]; moreover the index may be the same whether glucose or insulin is increased, despite a very different underlying pathology! 2) Clamp is usually performed at "euglycemic" glucose levels and very high insulin concentrations. This environment is physiologically irrelevant and introduces major artefacts such as sympathetic stimulation, increased bulk organ blood flow or activation of IGF-1 receptors to name a few. Since hepatic glucose production is blocked under these circumstances, the clamp procedure is eventually valid for comparing patients within a study but mostly unsuitable for mechanistic data interpretations. Alternatively the clamp is performed under hyperglycaemic conditions, which confronts the examinator to the problems linked to the peculiarities of intravenous glucose administration. Occasionally patients are investigated under so-called "isoglycemic" conditions, making comparisons between patients difficult because of their differing glucose levels.

Oral glucose tolerance test (OGTT) is widely used for evaluating glucose tolerance but is largely unphysiological in its classical form. Mixed meals are closer to the daily alimentary habits of patients but generate variable data both within and between patients.

These techniques, although having immensely augmented our knowledge of these pathologies, are nevertheless used "by default" due to the absence of better means and, accordingly their interpretation should be done with caution.

2.2.3. Skeletal Muscle Morphological and Functional Changes

Insulin resistance is considered to occur mostly in skeletal muscles and therefore the vast majority of studies on this parameter are directly or indirectly derived from this tissue. Skeletal muscles are composed of essentially three types of muscle fibers: highly oxidative, non oxidative and mixed fibers which can switch towards one of the other two subtypes under particular conditions. Illustrating the coupling between blood flow and metabolism, which permits fine adaptations of oxygen and nutrient delivery to local metabolic needs, the degree of fiber capillarization varies according to the fiber type: red fibers are surrounded by up to 8 capillaries, while white fibers can be surrounded by as little as 2-3 capillaries [31]. Reductions in absolute number of capillaries or in number of blood perfused capillaries will therefore limit nutrient supply, while an increase in muscle fiber diameter will increase the diffusion distances for incoming nutrients. It is thus easily understandable that changes in muscle fiber composition or size as well as in capillarization are direct confounding factors for microvascular or metabolic investigations. For evident reasons these morphological characteristics are little checked, despite the cardinal importance of this parameter! Indeed muscle fiber characteristics are linked to insulin sensitivity and glucose tolerance [32-34]. In NIDDM patients, the proportion of type 2b fibers is around 50% and capillary density is reduced [35, 36]. Importantly, increased number of type 2b fibers at the expense of oxidative fibers is seen in prediabetic, insulin resistant situations such as FDR [37], low birth weight [38], impaired glucose tolerance [39] or Turner syndrome [40]. Capillary rarefaction is also frequently reported in hypertension, even at very modest elevation in blood pressure [41].

Similarly, changes in skeletal muscle content of glucose transporters can be a factor strongly influencing insulin sensitivity measurements, even without functional defects in the capacity of remaining transporters. Thus IR could be a disease affecting a particular type of muscle, as has been suggested [42-44].

Ideally, thus, any study on microflow or glucose uptake in skeletal muscle should integrate a determination of muscle morphology to eliminate heavy confounding factors in the data interpretation…

3. PREDIABETES, DIABETES AND CARDIOVASCULAR DISEASES

3.1. Metabolic Syndrome/Insulin Resistance

Many studies have shown that subjects with MS and/or IR have an increased risk of developing NIDDM. Here again, however, the various definitions of MS used among studies show that differences in subject's profiles can be substantial. This comes from the integration-or not- of IR in the definitions, the number of parameters and the confounding factors described above. An illustrative example is found in a study on HIV-infected patients, where the absence of an increased waist/hip ratio prevents their classification as MS patients [45].The marked heterogeneity of these studies is increasingly recognized as a real problem and actually challenges even the notion of MS [46], even though all definitions capture the metabolic and vascular risks linked to MS [47-55].It is increasingly admitted that the simple components of the syndrome predict CVD as well as the various global MS definitions [56].

Despite the serious concerns linked to the definitions of MS, it is generally considered that IR is the main factor leading to CVD and NIDDM [3, 57]. In the study on the Turkish population, IR (+/-MS) was present in 57% of the metabolically abnormal population. One might add that other components of the MS may have synergistic effects with IR, explaining why the risk is highest if subjects present both IR and MS.

If one considers IR as the main cause of later diabetes and CVD, the question then is: "what is IR" ? One should recall here that IR is an observational definition, based on techniques to evaluate the efficacy of a given dose of insulin to stimulate glucose uptake by insulin sensitive tissues such as skeletal muscle and fat. The conclusions obtained from such studies are therefore quantitative but only indirectly qualitative and, therefore, explicative.

3.2. Cardiovascular Diseases

Prevalence of CVD is increased in MS, irrespective of MS definition [58]. A 15 year follow-up has confirmed the risk of CVD with a hazard ratio of 1.9, regardless of the presence of IGT or diabetes [59]. In men, the risk ratio is 2.88 for CVD [60]. In the general population IR is the prevalent predictor of CVD [61-63] and microalbuminuria (UAE>5μg/min) is another important associate of CVD, as strong as MS itself [64].

More data are available on MS subjects. Meta-analyzes clearly demonstrates the elevated risk, usually higher in women [65-67]. Each of the most used MS definitions capture this risk, which highlights its magnitude [56,68]. However a 13year follow-up in a Finnish population showed that MS is not more predictive than its individual components [56]. There are also different clusters of risk factors which generate variable risk ratio values [69]. Combined MS + ED further increase the risk, as shown in the recent NOMAS study [70]. It should however be pointed out that, in contrast to cardiac or cerebral vascular events, MS does not seem to predict peripheral vascular diseases in the absence of diabetes or microalbuminuria [71]. Individuals with MS present a high prevalence of subclinical atherosclerosis [72].

3.3. Searching for a Causal Common Denominator

Many mechanisms have been proposed to explain IR, from genetic to molecular biology, in the signalling pathways of the insulin receptor. It is, however, interesting to note that none of these individual mechanisms has been able to fully explain the phenomenon. Moreover, stimuli leading to IR by interfering with the defects are not common to all these subpopulations [see above]. Indeed not all subjects presenting with IR are overweight/obese, nor hyperlipidemic or hypertensive to name a few. Conversely all subjects being overweight/obese, dyslipidemic or hypertensive are not insulin resistant! From this simplistic view it appears that IR is not necessarily the only cause and that another [or other] factor[s] may be causally involved. Conceivably another parameter inherited or acquired and appearing very early in these subject's life, might be the trigger of IR and/or other metabolic parameters of MS; this parameter might, either per se or in combination with IR, lead to later development of diabetes and/or CVD.

It is unlikely that this hypothetical factor belongs to the actual list of parameters used to define MS. Assuming that a common denominator underlying this hypothesis exists; it should fulfil at least the following three criteria:

1. be common to a wide range of insulin resistant states
2. be present either before or concomitantly with IR, at very early stages of the metabolic disorder
3. be capable of inducing or aggravating IR or additional MS parameters

That vascular defect may underlie metabolic disorders characterizing prediabetes has been suggested at regular intervals [73-78]. The accumulation of supportive data in recent years has prompted us to propose, through this book, that **microcirculation** might be the factor we are looking for. In the following, therefore, we detail the arguments supporting this concept, in full awareness of the need for further proofs. In particular it will be shown that this relation between defects in nutritive blood flow and IR or MS parameters is at the least reciprocal.

4. PREDIABETES, DIABETES AND MICROCIRCULATION

A thorough look into the literature shows that microcirculation is indeed defective in prediabetic subjects. ED and IR are closely linked [79-81] and appear to function both ways [82, 83]. Because ED is only partly representative of microcirculation (see above), the examples described below are as good as possible focused on direct microvascular measurements in animals and humans, and preferentially on tests representing microcirculation rather than vessel reactivity in general.

4.1. Microvascular Defects are Present in IR/MS Situations

Metabolic Syndrome/Obesity

Nutritive perfusion is at the core of the metabolic effect of insulin since skeletal muscle stores glucose postprandially under the influence of the hormone. Defects in glucose and insulin delivery to muscle cells are therefore potential causes of downstream IR in the target tissue. The risk is higher in IGT than in IGT subjects because they exhibit more IR [84, 85]. Thus microvascular hyperemia to local skin heating was decreased in IGT and negatively correlated with insulin concentrations [86]. In a population "at risk", vasodilation to acetylcholine was blunted and endothelin levels increased if IGT was present; defective microvascular reactivity was related to systolic blood pressure, HDL cholesterol and HOMA-index [87].

In an animal model of MS, the fructose-fed rat, arteriolar damage was seen in the kidney [88]. In humans with MS a recent study showed abnormal microvascular reactivity while flow-mediated dilation (FMD) in the brachial artery was normal [89]. The ARIC study revealed that MS patients had retinal microangiopathy characterized by arteriolar narrowing and venular dilation [90], a finding conforted by the Funagata study in Japan [91]. ED is greater in MS and increases with each additional criterion of the ATP-III definition [92]. In pigs, obesity was accompanied by coronary ED and oxidative stress well before IR could be measured [93]. In obesity vasodilation to acetylcholine or insulin was blunted in skeletal muscles [94]. Defective capillary recruitment, a process which is cardinal for complete nutrient delivery, was reported in obese patients [95-97]. It is of interest to note that already adolescent, obese infants exhibit ED, with forearm blood flow responses correlating with IR [98]. Finally, blood viscosity and fibrinogen were increased in obese patients and also linked to IR [99]. The Framingham Offspring Study showed that obesity was associated with a prothrombotic state and impaired fibrinolysis [100]. Complete reviews of this question have recently appeared [Frisbee, this book][101-103]. Very importantly, it must be noted that several parameters of the microvascular physiology were abnormal in MS patients with normoglycemia [104].

Hypertension

Hypertension [HT] is another well-known insulin resistant pathology. THE VALSIM study showed that MS was linked to the prevalence of HT and high blood pressure was the most frequent MS component [105]. The hypothesis has been raised about HT being a microvascular disease [106]. In asymptomatic subjects with essential HT, reactive hyperemia was decreased [107]. The microvascular defect is not only manifested by reduced vasodilation but eventually reduced microcirculation as shown in mild HT and correlates with IR [108]. As will be seen later, this may have consequences! Another study failed to find this correlation but found fasting glycemia to be linked with reduced capillary density and blood flow velocity in capillaries [109]. This question has been recently reviewed [110].

To these frequent categories of patients we must add a large series of diseases which exhibit a high prevalence of IR.

Polycystic Ovary Syndrome

Many women with polycystic ovary syndrome (PCOS) are insulin resistant and this pathology is associated with increased cardiovascular risk [111-113]. Leg blood flow increases to insulin were impaired in PCOS patients [114].This population shows defective microvascular reactivity [115] and the defect was reported to occur very early in women with a normal metabolic profile [116]. This result has however not been confirmed in another study which advocated obesity as the determining factor [117]. PCOS is also associated with platelet and endothelial dysfunction in both lean and overweight patients [118] as well as with reduced fibrinolysis [119,120].

Sleep Disorders/ Sleep Apnea

Sleep disordered breathing (SDB), and more particularly obstructive sleep apnea (OSA) is an extremely common complication [121] which has long been considered as a passive consequence of overweight/obesity. The Sleep Heart Health Study has shown the correlation between repeated hypoxemia (due to OSA) and impaired glucose tolerance, independently of age, gender, BMI or waist circumference [122]. Recent investigations, however, point to a bidirectional relationship between vascular abnormalities and IR [123,124]. Indeed SBD can induce IR independently of obesity [125-127]. Thus there seems to exist a reciprocal and causal link between IR and SDB [128,129]. Fat diet in rats also causes OSA [130]. Patients affected by OSA, even children [131] develop CVD [132]. In mild HT the presence of OSA increases microvascular impairment [133]. Increased OSA is found in PCOS patients [134] and considered now as novel risk factor for MS [135]. Abdominal fat is involved and could be the source of inflammatory factors impacting on the vascular bed. Chronic sympathetic stimulation, inflammation and oxidative stress, generated by repeated posthypoxic reoxygenation episodes are likely factors impairing vascular reactivity [136-138]. Very interestingly simulation of this phenomenon by submitting rats to repetitive hypoxia leads to IR and microvascular abnormalities and might therefore represent a good model to study more in depth the relations between microvascular disturbances and IR [139-141]. Histological studies showed increased capillarization in tibialis anterior muscles, probably as a reactive tentative to compensate for the reduction in aerobic capacity [142]. In soft palate muscles, which are involved in snoring and OSA, capillarization was reduced, however [143]. Defects linked to OSA are not improved by blockade of the autonomic nervous system [144] and IR is not improved even by an intensive use of CPAP masks, despite a decrease in glycated haemoglobin [145]. SDB is in our opinion a very interesting situation to further elucidate how they are linked to IR and we have indeed hypothesized that microcirculation might be the linker [124].

Hepatic Steatosis

Metabolic changes in liver constitute a group of complications termed NAFLD, comprising non-alcoholic steatosis (NASH), whose prevalence is extremely high and seems strongly associated with IR, MS and NIDDM [146]. It is considered as a very early manifestation of IR and it was found that 80% of patients with NASH are insulin resistant while 68% had MS [147-149]. Elevated hepatic enzymes (GGT, ALT) are strong predictors of MS [150]. These patients are at elevated risk of developing CVD [151-153], since the liver liberates proatherogenic and inflammatory factors [154]. Fatty liver disease is linked to deficient hepatic microcirculation, forming a local vicious circle [155].

Acromegaly

Acromegaly is often accompanied by hyperinsulinemia, hypertension and IR [156]. These patients have early vascular modifications, in particular increased arterial stiffness and reduced flow-mediated blood flow; intima media thickness defects are not improved by curing the disease [157]. Reduced endothelium-dependent vasodilatation accompanies increased sympathetic vasoconstriction [158] and heterogeneous distribution of cardiac output is found in acromegalics [159]. Increased fibrinogen, tPA and PAI-1 also reflect a hypofibrinolytic state [160].

Iron Overload Diseases

Hereditary hemochromatosis patients have a high prevalence of abnormal glucose homeostasis and diabetes. Those with hypercholesterolemia and glucose intolerance have decreased insulin secretion responses but increased insulin sensitivity [161]. In this population impaired endothelial function and increased intima media thickness can be improved by iron depletion [162,163].

In beta-thalassemia [but not in thalassemia intermedia] abnormal glucose tolerance and persistent IR are common [164,165]. Acquired hypothyroidism may add to this situation [166]. In these patients markers of endothelial activation are elevated and activated blood cells may cause disturbances through the vascular bed [167]. Enhanced levels of von Willebrand factor [vWF] and adhesion molecules reflect endothelial injury, which could be involved in altered renal function manifested here as tubulointerstitial injury [158].

Hyperferritinemia in middle-aged men is characterized by a high rate of MS and ferritin levels appear to be positively associated with IR [169]. This was also concluded from an epidemiological study [170].

HIV Infection

AIDS is another disease where many patients exhibit IR and hyperlipidemia. Many patients have at least 2 components of MS and NIDDM prevalence is high among these individuals [45]. Treatment with antiretroviral agents was shown to aggravate IR, leading to glucose intolerance and diabetes [171,172]. ED was massively caused by Indinavir therapy [173] but it has recently been reported that newer agents like Atazanavir or Lopinavir might not cause ED, thereby potentially eliminating the superimposed risk [174]. Reactive hyperemia was also reduced [175]. A review on endothelial dysfunction in HIV infection can be found [176]. The hemorheological abnormalities [177] can also be seen in HIV patient's retina, where increased red cell aggregation and leucocyte rigidity underlie reductions in microvascular blood flow [178]. However, in the skin capillary perfusion has been reported to be increased [179]. Finally HIV-1Tat is able to activate apoptosis of microvascular endothelial cells [180].

Thyroid Disorders

Disorders of the thyroid function are intrinsically associated with both vascular and metabolic disturbances [181,182]. In subjects with hypothyroidism TSH levels correlated inversely with endothelium-dependent vasodilation, even in those with "high normal "values [183]. In addition to reduced vasodilation, a decrease in constrictory vessel reaction to sympathetic agonists was also noted [184].

Alzheimer Disease

Alzheimer disease is linked to MS, possibly involving a vascular component [185,186]. Interestingly, increases in insulin concentrations to levels found in IR stimulates the formation of beta-amyloid and inflammatory factors [185]. In contrast to Binswanger disease, cortical microvasculature exhibits morphological abnormalities such as reduced density and narrowing in Alzheimer brains [187]. The [(beta (4)25-35) protein induces vasoconstriction and antivasodilating effects in microvessels [188]. Thrombocytic microangiopathy has also been described [189]. Blood rheology is clearly modified already at early stages of Alzheimer disease, possibly as a consequence of exaggerated oxidative stress [190].

Hyperdynamic Circulation

Hyperdynamic circulation is a situation where heart rate, pulse wave velocity (PWV) and arterial stiffness are increased, frequently because of increased intima media thickness [191,192]. Epidemiological studies show that many patients with MS have increased IMT [193]. Elevated PWV is independently correlated with MS [194-197]. Normally acute insulin elevations in blood such as during postmeal counterbalance the augmentation index and this is apparently blunted in IR [199,200]. Very interestingly, ED, increased intima/media thickness and increased stiffness are found independently in FDRs of diabetic patients [200]. Hyperdynamic circulation is closely linked to several indices of MS and predicts diabetes [201]. Offsprings of parents with hyperdynamic circulation have higher BMI, skinfold thickness and waist/hip ratio as well as accelerated heart rate [202]. In adolescents [the Bogalusa Heart Study] hyperdynamic circulation was associated with triglycerides and IR in boys, independently of age, race and obesity, supporting the concept of an inherited defect [203].

Heart and Brain Infarction

Postinfarction: postischemic states are frequently characterized by peripheral motor disturbances of either neurologic or vascular origin. Microcirculation plays a prominent role in the immediate postischemic recirculation of infracted tissues [204,205] and largely determines survival or long term damaging consequences. The prevalence of IR was as high as 61% in chronic heart failure (CHF) patients [206]. In non diabetics with acute myocardial infarction, IR at 4 months correlated with leptin levels and contributed to later restenosis [207]. Survivors of a first myocardial infarction have a two (men)- to fivefold (women) increase in risk of developing NIDDM within the following 5 years [208]. In rats the resting diameter of A3 and A4 was reduced after experimental myocardial infarction and dilation to adenosine was attenuated: electrical stimulation of skeletal muscle corrected the basal modification but not the microvascular reactivity [209]. The proportion of capillaries containing red cells was reduced in the spinotrapezius muscles of CHF rats [210]. Capillary involutions were reported in plantaris (white) but not in soleus (red) muscle of CHF rats [211] as was capillary rarefaction in CHF rabbits [212]. On the other hand reduced levels of antioxidants and increases in iNOS and nNOS were found in soleus but not in white muscle. In humans with CHF, forearm blood flow (large vessels) was the highest in those patients having high insulin and IR, which might indicate an imbalance in the regulation between large and small vessel vasomotricity [213].

Stroke patients frequently present hemiparesis and abnormal glucose metabolism is extremely high over 3 years poststroke [214]. In these patients capillarization is decreased in hemiparetic muscles, to an extent similar to non-stroke subjects with impaired glucose tolerance and capillary density correlates inversely with the 120min glucose levels after OGTT [215].

Varia

Finally, one should cite some less frequent diseases which show similar characteristics. Behçet disease is associated with IR [216] and structural modifications (microaneurysms, megacapillaries, loops) are present in the microvasculature [217]. In Lupus erythematosus, prevalence of MS is high [218] and particularly associated with high levels of oxidized LDL. Arterial stiffness, intima media thickness and early atherosclerosis are also reported [219]. Gout is also associated with increased prevalence of MS [220].

4.2. Microvascular Defects are Present in "At Risk" Subjects

Here we define subjects "at risk" as those who have inherited risk factors by their genetic background or acquired these factors early in life such as during pregnancy.

In spontaneously hypertensive rats the dilating response to insulin was already blunted in 5 week old animals, i.e. before HT was measurable [221].

First degree relatives (FDRs), also termed offsprings, of diabetic parents are a well-known population presenting IR and elevated risk of developing NIDDM and/or CVD even in young lean individuals [222]. Familial history of diabetes is indeed a major determinant of ED in offsprings [223] as well as maternal BMI and low physical activity [224]. These subjects may appear perfectly healthy for decades, however. Nevertheless clinical investigations show abnormal responses in ED [200,225] or more so in specific microvascular measurements [226]. Forearm blood flow increase is impaired while the M value, an indicator of peripheral insulin resistance, is reduced [227,228]. The reduced microvascular dilating capacity is correlated with IR and very particularly to PAI-1, which is increased in these individuals [229,230]. In the Framingham Offspring Study, FDRs exhibited reductions in flow-mediated dilation and reactive hyperemia, signs of defective microvascular reactivity. 51% had subclinical atherosclerosis [72]; obese offsprings have also abnormal hemostasis [100]. Low grade inflammation represents another possible cause [231,232]. Offsprings of parents with only MS have high values of TNFα and low HDL, two major cardiovascular risk factors [233]. FDRs of diabetic parents have also elevated TNFα [234]. Interestingly familial history of obesity is only weakly associated with MS in FDRs [235][236], in contrast to history of HT or diabetes. Offsprings of hypertensive parents are more IR [237] and a recent study has even suggested that MS was associated with familial history of CVD but not of diabetes! [238]. Genetic mutations in eNOS have been identified, which could partly explain the defects in vascular reactivity; they are linked to IR and intima media thickness [IMT], even in non-diabetic subjects [239,240]. Similar data exist for EDHF, the equivalent of NO in the tiniest vessels [241].

Finally this population exhibits a clustering of fibrinolytic risk factors [242]. Arterial stiffness, IMT and accelerated heart arte with increased pulse wave velocity (PWV) are closely associated with IR and MS [200,243,244]. Offsprings with increased carotid-femoral PWV show blunted microvascular reactivity, in excess of changes in conventional CV risk factors including HT [245]. Even offsprings of only one parent with HT show increased PWV [246]. The Tecumseh Offspring Study showed that parental hyperdynamic circulation predicted IR in FDRs.

Fetal growth is linked to metabolic and vascular disorders in adult life [247], more particularly if fast postnatal growth is promoted ['catch-up growth'] [248,249]. A 32 year follow-up in Sweden showed the inverse relationship between birth weight and diabetes incidence [250]. In children 2-47months of age, percent body fat is higher at any weight in small for gestational age (SGA)-born individuals [251]. In young overweight children, SGA adds to the risk to develop MS [252]. In 9 year old children increased arterial stiffness has been observed [253]. Offspring birth weight is inversely correlated to CVD mortality in their parents [254], as well as with their fasting insulinemia and heart rate [4]. In SGA children ED is present and the microvascular dilation was found abnormal as early as 3 months of age [255]. Even at 3days after delivery acetylcholine-mediated vasodilation was reduced [256].

Gestational diabetes (GDM) is frequently associated with later development of glucose intolerance [257], MS [258,259], NIDDM [260] and CVD; this is not only occurring in mothers but also in their children [261-263]. A twofold increase in risk of GDM is itself related to maternal low birth weight [264]. Increased arterial stiffness and reduced vasodilation to acetylcholine or to heat [265,266] are observed. Defects in maximal microvascular hyperaemic response are reported, which are not explained by aspects of ED determined by the other techniques, supporting the concept of specific disturbances in the microvasculature, adding to those found in larger vessels [267]. Elevated CRP and PAI-1 levels as well as increased conduit vessel stiffness are also described [268]. In this pathology ADMA has been suggested to be more particularly involved, since blood ADMA levels were related to the progressive deterioration of glucose tolerance after 3years following GDM [263,269]. Offsprings of GDM mothers have a higher prevalence of MS, whether large or small for gestational age [262,270].

Preeclampsia is another complication of pregnancy. Women with a history of preeclampsia develop a reduced sensitivity to insulin and a MS profile [271,272]. These patients are indeed at higher risk for developing CVD [273-275]. Endothelium-dependent microvascular reactivity is paradoxically increased, albeit reflecting an abnormal endothelial function [276].

4.3. The Link in Healthy Populations

Submitting healthy animals or persons to physical inactivity very rapidly leads to vascular and metabolic disturbances. In rats it increases in vascular NADPH oxidase, production of reactive oxygen species, reductions in citrate synthase as well as to ED and atherosclerosis [277,278]. In humans physical inactivity in healthy volunteers leads to IR and microvascular dysfunction as early as day 3, i.e. at times when neither inflammation nor conduit artery changes could be observed [279]. This important result suggests that both IR and microvascular defects are rapidly developing processes which occur concomitantly.

Moreover it is fascinating to observe that even under resting conditions in healthy young people, direct visualization of microvessels by skin videomicroscopy revealed an association between the capacity of the microvascular bed to recruit additional capillaries on the one hand and insulin sensitivity within the physiological range on the other hand. Microvascular function was strongly related to both, suggesting a bridging role [280].

5. CONCLUSION

In conclusion, a thorough analysis of the literature reveals that , without any doubt, insulin resistance and microvascular dysfunction are closely and systematically correlated as shown in most various clinical situations of IR or MS (Table 1). Despite the relatively low number of investigations, it is evident that microvascular abnormalities are seen very early, before other components of the MS are increased. Moreover several interesting clinical situations show that they can be observed without the presence of concomitant, traditional MS components. Thus, this connection between microcirculation and insulin sensitivity is probably intrinsic. It is puzzling that microvascular disorders are found in all these various situations linked to CVDs and/or diabetes later in life, which inevitably raises the crucial question of reciprocity and causality. In the next paragraphs we will analyze how insulin itself is involved in microcirculation and address this cardinal question as to whether abnormalities in microvascular reactivity and nutritive flow distribution can generate or aggravate IR and, if so, by which mechanisms.

Subjects/Patients	INS-RES/MS	μ VASC DYSF
Obesity	+	+
Hypertension	+	+
Hyperdynamic circulation (PWV)	+	+
Gestational diabetes	+	+
Preeclampsia	+	+
Obstructive sleep apnea	+	+
Low birth weight (SGA)	+	+
Acromegaly	+	+
PCOS	+	+
Thyroid disorders	+	+
NASH	+	+
Thalassemia	+	+
Chronic heart failure	+	+
Post MI/post stroke	+	+
Hemochromatosis	+	+
HIV	+	+
Offspring of T2DM	+	+
Offspring of HT	+	+
Offspring of hyperdynamic circulation	+	+
Offspring of peripheral vascular disease	+	+
Beyçet disease	+	+

6. REFERENCES

[1]   Narayan KM, Boyle JP, Thompson TJ, Sorensen SW, Williamson DF. Lifetime risk for diabetes mellitus in the United States. JAMA 2003 Oct 8; 290(14): 1884-90.

[2]   Ford ES, Li C, Sattar N. Metabolic syndrome and incident diabetes: current state of the evidence. Diabetes Care 2008 Sep; 31(9): 1898-904.

[3]   Meigs JB, Rutter MK, Sullivan LM, Fox CS, D'Agostino RB, Sr., Wilson PW. Impact of insulin resistance on risk of type 2 diabetes and cardiovascular disease in people with metabolic syndrome. Diabetes Care 2007 May; 30(5): 12 19-25.

[4]   Stern MP. Diabetes and cardiovascular disease. The "common soil" hypothesis. Diabetes 1995 Apr; 44(4): 369-74.

[5]   Jarrett RJ. The cardiovascular risk associated with impaired glucose tolerance. Diabet Med 1996; 13(3 Suppl 2): S15-9.

[6]   Ardern CI, Janssen I. Metabolic syndrome and its association with morbidity and mortality. Appl Physiol Nutr Metab 2007 Feb; 32(1): 33-45.

[7]   Razzouk L, Muntner P. Ethnic, gender, and age-related differences in patients with the metabolic syndrome. Curr Hypertens Rep 2009 Apr; 11(2): 127-32.

[8]   Kahn R, Buse J, Ferrannini E, Stern M. The metabolic syndrome: time for a critical appraisal: joint statement from the American Diabetes Association and the European Association for the Study of Diabetes. Diabetes Care 2005 Sep; 28(9): 2289-304.

[9]   Raji A, Gerhard-Herman MD, Warren M, Silverman SG, Raptopoulos V, Mantzoros CS, *et al.* Insulin resistance and vascular dysfunction in nondiabetic Asian Indians. J Clin Endocrinol Metab 2004 Aug; 89(8): 3965-72.

[10]   Lteif AA, Han K, Mather KJ. Obesity, insulin resistance, and the metabolic syndrome: determinants of endothelial dysfunction in whites and blacks. Circulation 2005 Jul 5; 112(1): 32-8.

[11]   Sumner AE. The relationship of body fat to metabolic disease: influence of sex and ethnicity. Gend Med 2008 Dec; 5(4): 361-71.

[12]   Meis SB, Schuster D, Gaillard T, Osei K. Metabolic syndrome in nondiabetic, obese, first-degree relatives of African American patients with type 2 diabetes: African American triglycerides-HDL-C and insulin resistance paradox. Ethn Dis 2006 Autumn; 16(4): 830-6.

[13]   Reimann M, Schutte AE, Malan NT, Schwarz PE, Benndorf RA, Schulze F, *et al.* Asymmetric dimethylarginine is associated with parameters of glucose metabolism in Caucasian but not in African women from South Africa. Exp Clin Endocrinol Diabetes 2007 Oct; 115(9): 600-5.

[14]   Garcia RG, Perez M, Maas R, Schwedhelm E, Boger RH, Lopez-Jaramillo P. Plasma concentrations of asymmetric dimethylarginine (ADMA) in metabolic syndrome. Int J Cardiol 2007 Nov 15; 122(2): 176-8.

[15]   Meigs JB, Wilson PW, Fox CS, Vasan RS, Nathan DM, Sullivan LM, *et al.* Body mass index, metabolic syndrome, and risk of type 2 diabetes or cardiovascular disease. J Clin Endocrinol Metab 2006 Aug; 91(8): 2906-12.

[16]   Mikhail N. The metabolic syndrome: insulin resistance. Curr Hypertens Rep 2009 Apr; 11(2): 156-8.

[17]   Onat A, Hergenc G, Turkmen S, Yazici M, Sari I, Can G. Discordance between insulin resistance and metabolic syndrome: features and associated cardiovascular risk in adults with normal glucose regulation. Metabolism 2006 Apr; 55(4): 445-52.

[18]   Sandberg K. The metabolic syndrome: racist, sexist, or both? Gend Med 2008 Dec; 5(4): 372-3.

[19]   Hunt KJ, Williams K, Hazuda HP, Stern MP, Haffner SM. The metabolic syndrome and the impact of diabetes on coronary heart disease mortality in women and men: the San Antonio Heart Study. Ann Epidemiol 2007 Nov; 17(11): 870-7.

[20]   Regitz-Zagrosek V, Lehmkuhl E, Mahmoodzadeh S. Gender aspects of the role of the metabolic syndrome as a risk factor for cardiovascular disease. Gend Med 2007; 4 Suppl B: S162-77.

[21]   Skilton MR, Lai NT, Griffiths KA, Molyneaux LM, Yue DK, Sullivan DR, *et al.* Meal-related increases in vascular reactivity are impaired in older and diabetic adults: insights into roles of aging and insulin in vascular flow. Am J Physiol Heart Circ Physiol 2005 Mar; 288(3): H1404-10.

[22]   Wendelhag I, Fagerberg B, Hulthe J, Bokemark L, Wikstrand J. Endothelium-dependent flow-mediated vasodilatation, insulin resistance and the metabolic syndrome in 60-year-old men. J Intern Med 2002 Oct; 252(4): 305-13.

[23]   Wright CI, Scholten HJ, Schilder JC, Elsen BM, Hanselaar W, Kroner CI, *et al.* Arterial stiffness, endothelial function and microcirculatory reactivity in healthy young males. Clin Physiol Funct Imaging 2008 Sep; 28(5): 299-306.

[24]   Wiernsperger N. Defects in microvascular haemodynamics during prediabetes: contributor or epiphenomenon? Diabetologia 2000 Nov; 43(11): 1439-48.

[25]   Ghiadoni L, Versari D, Giannarelli C, Faita F, Taddei S. Non-invasive diagnostic tools for investigating endothelial dysfunction. Curr Pharm Des 2008; 14(35): 3715-22.

[26]   Muniyappa R, Lee S, Chen H, Quon MJ. Current approaches for assessing insulin sensitivity and resistance in vivo: advantages, limitations, and appropriate usage. Am J Physiol Endocrinol Metab 2008 Jan; 294(1): E15-26.

[27]   Lott ME, Hogeman C, Herr M, Bhagat M, Kunselman A, Sinoway LI. Vasoconstrictor responses in the upper and lower limbs to increases in transmural pressure. J Appl Physiol 2009 Jan; 106(1): 302-10.

[28]   Proctor DN, Newcomer SC. Is there a difference in vascular reactivity of the arms and legs? Med Sci Sports Exerc 2006 Oct; 38(10): 18 19-28.

[29]   Turner J, Belch JJ, Khan F. Current concepts in assessment of microvascular endothelial function using laser Doppler imaging and iontophoresis. Trends Cardiovasc Med 2008 May; 18(4): 109-16.

[30]   Mather K. Surrogate measures of insulin resistance: of rats, mice, and men. Am J Physiol Endocrinol Metab 2009 Feb; 296(2): E398-9.

[31]   Gray SD, Renkin EM, Mangseth G. Distribution of capillaries to fibers of different types in mixed muscle. Bibl Anat 1977(15 Pt 1): 535-8.

[32]   Lillioja S, Young AA, Culter CL, Ivy JL, Abbott WG, Zawadzki JK, *et al.* Skeletal muscle capillary density and fiber type are possible determinants of in vivo insulin resistance in man. J Clin Invest 1987 Aug; 80(2): 415-24.

[33]   Hernandez N, Torres SH, Vera O, De Sanctis JB, Flores E. Muscle fiber composition and capillarization in relation to metabolic alterations in hypertensive men. J Med 2001; 32(1-2): 67-82.

[34]   Lithell H, Lindgarde F, Hellsing K, Lundqvist G, Nygaard E, Vessby B, *et al.* Body weight, skeletal muscle morphology, and enzyme activities in relation to fasting serum insulin concentration and glucose tolerance in 48-year-old men. Diabetes 1981 Jan; 30(1): 19-25.

[35]   Marin P, Andersson B, Krotkiewski M, Bjorntorp P. Muscle fiber composition and capillary density in women and men with NIDDM. Diabetes Care 1994 May; 17(5): 382-6.

[36]   Oberbach A, Bossenz Y, Lehmann S, Niebauer J, Adams V, Paschke R, *et al.* Altered fiber distribution and fiber-specific glycolytic and oxidative enzyme activity in skeletal muscle of patients with type 2 diabetes. Diabetes Care 2006 Apr; 29(4): 895-900.

[37] Nyholm B, Qu Z, Kaal A, Pedersen SB, Gravholt CH, Andersen JL, *et al.* Evidence of an increased number of type IIb muscle fibers in insulin-resistant first-degree relatives of patients with NIDDM. Diabetes 1997 Nov; 46(11): 1822-8.

[38] Jensen CB, Storgaard H, Madsbad S, Richter EA, Vaag AA. Altered skeletal muscle fiber composition and size precede whole-body insulin resistance in young men with low birth weight. J Clin Endocrinol Metab 2007 Apr; 92(4): 1530-4.

[39] Toft I, Bonaa KH, Lindal S, Jenssen T. Insulin kinetics, insulin action, and muscle morphology in lean or slightly overweight persons with impaired glucose tolerance. Metabolism 1998 Jul; 47(7): 848-54.

[40] Gravholt CH, Nyholm B, Saltin B, Schmitz O, Christiansen JS. Muscle fiber composition and capillary density in Turner syndrome: evidence of increased muscle fiber size related to insulin resistance. Diabetes Care 2001 Sep; 24(9): 1668-73.

[41] Cheng C, Daskalakis C, Falkner B. Capillary rarefaction in treated and untreated hypertensive subjects. Ther Adv Cardiovasc Dis 2008 Apr; 2(2): 79-88.

[42] Gaster M, Staehr P, Beck-Nielsen H, Schroder HD, Handberg A. GLUT4 is reduced in slow muscle fibers of type 2 diabetic patients: is insulin resistance in type 2 diabetes a slow, type 1 fiber disease? Diabetes 2001 Jun; 50(6): 1324-9.

[43] Halseth AE, Bracy DP, Wasserman DH. Functional limitations to glucose uptake in muscles comprised of different fiber types. Am J Physiol Endocrinol Metab 2001 Jun; 280(6): E994-9.

[44] Rush JW, Green HJ, Maclean DA, Code LM. Oxidative stress and nitric oxide synthase in skeletal muscles of rats with post-infarction, compensated chronic heart failure. Acta Physiol Scand 2005 Nov; 185(3): 211-8.

[45] Samaras K, Wand H, Law M, Emery S, Cooper D, Carr A. Prevalence of metabolic syndrome in HIV-infected patients receiving highly active antiretroviral therapy using International Diabetes Foundation and Adult Treatment Panel III criteria: associations with insulin resistance, disturbed body fat compartmentalization, elevated C-reactive protein, and [corrected] hypoadiponectinemia. Diabetes Care 2007 Jan; 30(1): 113-9.

[46] Cameron AJ, Zimmet PZ, Shaw JE, Alberti KG. The metabolic syndrome: in need of a global mission statement. Diabet Med 2009 Mar; 26(3): 306-9.

[47] de Simone G, Devereux RB, Chinali M, Best LG, Lee ET, Galloway JM, *et al.* Prognostic impact of metabolic syndrome by different definitions in a population with high prevalence of obesity and diabetes: the Strong Heart Study. Diabetes Care 2007 Jul; 30(7): 1851-6.

[48] de Zeeuw D, Bakker SJ. Does the metabolic syndrome add to the diagnosis and treatment of cardiovascular disease? Nat Clin Pract Cardiovasc Med 2008 Jul; 5 Suppl 1: S10-4.

[49] Daskalopoulou SS, Athyros VG, Kolovou GD, Anagnostopoulou KK, Mikhailidis DP. Definitions of metabolic syndrome: Where are we now? Curr Vasc Pharmacol 2006 Jul; 4(3): 185-97.

[50] Day C. Metabolic syndrome, or What you will: definitions and epidemiology. Diab Vasc Dis Res 2007 Mar; 4(1): 32-8.

[51] Ferrannini E, Iozzo P. Is insulin resistance atherogenic? A review of the evidence. Atheroscler Suppl 2006 Aug; 7(4): 5-10.

[52] Carlsson AC, Wandell PE, Halldin M, de Faire U, Hellenius ML. Is a Unified Definition of Metabolic Syndrome Needed? Comparison of Three Definitions of Metabolic Syndrome in 60-Year-Old Men and Women. Metab Syndr Relat Disord 2009 Mar 14.

[53] Li WJ, Xue H, Sun K, Song XD, Wang YB, Zhen YS, *et al.* Cardiovascular risk and prevalence of metabolic syndrome by differing criteria. Chin Med J (Engl) 2008 Aug 20; 121(16): 1532-6.

[54] Nilsson PM, Engstrom G, Hedblad B. The metabolic syndrome and incidence of cardiovascular disease in non-diabetic subjects--a population-based study comparing three different definitions. Diabet Med 2007 May; 24(5): 464-72.

[55] Yudkin JS. Insulin resistance and the metabolic syndrome--or the pitfalls of epidemiology. Diabetologia 2007 Aug; 50(8): 1576-86.

[56] Wang J, Ruotsalainen S, Moilanen L, Lepisto P, Laakso M, Kuusisto J. The metabolic syndrome predicts cardiovascular mortality: a 13-year follow-up study in elderly non-diabetic Finns. Eur Heart J 2007 Apr; 28(7): 857-64.

[57] Rutter MK, Meigs JB, Sullivan LM, D'Agostino RB, Sr., Wilson PW. Insulin resistance, the metabolic syndrome, and incident cardiovascular events in the Framingham Offspring Study. Diabetes 2005 Nov; 54(11): 3252-7.

[58] Athyros VG, Ganotakis ES, Elisaf MS, Liberopoulos EN, Goudevenos IA, Karagiannis A. Prevalence of vascular disease in metabolic syndrome using three proposed definitions. Int J Cardiol 2007 Apr 25; 117(2): 204-10.

[59] Noto D, Barbagallo CM, Cefalu AB, Falletta A, Sapienza M, Cavera G, *et al.* The metabolic syndrome predicts cardiovascular events in subjects with normal fasting glucose: results of a 15 years follow-up in a Mediterranean population. Atherosclerosis 2008 Mar; 197(1): 147-53.

[60] Wilson PW, D'Agostino RB, Parise H, Sullivan L, Meigs JB. Metabolic syndrome as a precursor of cardiovascular disease and type 2 diabetes mellitus. Circulation 2005 Nov 15; 112(20): 3066-72.

[61] Deveci E, Yesil M, Akinci B, Yesil S, Postaci N, Arikan E, *et al.* Evaluation of insulin resistance in normoglycemic patients with coronary artery disease. Clin Cardiol 2009 Jan; 32(1): 32-6.

[62]   Bonora E, Kiechl S, Willeit J, Oberhollenzer F, Egger G, Meigs JB, *et al.* Insulin resistance as estimated by homeostasis model assessment predicts incident symptomatic cardiovascular disease in caucasian subjects from the general population: the Bruneck study. Diabetes Care 2007 Feb; 30(2): 318-24.

[63]   Ford ES. Risks for all-cause mortality, cardiovascular disease, and diabetes associated with the metabolic syndrome: a summary of the evidence. Diabetes Care 2005 Jul; 28(7): 1769-78.

[64]   Klausen KP, Parving HH, Scharling H, Jensen JS. The association between metabolic syndrome, microalbuminuria and impaired renal function in the general population: impact on cardiovascular disease and mortality. J Intern Med 2007 Oct; 262(4): 470-8.

[65]   Galassi A, Reynolds K, He J. Metabolic syndrome and risk of cardiovascular disease: a meta-analysis. Am J Med 2006 Oct; 1 19(10): 812-9.

[66]   Gami AS, Witt BJ, Howard DE, Erwin PJ, Gami LA, Somers VK, *et al.* Metabolic syndrome and risk of incident cardiovascular events and death: a systematic review and meta-analysis of longitudinal studies. J Am Coll Cardiol 2007 Jan 30; 49(4): 403-14.

[67]   Hoang KC, Ghandehari H, Lopez VA, Barboza MG, Wong ND. Global coronary heart disease risk assessment of individuals with the metabolic syndrome in the U.S. Diabetes Care 2008 Jul; 31(7): 1405-9.

[68]   Qiao Q, Laatikainen T, Zethelius B, Stegmayr B, Eliasson M, Jousilahti P, *et al.* Comparison of definitions of metabolic syndrome in relation to the risk of developing stroke and coronary heart disease in Finnish and Swedish cohorts. Stroke 2009 Feb; 40(2): 337-43.

[69]   Hong D, Jaron D, Buerk DG, Barbee KA. Heterogeneous response of microvascular endothelial cells to shear stress. Am J Physiol Heart Circ Physiol 2006 Jun; 290(6): H2498-508.

[70]   Suzuki T, Hirata K, Elkind MS, Jin Z, Rundek T, Miyake Y, *et al.* Metabolic syndrome, endothelial dysfunction, and risk of cardiovascular events: the Northern Manhattan Study (NOMAS). Am Heart J 2008 Aug; 156(2): 405-10.

[71]   Wang J, Ruotsalainen S, Moilanen L, Lepisto P, Laakso M, Kuusisto J. Metabolic syndrome and incident end-stage peripheral vascular disease: a 14-year follow-up study in elderly Finns. Diabetes Care 2007 Dec; 30(12): 3099-104.

[72]   Ingelsson E, Sullivan LM, Murabito JM, Fox CS, Benjamin EJ, Polak JF, *et al.* Prevalence and prognostic impact of subclinical cardiovascular disease in individuals with the metabolic syndrome and diabetes. Diabetes 2007 Jun; 56(6): 1718-26.

[73]   Ganrot PO, Curman B, Kron B. Type 2 diabetes. Primary vascular disorder with metabolic symptoms? Med Hypotheses 1987 Sep; 24(1): 77-86.

[74]   Egan BM. Neurohumoral, hemodynamic and microvascular changes as mechanisms of insulin resistance in hypertension: a provocative but partial picture. Int J Obes 1991 Sep; 15 Suppl 2: 133-9.

[75]   Baron AD. Insulin and the vasculature--old actors, new roles. J Investig Med 1996 Oct; 44(8): 406-12.

[76]   Shoemaker JK, Bonen A. Vascular actions of insulin in health and disease. Can J Appl Physiol 1995 Jun; 20(2): 127-54.

[77]   Serne EH, de Jongh RT, Eringa EC, RG IJ, Stehouwer CD. Microvascular dysfunction: a potential pathophysiological role in the metabolic syndrome. Hypertension 2007 Jul; 50(1): 204-11.

[78]   Cleland SJ, Petrie JR, Ueda S, Elliott HL, Connell JM. Insulin as a vascular hormone: implications for the pathophysiology of cardiovascular disease. Clin Exp Pharmacol Physiol 1998 Mar-Apr; 25(3-4): 175-84.

[79]   Kearney MT, Duncan ER, Kahn M, Wheatcroft SB. Insulin resistance and endothelial cell dysfunction: studies in mammalian models. Exp Physiol 2008 Jan; 93(1): 158-63.

[80]   Cersosimo E, DeFronzo RA. Insulin resistance and endothelial dysfunction: the road map to cardiovascular diseases. Diabetes Metab Res Rev 2006 Nov-Dec; 22(6): 423-36.

[81]   Jansson PA. Endothelial dysfunction in insulin resistance and type 2 diabetes. J Intern Med 2007 Aug; 262(2): 173-83.

[82]   Han SH, Quon MJ, Koh KK. Reciprocal relationships between abnormal metabolic parameters and endothelial dysfunction. Curr Opin Lipidol 2007 Feb; 18(1): 58-65.

[83]   Kim JA, Montagnani M, Koh KK, Quon MJ. Reciprocal relationships between insulin resistance and endothelial dysfunction: molecular and pathophysiological mechanisms. Circulation 2006 Apr 18; 113(15): 1888-904.

[84]   Festa A, D'Agostino R, Jr., Hanley AJ, Karter AJ, Saad MF, Haffner SM. Differences in insulin resistance in nondiabetic subjects with isolated impaired glucose tolerance or isolated impaired fasting glucose. Diabetes 2004 Jun; 53(6): 1549-55.

[85]   Miyazaki Y, Akasaka H, Ohnishi H, Saitoh S, DeFronzo RA, Shimamoto K. Differences in insulin action and secretion, plasma lipids and blood pressure levels between impaired fasting glucose and impaired glucose tolerance in Japanese subjects. Hypertens Res 2008 Jul; 31(7): 1357-63.

[86]   Jaap AJ, Shore AC, Tooke JE. Relationship of insulin resistance to microvascular dysfunction in subjects with fasting hyperglycaemia. Diabetologia 1997 Feb; 40(2): 238-43.

[87]   Caballero AE, Arora S, Saouaf R, Lim SC, Smakowski P, Park JY, *et al.* Microvascular and macrovascular reactivity is reduced in subjects at risk for type 2 diabetes. Diabetes 1999 Sep; 48(9): 1856-62.

[88]   Sanchez-Lozada LG, Tapia E, Jimenez A, Bautista P, Cristobal M, Nepomuceno T, *et al.* Fructose-induced metabolic syndrome is associated with glomerular hypertension and renal microvascular damage in rats. Am J Physiol Renal Physiol 2007 Jan; 292(1): F423-9.

[89]   Title LM, Lonn E, Charbonneau F, Fung M, Mather KJ, Verma S, *et al.* Relationship between brachial artery flow-mediated dilatation, hyperemic shear stress, and the metabolic syndrome. Vasc Med 2008 Nov; 13(4): 263-70.

[90]   Wong TY, Duncan BB, Golden SH, Klein R, Couper DJ, Klein BE, *et al.* Associations between the metabolic syndrome and retinal microvascular signs: the Atherosclerosis Risk In Communities study. Invest Ophthalmol Vis Sci 2004 Sep; 45(9): 2949-54.

[91]   Kawasaki R, Tielsch JM, Wang JJ, Wong TY, Mitchell P, Tano Y, *et al.* The metabolic syndrome and retinal microvascular signs in a Japanese population: the Funagata study. Br J Ophthalmol 2008 Feb; 92(2): 161-6.

[92]   Melikian N, Chowienczyk P, MacCarthy PA, Williams IL, Wheatcroft SB, Sherwood R, *et al.* Determinants of endothelial function in asymptomatic subjects with and without the metabolic syndrome. Atherosclerosis 2008 Mar; 197(1): 375-82.

[93]   Galili O, Versari D, Sattler KJ, Olson ML, Mannheim D, McConnell JP, *et al.* Early experimental obesity is associated with coronary endothelial dysfunction and oxidative stress. Am J Physiol Heart Circ Physiol 2007 Feb; 292(2): H904-11.

[94]   Steinberg HO, Chaker H, Leaming R, Johnson A, Brechtel G, Baron AD. Obesity/insulin resistance is associated with endothelial dysfunction. Implications for the syndrome of insulin resistance. J Clin Invest 1996 Jun 1; 97(11): 2601-10.

[95]   de Jongh RT, Clark AD, RG IJ, Serne EH, de Vries G, Stehouwer CD. Physiological hyperinsulinaemia increases intramuscular microvascular reactive hyperaemia and vasomotion in healthy volunteers. Diabetologia 2004 Jun; 47(6): 978-86.

[96]   Jonk AM, Houben AJ, de Jongh RT, Serne EH, Schaper NC, Stehouwer CD. Microvascular dysfunction in obesity: a potential mechanism in the pathogenesis of obesity-associated insulin resistance and hypertension. Physiology (Bethesda) 2007 Aug; 22: 252-60.

[97]   silva E, Genelhu,V, Tibirica,EV, Duarte,SF, Santos,LJ, Valenca,DT, Pina,RS, Caramuru,EP, Celoria,BM, Figueiredo,DP, Francischetti,EA, editor. Evaluation of the microvascular function in metabolic syndrome: relevance for the metabolic risk profile associated with obesity. Diab Vasc Dis Res; 2007.

[98]   Rocchini AP, Moorehead C, Katch V, Key J, Finta KM. Forearm resistance vessel abnormalities and insulin resistance in obese adolescents. Hypertension 1992 Jun; 19(6 Pt 2): 615-20.

[99]   Sola E, Vaya A, Simo M, Hernandez-Mijares A, Morillas C, Espana F, *et al.* Fibrinogen, plasma viscosity and blood viscosity in obesity. Relationship with insulin resistance. Clin Hemorheol Microcirc 2007; 37(4): 309-18.

[100]   Rosito GA, D'Agostino RB, Massaro J, Lipinska I, Mittleman MA, Sutherland P, *et al.* Association between obesity and a prothrombotic state: the Framingham Offspring Study. Thromb Haemost 2004 Apr; 91(4): 683-9.

[101]   Frisbee JC. Obesity, insulin resistance, and microvessel density. Microcirculation 2007 Jun-Jul; 14(4-5): 289-98.

[102]   Wiernsperger N, Nivoit P, De Aguiar LG, Bouskela E. Microcirculation and the metabolic syndrome. Microcirculation 2007 Jun-Jul; 14(4-5): 403-38.

[103]   Wiernsperger N, Nivoit P, Bouskela E. Microcirculation in obesity: an unexplored domain. An Acad Bras Cienc 2007 Dec; 79(4): 617-38.

[104]   Kraemer-Aguiar LG, Laflor CM, Bouskela E. Skin microcirculatory dysfunction is already present in normoglycemic subjects with metabolic syndrome. Metabolism 2008 Dec; 57(12): 1740-6.

[105]   Fiuza M, Cortez-Dias N, Martins S, Belo A. Metabolic syndrome in Portugal: prevalence and implications for cardiovascular risk--results from the VALSIM Study. Rev Port Cardiol 2008 Dec; 27(12): 1495-529.

[106]   Feihl F, Liaudet L, Waeber B, Levy BI. Hypertension: a disease of the microcirculation? Hypertension 2006 Dec; 48(6): 1012-7.

[107]   Kullo IJ, Malik AR, Santos S, Ehrsam JE, Turner ST. Association of cardiovascular risk factors with microvascular and conduit artery function in hypertensive subjects. Am J Hypertens 2007 Jul; 20(7): 735-42.

[108]   Nazzaro P, Vulpis V, Schirosi G, Serio G, Battista L, Lucivero V, *et al.* Microvascular impairment is associated with insulin resistance in euglycemic mild hypertensives. Am J Hypertens 2008 Apr; 21(4): 432-7.

[109]   Irving RJ, Walker BR, Noon JP, Watt GC, Webb DJ, Shore AC. Microvascular correlates of blood pressure, plasma glucose, and insulin resistance in health. Cardiovasc Res 2002 Jan; 53(1): 271-6.

[110]   de Jongh RT, Serne EH, RG IJ, Stehouwer CD. Microvascular function: a potential link between salt sensitivity, insulin resistance and hypertension. J Hypertens 2007 Sep; 25(9): 1887-93.

[111]   Giallauria F, Orio F, Palomba S, Lombardi G, Colao A, Vigorito C. Cardiovascular risk in women with polycystic ovary syndrome. J Cardiovasc Med (Hagerstown) 2008 Oct; 9(10): 987-92.

[112]   Legro RS. Polycystic ovary syndrome and cardiovascular disease: a premature association? Endocr Rev 2003 Jun; 24(3): 302-12.

[113]   Macut D, Micic D, Cvijovic G, Sumarac M, Kendereski A, Zoric S, *et al.* Cardiovascular risk in adolescent and young adult obese females with polycystic ovary syndrome (PCOS). J Pediatr Endocrinol Metab 2001; 14 Suppl 5: 1353-59; discussion 65.

[114]   Paradisi G, Steinberg HO, Hempfling A, Cronin J, Hook G, Shepard MK, *et al.* Polycystic ovary syndrome is associated with endothelial dysfunction. Circulation 2001 Mar 13; 103(10): 1410-5.

[115]   Lakhani K, Leonard A, Seifalian AM, Hardiman P. Microvascular dysfunction in women with polycystic ovary syndrome. Hum Reprod 2005 Nov; 20(11): 32 19-24.

[116]   Alexandraki K, Protogerou AD, Papaioannou TG, Piperi C, Mastorakos G, Lekakis J, *et al.* Early microvascular and macrovascular dysfunction is not accompanied by structural arterial injury in polycystic ovary syndrome. Hormones (Athens) 2006 Apr-Jun; 5(2): 126-36.

[117]   Ketel IJ, Stehouwer CD, Serne EH, Korsen TJ, Hompes PG, Smulders YM, *et al.* Obese but not normal-weight women with polycystic ovary syndrome are characterized by metabolic and microvascular insulin resistance. J Clin Endocrinol Metab 2008 Sep; 93(9): 3365-72.

[118]   Rajendran S, Willoughby SR, Chan WP, Liberts EA, Heresztyn T, Saha M, *et al.* Polycystic ovary syndrome is associated with severe platelet and endothelial dysfunction in both obese and lean subjects. Atherosclerosis 2008 Sep 17.

[119]   Oral B, Mermi B, Dilek M, Alanoglu G, Sutcu R. Thrombin activatable fibrinolysis inhibitor and other hemostatic parameters in patients with polycystic ovary syndrome. Gynecol Endocrinol 2009 Feb; 25(2): 110-6.

[120]   Atiomo WU, Bates SA, Condon JE, Shaw S, West JH, Prentice AG. The plasminogen activator system in women with polycystic ovary syndrome. Fertil Steril 1998 Feb; 69(2): 236-41.

[121]   Jennum P, Riha RL. Epidemiology of sleep apnoea/hypopnoea syndrome and sleep-disordered breathing. Eur Respir J 2009 Apr; 33(4): 907-14.

[122]   Punjabi NM, Shahar E, Redline S, Gottlieb DJ, Givelber R, Resnick HE. Sleep-disordered breathing, glucose intolerance, and insulin resistance: the Sleep Heart Health Study. Am J Epidemiol 2004 Sep 15; 160(6): 521-30.

[123]   Bonsignore MR, Zito A. Metabolic effects of the obstructive sleep apnea syndrome and cardiovascular risk. Arch Physiol Biochem 2008 Oct; 114(4): 255-60.

[124]   Wiernsperger N, Nivoit P, Bouskela E. Obstructive sleep apnea and insulin resistance: a role for microcirculation? Clinics 2006 Jun; 61(3): 253-66.

[125]   Knutson KL, Spiegel K, Penev P, Van Cauter E. The metabolic consequences of sleep deprivation. Sleep Med Rev 2007 Jun; 11(3): 163-78.

[126]   Makino S, Handa H, Suzukawa K, Fujiwara M, Nakamura M, Muraoka S, *et al.* Obstructive sleep apnoea syndrome, plasma adiponectin levels, and insulin resistance. Clin Endocrinol (Oxf) 2006 Jan; 64(1): 12-9.

[127]   Punjabi NM, Beamer BA. Alterations in Glucose Disposal in Sleep-disordered Breathing. Am J Respir Crit Care Med 2009 Feb 1; 179(3): 235-40.

[128]   Theorell-Haglow J, Berne C, Janson C, Lindberg E. Obstructive sleep apnoea is associated with decreased insulin sensitivity in females. Eur Respir J 2008 May; 31(5): 1054-60.

[129]   Vgontzas AN, Bixler EO, Chrousos GP. Metabolic disturbances in obesity versus sleep apnoea: the importance of visceral obesity and insulin resistance. J Intern Med 2003 Jul; 254(1): 32-44.

[130]   Ramadan W, Dewasmes G, Petitjean M, Wiernsperger N, Delanaud S, Geloen A, *et al.* Sleep apnea is induced by a high-fat diet and reversed and prevented by metformin in non-obese rats. Obesity (Silver Spring) 2007 Jun; 15(6): 1409-18.

[131]   Bhattacharjee R, Kheirandish-Gozal L, Pillar G, Gozal D. Cardiovascular complications of obstructive sleep apnea syndrome: evidence from children. Prog Cardiovasc Dis 2009 Mar-Apr; 51(5): 416-33.

[132]   Pack AI, Gislason T. Obstructive sleep apnea and cardiovascular disease: a perspective and future directions. Prog Cardiovasc Dis 2009 Mar-Apr; 51(5): 434-51.

[133]   Nazzaro P, Schirosi G, Clemente R, Battista L, Serio G, Boniello E, *et al.* Severe obstructive sleep apnoea exacerbates the microvascular impairment in very mild hypertensives. Eur J Clin Invest 2008 Oct; 38(10): 766-73.

[134]   Tasali E, Van Cauter E, Ehrmann DA. Polycystic Ovary Syndrome and Obstructive Sleep Apnea. Sleep Med Clin 2008 Mar; 3(1): 37-46.

[135]   Tasali E, Ip MS. Obstructive sleep apnea and metabolic syndrome: alterations in glucose metabolism and inflammation. Proc Am Thorac Soc 2008 Feb 15; 5(2): 207-17.

[136]   Atkeson A, Yeh SY, Malhotra A, Jelic S. Endothelial function in obstructive sleep apnea. Prog Cardiovasc Dis 2009 Mar-Apr; 51(5): 351-62.

[137]   Lavie L. Oxidative stress--a unifying paradigm in obstructive sleep apnea and comorbidities. Prog Cardiovasc Dis 2009 Jan-Feb; 51(4): 303-12.

[138]   Wolf J, Lewicka J, Narkiewicz K. Obstructive sleep apnea: an update on mechanisms and cardiovascular consequences. Nutr Metab Cardiovasc Dis 2007 Mar; 17(3): 233-40.

[139]   Nacher M, Serrano-Mollar A, Farre R, Panes J, Segui J, Montserrat JM. Recurrent obstructive apneas trigger early systemic inflammation in a rat model of sleep apnea. Respir Physiol Neurobiol 2007 Jan 15; 155(1): 93-6.

[140]   Iiyori N, Alonso LC, Li J, Sanders MH, Garcia-Ocana A, O'Doherty RM, *et al.* Intermittent hypoxia causes insulin resistance in lean mice independent of autonomic activity. Am J Respir Crit Care Med 2007 Apr 15; 175(8): 851-7.

[141]   Bertuglia S, Reiter RJ. Melatonin reduces microvascular damage and insulin resistance in hamsters due to chronic intermittent hypoxia. J Pineal Res 2009 Apr; 46(3): 307-13.

[142]   Wahlin Larsson B, Kadi F, Ulfberg J, Piehl Aulin K. Skeletal muscle morphology and aerobic capacity in patients with obstructive sleep apnoea syndrome. Respiration 2008; 76(1): 21-7.

[143]   Stal PS, Lindman R, Johansson B. Capillary supply of the soft palate muscles is reduced in long-term habitual snorers. Respiration 2009; 77(3): 303-10.

[144]   O'Donnell CP. Metabolic consequences of intermittent hypoxia. Adv Exp Med Biol 2007; 618: 41-9.

[145] Steiropoulos P, Papanas N, Nena E, Tsara V, Fitili C, Tzouvelekis A, *et al.* Markers of glycemic control and insulin resistance in non-diabetic patients with Obstructive Sleep Apnea Hypopnea Syndrome: Does adherence to CPAP treatment improve glycemic control? Sleep Med 2009 Feb 20.

[146] Clark JM. The epidemiology of nonalcoholic fatty liver disease in adults. J Clin Gastroenterol 2006 Mar; 40 Suppl 1: S5-10.

[147] Abdeen MB, Chowdhury NA, Hayden MR, Ibdah JA. Nonalcoholic steatohepatitis and the cardiometabolic syndrome. J Cardiometab Syndr 2006 Winter; 1(1): 36-40.

[148] Abdelmalek MF, Diehl AM. Nonalcoholic fatty liver disease as a complication of insulin resistance. Med Clin North Am 2007 Nov; 91(6): 1125-49, ix.

[149] Amarapurkar DN, Patel ND. Prevalence of metabolic syndrome in non-diabetic and non-cirrhotic patients with non-alcoholic steatohepatitis. Trop Gastroenterol 2004 Jul-Sep; 25(3): 125-9.

[150] Andre P, Balkau B, Vol S, Charles MA, Eschwege E. Gamma-glutamyltransferase activity and development of the metabolic syndrome (International Diabetes Federation Definition) in middle-aged men and women: Data from the Epidemiological Study on the Insulin Resistance Syndrome (DESIR) cohort. Diabetes Care 2007 Sep; 30(9): 2355-61.

[151] Misra VL, Khashab M, Chalasani N. Nonalcoholic fatty liver disease and cardiovascular risk. Curr Gastroenterol Rep 2009 Feb; 11(1): 50-5.

[152] Montecucco F, Mach F. Does non-alcoholic fatty liver disease (NAFLD) increase cardiovascular risk? Endocr Metab Immune Disord Drug Targets 2008 Dec; 8(4): 301-7.

[153] Santoliquido A, Di Campli C, Miele L, Gabrieli ML, Forgione A, Zocco MA, *et al.* Hepatic steatosis and vascular disease. Eur Rev Med Pharmacol Sci 2005 Sep-Oct; 9(5): 269-71.

[154] Targher G, Marra F, Marchesini G. Increased risk of cardiovascular disease in non-alcoholic fatty liver disease: causal effect or epiphenomenon? Diabetologia 2008 Nov; 51(11): 1947-53.

[155] Farrell GC, Teoh NC, McCuskey RS. Hepatic microcirculation in fatty liver disease. Anat Rec (Hoboken) 2008 Jun; 291(6): 684-92.

[156] Slowinska-Srzednicka J, Zgliczynski S, Soszynski P, Zgliczynski W, Jeske W. High blood pressure and hyperinsulinaemia in acromegaly and in obesity. Clin Exp Hypertens A 1989; 11(3): 407-25.

[157] Brevetti G, Marzullo P, Silvestro A, Pivonello R, Oliva G, di Somma C, *et al.* Early vascular alterations in acromegaly. J Clin Endocrinol Metab 2002 Jul; 87(7): 3174-9.

[158] Maison P, Demolis P, Young J, Schaison G, Giudicelli JF, Chanson P. Vascular reactivity in acromegalic patients: preliminary evidence for regional endothelial dysfunction and increased sympathetic vasoconstriction. Clin Endocrinol (Oxf) 2000 Oct; 53(4): 445-51.

[159] Chanson P, Megnien JL, del Pino M, Coirault C, Merli I, Houdouin L, *et al.* Decreased regional blood flow in patients with acromegaly. Clin Endocrinol (Oxf) 1998 Dec; 49(6): 725-31.

[160] Erem C, Nuhoglu I, Kocak M, Yilmaz M, Sipahi ST, Ucuncu O, *et al.* Blood coagulation and fibrinolysis in patients with acromegaly: increased plasminogen activator inhibitor-1 (PAI-1), decreased tissue factor pathway inhibitor (TFPI), and an inverse correlation between growth hormone and TFPI. Endocrine 2008 Nov 18.

[161] McClain DA, Abraham D, Rogers J, Brady R, Gault P, Ajioka R, *et al.* High prevalence of abnormal glucose homeostasis secondary to decreased insulin secretion in individuals with hereditary haemochromatosis. Diabetologia 2006 Jul; 49(7): 1661-9.

[162] Gaenzer H, Marschang P, Sturm W, Neumayr G, Vogel W, Patsch J, *et al.* Association between increased iron stores and impaired endothelial function in patients with hereditary hemochromatosis. J Am Coll Cardiol 2002 Dec 18; 40(12): 2189-94.

[163] Lekakis J, Papamicheal C, Stamatelopoulos K, Cimponeriu A, Voutsas A, Vemmos K, *et al.* Hemochromatosis associated with endothelial dysfunction: evidence for the role of iron stores in early atherogenesis. Vasc Med 1999; 4(3): 147-8.

[164] Khalifa AS, Salem M, Mounir E, El-Tawil MM, El-Sawy M, Abd Al-Aziz MM. Abnormal glucose tolerance in Egyptian beta-thalassemic patients: possible association with genotyping. Pediatr Diabetes 2004 Sep; 5(3): 126-32.

[165] Messina MF, Lombardo F, Meo A, Miceli M, Wasniewska M, Valenzise M, *et al.* Three-year prospective evaluation of glucose tolerance, beta-cell function and peripheral insulin sensitivity in non-diabetic patients with thalassemia major. J Endocrinol Invest 2002 Jun; 25(6): 497-501.

[166] Toumba M, Sergis A, Kanaris C, Skordis N. Endocrine complications in patients with Thalassaemia Major. Pediatr Endocrinol Rev 2007 Dec; 5(2): 642-8.

[167] Kyriakou DS, Alexandrakis MG, Kyriakou ES, Liapi D, Kourelis TV, Passam F, *et al.* Activated peripheral blood and endothelial cells in thalassemia patients. Ann Hematol 2001 Oct; 80(10): 577-83.

[168] Butthep P, Nuchprayoon I, Futrakul N. Endothelial injury and altered hemodynamics in thalassemia. Clin Hemorheol Microcirc 2004; 31(4): 287-93.

[169] Brudevold R, Hole T, Hammerstrom J. Hyperferritinemia is associated with insulin resistance and fatty liver in patients without iron overload. PLoS ONE 2008; 3(10): e3547.

[170] Vari IS, Balkau B, Kettaneh A, Andre P, Tichet J, Fumeron F, *et al.* Ferritin and transferrin are associated with metabolic syndrome abnormalities and their change over time in a general population: Data from an Epidemiological Study on the Insulin Resistance Syndrome (DESIR). Diabetes Care 2007 Jul; 30(7): 1795-801.

[171] Aboud M, Elgalib A, Kulasegaram R, Peters B. Insulin resistance and HIV infection: a review. Int J Clin Pract 2007 Mar; 61(3): 463-72.

[172] Filardi PP, Paolillo S, Marciano C, Iorio A, Losco T, Marsico F, *et al.* Cardiovascular effects of antiretroviral drugs: clinical review. Cardiovasc Hematol Disord Drug Targets 2008 Dec; 8(4): 238-44.

[173] Shankar SS, Dube MP. Clinical aspects of endothelial dysfunction associated with human immunodeficiency virus infection and antiretroviral agents. Cardiovasc Toxicol 2004; 4(3): 261-9.

[174] Dube MP, Shen C, Greenwald M, Mather KJ. No impairment of endothelial function or insulin sensitivity with 4 weeks of the HIV protease inhibitors atazanavir or lopinavir-ritonavir in healthy subjects without HIV infection: a placebo-controlled trial. Clin Infect Dis 2008 Aug 15; 47(4): 567-74.

[175] Monsuez JJ, Dufaux J, Vittecoq D, Vicaut E. Reduced reactive hyperemia in HIV-infected patients. J Acquir Immune Defic Syndr 2000 Dec 15; 25(5): 434-42.

[176] Chi D, Henry J, Kelley J, Thorpe R, Smith JK, Krishnaswamy G. The effects of HIV infection on endothelial function. Endothelium 2000; 7(4): 223-42.

[177] Monsuez JJ, Dufaux J, Vittecoq D, Flaud P, Vicaut E. Hemorheology in asymptomatic HIV-infected patients. Clin Hemorheol Microcirc 2000; 23(1): 59-66.

[178] Dadgostar H, Holland GN, Huang X, Tufail A, Kim A, Fisher TC, *et al.* Hemorheologic abnormalities associated with HIV infection: in vivo assessment of retinal microvascular blood flow. Invest Ophthalmol Vis Sci 2006 Sep; 47(9): 3933-8.

[179] Maggi P, Bellacosa C, Grattagliano V, Pastore G, Lapadula G. Functional impairments of microcirculation in HIV-positive patients: a laser Doppler fluxometry-based investigation. HIV Clin Trials 2008 Nov-Dec; 9(6): 428-33.

[180] Park IW, Ullrich CK, Schoenberger E, Ganju RK, Groopman JE. HIV-1 Tat induces microvascular endothelial apoptosis through caspase activation. J Immunol 2001 Sep 1; 167(5): 2766-71.

[181] Fernandez-Real JM, Lopez-Bermejo A, Castro A, Casamitjana R, Ricart W. Thyroid function is intrinsically linked to insulin sensitivity and endothelium-dependent vasodilation in healthy euthyroid subjects. J Clin Endocrinol Metab 2006 Sep; 91(9): 3337-43.

[182] Stanicka S, Vondra K, Pelikanova T, Vlcek P, Hill M, Zamrazil V. Insulin sensitivity and counter-regulatory hormones in hypothyroidism and during thyroid hormone replacement therapy. Clin Chem Lab Med 2005; 43(7): 715-20.

[183] Lekakis J, Papamichael C, Alevizaki M, Piperingos G, Marafelia P, Mantzos J, *et al.* Flow-mediated, endothelium-dependent vasodilation is impaired in subjects with hypothyroidism, borderline hypothyroidism, and high-normal serum thyrotropin (TSH) values. Thyroid 1997 Jun; 7(3): 411-4.

[184] Vargas F, Moreno JM, Rodriguez-Gomez I, Wangensteen R, Osuna A, Alvarez-Guerra M, *et al.* Vascular and renal function in experimental thyroid disorders. Eur J Endocrinol 2006 Feb; 154(2): 197-212.

[185] Craft S. Insulin resistance syndrome and Alzheimer disease: pathophysiologic mechanisms and therapeutic implications. Alzheimer Dis Assoc Disord 2006 Oct-Dec; 20(4): 298-301.

[186] Milionis HJ, Florentin M, Giannopoulos S. Metabolic syndrome and Alzheimer's disease: a link to a vascular hypothesis? CNS Spectr 2008 Jul; 13(7): 606-13.

[187] Kitaguchi H, Ihara M, Saiki H, Takahashi R, Tomimoto H. Capillary beds are decreased in Alzheimer's disease, but not in Binswanger's disease. Neurosci Lett 2007 May 1; 417(2): 128-31.

[188] Khalil Z, Chen H, Helme RD. Mechanisms underlying the vascular activity of beta-amyloid protein fragment (beta A(4)25-35) at the level of skin microvasculature. Brain Res 1996 Oct 14; 736(1-2): 206-16.

[189] Maslo C, Peraldi MN, Desenclos JC, Mougenot B, Cywiner-Golenzer C, Chatelet FP, *et al.* Thrombotic microangiopathy and cytomegalovirus disease in patients infected with human immunodeficiency virus. Clin Infect Dis 1997 Mar; 24(3): 350-5.

[190] Chang CY, Liang HJ, Chow SY, Chen SM, Liu DZ. Hemorheological mechanisms in Alzheimer's disease. Microcirculation 2007 Aug; 14(6): 627-34.

[191] Guize L, Pannier B, Thomas F, Bean K, Jego B, Benetos A. Recent advances in metabolic syndrome and cardiovascular disease. Arch Cardiovasc Dis 2008 Sep; 101(9): 577-83.

[192] Kovaite M, Petrulioniene Z, Ryliskyte L, Badariene J, Dzenkeviciute V, Cypiene A, *et al.* Systemic assessment of arterial wall structure and function in metabolic syndrome. Proc West Pharmacol Soc 2007; 50: 123-30.

[193] Adolphe A, Cook LS, Huang X. A cross-sectional study of intima-media thickness, ethnicity, metabolic syndrome, and cardiovascular risk in 2268 study participants. Mayo Clin Proc 2009 Mar; 84(3): 221-8.

[194] Achimastos AD, Efstathiou SP, Christoforatos T, Panagiotou TN, Stergiou GS, Mountokalakis TD. Arterial stiffness: determinants and relationship to the metabolic syndrome. Angiology 2007 Feb-Mar; 58(1): 11-20.

[195] Ghiadoni L, Penno G, Giannarelli C, Plantinga Y, Bernardini M, Pucci L, *et al.* Metabolic syndrome and vascular alterations in normotensive subjects at risk of diabetes mellitus. Hypertension 2008 Feb; 51(2): 440-5.

[196] Nam JS, Park JS, Cho MH, Jee SH, Lee HS, Ahn CW, *et al.* The association between pulse wave velocity and metabolic syndrome and adiponectin in patients with impaired fasting glucose: cardiovascular risks and adiponectin in IFG. Diabetes Res Clin Pract 2009 May; 84(2): 145-51.

[197] Zhe XW, Zeng J, Tian XK, Chen W, Gu Y, Cheng LT, *et al.* Pulse wave velocity is associated with metabolic syndrome components in CAPD patients. Am J Nephrol 2008; 28(4): 641-6.

[198] Westerbacka J, Yki-Jarvinen H. Arterial stiffness and insulin resistance. Semin Vasc Med 2002 May; 2(2): 157-64.

[199] Yki-Jarvinen H, Westerbacka J. Insulin resistance, arterial stiffness and wave reflection. Adv Cardiol 2007; 44: 252-60.

[200]   Scuteri A, Tesauro M, Rizza S, Iantorno M, Federici M, Lauro D, *et al.* Endothelial function and arterial stiffness in normotensive normoglycemic first-degree relatives of diabetic patients are independent of the metabolic syndrome. Nutr Metab Cardiovasc Dis 2008 Jun; 18(5): 349-56.

[201]   Stern MP, Morales PA, Haffner SM, Valdez RA. Hyperdynamic circulation and the insulin resistance syndrome ("syndrome X"). Hypertension 1992 Dec; 20(6): 802-8.

[202]   Palatini P, Vriz O, Nesbitt S, Amerena J, Majahalme S, Valentini M, *et al.* Parental hyperdynamic circulation predicts insulin resistance in offspring: The Tecumseh Offspring Study. Hypertension 1999 Mar; 33(3): 769-74.

[203]   Jiang ZY, Lin YW, Clemont A, Feener EP, Hein KD, Igarashi M, *et al.* Characterization of selective resistance to insulin signaling in the vasculature of obese Zucker (fa/fa) rats. J Clin Invest 1999 Aug; 104(4): 447-57.

[204]   Sambuceti G, L'Abbate A, Marzilli M. Why should we study the coronary microcirculation? Am J Physiol Heart Circ Physiol 2000 Dec; 279(6): H2581-4.

[205]   Wu KC, Zerhouni EA, Judd RM, Lugo-Olivieri CH, Barouch LA, Schulman SP, *et al.* Prognostic significance of microvascular obstruction by magnetic resonance imaging in patients with acute myocardial infarction. Circulation 1998 Mar 3; 97(8): 765-72.

[206]   AlZadjali MA, Godfrey V, Khan F, Choy A, Doney AS, Wong AK, *et al.* Insulin resistance is highly prevalent and is associated with reduced exercise tolerance in nondiabetic patients with heart failure. J Am Coll Cardiol 2009 Mar 3; 53(9): 747-53.

[207]   Nishio K, Shigemitsu M, Kusuyama T, Fukui T, Kawamura K, Itoh S, *et al.* Insulin resistance in nondiabetic patients with acute myocardial infarction. Cardiovasc Revasc Med 2006 Apr-Jun; 7(2): 54-60.

[208]   Pajunen P, Koukkunen H, Ketonen M, Jerkkola T, Immonen-Raiha P, Karja-Koskenkari P, *et al.* Five-year risk of developing clinical diabetes after first myocardial infarction; the FINAMI study. Diabet Med 2005 Oct; 22(10): 1334-7.

[209]   Thomas DP, Hudlicka O. Arteriolar reactivity and capillarization in chronically stimulated rat limb skeletal muscle post-MI. J Appl Physiol 1999 Dec; 87(6): 2259-65.

[210]   Richardson TE, Kindig CA, Musch TI, Poole DC. Effects of chronic heart failure on skeletal muscle capillary hemodynamics at rest and during contractions. J Appl Physiol 2003 Sep; 95(3): 1055-62.

[211]   Xu L, Poole DC, Musch TI. Effect of heart failure on muscle capillary geometry: implications for 02 exchange. Med Sci Sports Exerc 1998 Aug; 30(8): 1230-7.

[212]   Nusz DJ, White DC, Dai Q, Pippen AM, Thompson MA, Walton GB, *et al.* Vascular rarefaction in peripheral skeletal muscle after experimental heart failure. Am J Physiol Heart Circ Physiol 2003 Oct; 285(4): H1554-62.

[213]   Houghton AR, Harrison M, Perry AJ, Evans AJ, Cowley AJ. Endogenous insulin and insulin sensitivity. An important determinant of skeletal muscle blood flow in chronic heart failure? Eur Heart J 1998 Mar; 19(3): 476-80.

[214]   Ivey FM, Ryan AS, Hafer-Macko CE, Garrity BM, Sorkin JD, Goldberg AP, *et al.* High prevalence of abnormal glucose metabolism and poor sensitivity of fasting plasma glucose in the chronic phase of stroke. Cerebrovasc Dis 2006; 22(5-6): 368-71.

[215]   Prior SJ, McKenzie MJ, Joseph LJ, Ivey FM, Macko RF, Hafer-Macko CE, *et al.* Reduced skeletal muscle capillarization and glucose intolerance. Microcirculation 2009 Apr; 16(3): 203-12.

[216]   Erdem H, Dinc A, Pay S, Simsek I, Turan M. Peripheral insulin resistance in patients with Behcet's disease. J Eur Acad Dermatol Venereol 2006 Apr; 20(4): 391-5.

[217]   Pasqui AL, Pastorelli M, Puccetti L, Beerman U, Biagi F, Camarri A, *et al.* Microvascular assessment in Behcet disease: videocapillaroscopic study. Int J Tissue React 2003; 25(3): 105-15.

[218]   Vadacca M, Margiotta D, Rigon A, Cacciapaglia F, Coppolino G, Amoroso A, *et al.* Adipokines and systemic lupus erythematosus: relationship with metabolic syndrome and cardiovascular disease risk factors. J Rheumatol 2009 Feb; 36(2): 295-7.

[219]   Cacciapaglia F, Zardi E, Coppolino G, Buzzulini F, Margiotta D, Arcarese L, *et al.* Stiffness parameters, intima-media thickness and early atherosclerosis in systemic lupus erythematosus patients. Lupus 2009; 18(3): 249-56.

[220]   Rho YH, Choi SJ, Lee YH, Ji JD, Choi KM, Baik SH, *et al.* The prevalence of metabolic syndrome in patients with gout: a multicenter study. J Korean Med Sci 2005 Dec; 20(6): 1029-33.

[221]   Lembo G, Iaccarino G, Vecchione C, Rendina V, Trimarco B. Insulin modulation of vascular reactivity is already impaired in prehypertensive spontaneously hypertensive rats. Hypertension 1995 Aug; 26(2): 290-3.

[222]   Straczkowski M, Kowalska I, Stepien A, Dzienis-Straczkowska S, Szelachowska M, Kinalska I, *et al.* Insulin resistance in the first-degree relatives of persons with type 2 diabetes. Med Sci Monit 2003 May; 9(5): CR186-90.

[223]   Goldfine AB, Beckman JA, Betensky RA, Devlin H, Hurley S, Varo N, *et al.* Family history of diabetes is a major determinant of endothelial function. J Am Coll Cardiol 2006 Jun 20; 47(12): 2456-61.

[224]   Ekelund U, Anderssen S, Andersen LB, Riddoch CJ, Sardinha LB, Luan J, *et al.* Prevalence and correlates of the metabolic syndrome in a population-based sample of European youth. Am J Clin Nutr 2009 Jan; 89(1): 90-6.

[225]   Balletshofer BM, Rittig K, Enderle MD, Volk A, Maerker E, Jacob S, *et al.* Endothelial dysfunction is detectable in young normotensive first-degree relatives of subjects with type 2 diabetes in association with insulin resistance. Circulation 2000 Apr 18; 101(15): 1780-4.

[226]   Jorneskog G, Kalani M, Kuhl J, Bavenholm P, Katz A, Allerstrand G, *et al.* Early microvascular dysfunction in healthy normal-weight males with heredity for type 2 diabetes. Diabetes Care 2005 Jun; 28(6): 1495-7.

[227]   McSorley PT, Bell PM, Young IS, Atkinson AB, Sheridan B, Fee JP, *et al.* Endothelial function, insulin action and cardiovascular risk factors in young healthy adult offspring of parents with Type 2 diabetes: effect of vitamin E in a randomized double-blind, controlled clinical trial. Diabet Med 2005 Jun; 22(6): 703-10.

[228]   Sonne MP, Hojbjerre L, Alibegovic AA, Vaag A, Stallknecht B, Dela F. Impaired endothelial function and insulin action in first-degree relatives of patients with type 2 diabetes mellitus. Metabolism 2009 Jan; 58(1): 93-101.

[229]   Lee BC, Shore AC, Humphreys JM, Lowe GD, Rumley A, Clark PM, *et al.* Skin microvascular vasodilatory capacity in offspring of two parents with Type 2 diabetes. Diabet Med 2001 Jul; 18(7): 541-5.

[230]   Gurlek A, Bayraktar M, Kirazli S. Increased plasminogen activator inhibitor-1 activity in offspring of type 2 diabetic patients: lack of association with plasma insulin levels. Diabetes Care 2000 Jan; 23(1): 88-92.

[231]   Ruotsalainen E, Vauhkonen I, Salmenniemi U, Pihlajamaki J, Punnonen K, Kainulainen S, *et al.* Markers of endothelial dysfunction and low-grade inflammation are associated in the offspring of type 2 diabetic subjects. Atherosclerosis 2008 Mar; 197(1): 271-7.

[232]   Tesauro M, Rizza S, Iantorno M, Campia U, Cardillo C, Lauro D, *et al.* Vascular, metabolic, and inflammatory abnormalities in normoglycemic offspring of patients with type 2 diabetes mellitus. Metabolism 2007 Mar; 56(3): 413-9.

[233]   Maumus S, Marie B, Siest G, Visvikis-Siest S. A prospective study on the prevalence of metabolic syndrome among healthy french families: two cardiovascular risk factors (HDL cholesterol and tumor necrosis factor-alpha) are revealed in the offspring of parents with metabolic syndrome. Diabetes Care 2005 Mar; 28(3): 675-82.

[234]   Maltezos E, Papazoglou D, Exiara T, Papazoglou L, Karathanasis E, Christakidis D, *et al.* Tumour necrosis factor-alpha levels in non-diabetic offspring of patients with type 2 diabetes mellitus. J Int Med Res 2002 Nov-Dec; 30(6): 576-83.

[235]   Hunt KJ, Heiss G, Sholinsky PD, Province MA. Familial history of metabolic disorders and the multiple metabolic syndrome: the NHLBI family heart study. Genet Epidemiol 2000 Dec; 19(4): 395-409.

[236]   Lazarin MA, Bennini JR, Pereira CL, Astiarraga BD, Ferrannini E, Muscelli E. Normal insulin sensitivity in lean offspring of obese parents. Obes Res 2004 Apr; 12(4): 621-6.

[237]   Chen HS, Hwu CM, Kwok CF, Shih KC, Hsiao LC, Lee SH, *et al.* Insulin sensitivity in normotensive offspring of hypertensive parents. Horm Metab Res 2000 Mar; 32(3): 110-4.

[238]   Dunkley AJ, Taub NA, Davies MJ, Stone MA, Khunti K. Is having a family history of type 2 diabetes or cardiovascular disease a predictive factor for metabolic syndrome? Prim Care Diabetes 2009 Feb; 3(1): 49-56.

[239]   Ohtoshi K, Yamasaki Y, Gorogawa S, Hayaishi-Okano R, Node K, Matsuhisa M, *et al.* Association of (-)786T-C mutation of endothelial nitric oxide synthase gene with insulin resistance. Diabetologia 2002 Nov; 45(11): 1594-601.

[240]   Rizza S, Tesauro M, Cardellini M, Menghini R, Bellia A, Marini MA, *et al.* Insulin resistance and increased intimal medial thickness in glucose tolerant offspring of type 2 diabetic subjects carrying the D298D genotype of endothelial nitric oxide synthase. Arterioscler Thromb Vasc Biol 2006 Feb; 26(2): 431-2.

[241]   Ohtoshi K, Kaneto H, Node K, Nakamura Y, Shiraiwa T, Matsuhisa M, *et al.* Association of soluble epoxide hydrolase gene polymorphism with insulin resistance in type 2 diabetic patients. Biochem Biophys Res Commun 2005 May 27; 331(1): 347-50.

[242]   Parry DJ, Grant PJ, Scott DJ. Fibrinolytic risk factor clustering and insulin resistance in healthy male relatives of men with intermittent claudication. Br J Surg 2006 Mar; 93(3): 315-24.

[243]   Anderwald C, Pfeiler G, Nowotny P, Anderwald-Stadler M, Krebs M, Bischof MG, *et al.* Glucose turnover and intima media thickness of internal carotid artery in type 2 diabetes offspring. Eur J Clin Invest 2008 Apr; 38(4): 227-37.

[244]   Lee JW, Lee DC, Im JA, Shim JY, Kim SM, Lee HR. Insulin resistance is associated with arterial stiffness independent of obesity in male adolescents. Hypertens Res 2007 Jan; 30(1): 5-11.

[245]   Mitchell GF, Vita JA, Larson MG, Parise H, Keyes MJ, Warner E, *et al.* Cross-sectional relations of peripheral microvascular function, cardiovascular disease risk factors, and aortic stiffness: the Framingham Heart Study. Circulation 2005 Dec 13; 112(24): 3722-8.

[246]   Kyvelou SM, Vyssoulis GP, Karpanou EA, Adamopoulos DN, Gialernios TP, Spanos PG, *et al.* Arterial hypertension parental burden affects arterial stiffness and wave reflection to the aorta in young offsprings. Int J Cardiol 2009 Jan 26.

[247]   Barker DJ, Osmond C, Simmonds SJ, Wield GA. The relation of small head circumference and thinness at birth to death from cardiovascular disease in adult life. BMJ 1993 Feb 13; 306(6875): 422-6.

[248]   Vaag A. Low birth weight and early weight gain in the metabolic syndrome: consequences for infant nutrition. Int J Gynaecol Obstet 2009 Mar; 104 Suppl 1: S32-4.

[249]   Fagerberg B, Bondjers L, Nilsson P. Low birth weight in combination with catch-up growth predicts the occurrence of the metabolic syndrome in men at late middle age: the Atherosclerosis and Insulin Resistance study. J Intern Med 2004 Sep; 256(3): 254-9.

[250]   Lapidus L, Andersson SW, Bengtsson C, Bjorkelund C, Rossander-Hulthen L, Lissner L. Weight and length at birth and their relationship to diabetes incidence and all-cause mortality--a 32-year follow-up of the population study of women in Gothenburg, Sweden. Prim Care Diabetes 2008 Sep; 2(3): 127-33.

[251]   Hediger ML, Overpeck MD, Kuczmarski RJ, McGlynn A, Maurer KR, Davis WW. Muscularity and fatness of infants and young children born small- or large-for-gestational-age. Pediatrics 1998 Nov; 102(5): E60.

[252]   Reinehr T, Kleber M, Toschke AM. Small for gestational age status is associated with metabolic syndrome in overweight children. Eur J Endocrinol 2009 Apr; 160(4): 579-84.

[253]   Martin H, Hu J, Gennser G, Norman M. Impaired endothelial function and increased carotid stiffness in 9-year-old children with low birthweight. Circulation 2000 Nov 28; 102(22): 2739-44.

[254]   Smith GD, Sterne J, Tynelius P, Lawlor DA, Rasmussen F. Birth weight of offspring and subsequent cardiovascular mortality of the parents. Epidemiology 2005 Jul; 16(4): 563-9.

[255]   Goh KL, Shore AC, Quinn M, Tooke JE. Impaired microvascular vasodilatory function in 3-month-old infants of low birth weight. Diabetes Care 2001 Jun; 24(6): 1102-7.

[256]   Martin H, Gazelius B, Norman M. Impaired acetylcholine-induced vascular relaxation in low birth weight infants: implications for adult hypertension? Pediatr Res 2000 Apr; 47(4 Pt 1): 457-62.

[257]   Albareda M, Caballero A, Badell G, Rodriguez-Espinosa J, Ordonez-Llanos J, de Leiva A, et al. Metabolic syndrome at follow-up in women with and without gestational diabetes mellitus in index pregnancy. Metabolism 2005 Aug; 54(8): 1115-21.

[258]   Byberg L, McKeigue PM, Zethelius B, Lithell HO. Birth weight and the insulin resistance syndrome: association of low birth weight with truncal obesity and raised plasminogen activator inhibitor-1 but not with abdominal obesity or plasma lipid disturbances. Diabetologia 2000 Jan; 43(1): 54-60.

[259]   Lauenborg J, Mathiesen E, Hansen T, Glumer C, Jorgensen T, Borch-Johnsen K, et al. The prevalence of the metabolic syndrome in a danish population of women with previous gestational diabetes mellitus is three-fold higher than in the general population. J Clin Endocrinol Metab 2005 Jul; 90(7): 4004-10.

[260]   Cheung NW, Helmink D. Gestational diabetes: the significance of persistent fasting hyperglycemia for the subsequent development of diabetes mellitus. J Diabetes Complications 2006 Jan-Feb; 20(1): 21-5.

[261]   Banerjee M, Cruickshank JK. Pregnancy as the prodrome to vascular dysfunction and cardiovascular risk. Nat Clin Pract Cardiovasc Med 2006 Nov; 3(11): 596-603.

[262]   Damm P. Future risk of diabetes in mother and child after gestational diabetes mellitus. Int J Gynaecol Obstet 2009 Mar; 104 Suppl 1: S25-6.

[263]   Pleiner J, Mittermayer F, Langenberger H, Winzer C, Schaller G, Pacini G, et al. Impaired vascular nitric oxide bioactivity in women with previous gestational diabetes. Wien Klin Wochenschr 2007; 1 19(15-16): 483-9.

[264]   Seghieri G, Anichini R, De Bellis A, Alviggi L, Franconi F, Breschi MC. Relationship between gestational diabetes mellitus and low maternal birth weight. Diabetes Care 2002 Oct; 25(10): 1761-5.

[265]   Hu J, Norman M, Wallensteen M, Gennser G. Increased large arterial stiffness and impaired acetylcholine induced skin vasodilatation in women with previous gestational diabetes mellitus. Br J Obstet Gynaecol 1998 Dec; 105(12): 1279-87.

[266]   Middlebrooke AR, Armstrong N, Welsman JR, Shore AC, Clark P, MacLeod KM. Does aerobic fitness influence microvascular function in healthy adults at risk of developing Type 2 diabetes? Diabet Med 2005 Apr; 22(4): 483-9.

[267]   Hannemann MM, Liddell WG, Shore AC, Clark PM, Tooke JE. Vascular function in women with previous gestational diabetes mellitus. J Vasc Res 2002 Jul-Aug; 39(4): 311-9.

[268]   Heitritter SM, Solomon CG, Mitchell GF, Skali-Ounis N, Seely EW. Subclinical inflammation and vascular dysfunction in women with previous gestational diabetes mellitus. J Clin Endocrinol Metab 2005 Jul; 90(7): 3983-8.

[269]   Mittermayer F, Kautzky-Willer A, Winzer C, Krzyzanowska K, Prikoszovich T, Demehri S, et al. Elevated concentrations of asymmetric dimethylarginine are associated with deterioration of glucose tolerance in women with previous gestational diabetes mellitus. J Intern Med 2007 Apr; 261(4): 392-8.

[270]   Akinci B, Celtik A, Yener S, Yesil S. Prediction of developing metabolic syndrome after gestational diabetes mellitus. Fertil Steril 2009 Jan 13.

[271]   Isezuo SA, Ekele BA. Comparison of metabolic syndrome variables among pregnant women with and without eclampsia. J Natl Med Assoc 2008 Sep; 100(9): 1059-62.

[272]   Soonthornpun K, Soonthornpun S, Wannaro P, Setasuban W, Thamprasit A. Insulin resistance in women with a history of severe pre-eclampsia. J Obstet Gynaecol Res 2009 Feb; 35(1): 55-9.

[273]   Harskamp RE, Zeeman GG. Preeclampsia: at risk for remote cardiovascular disease. Am J Med Sci 2007 Oct; 334(4): 291-5.

[274]   Rodie VA, Freeman DJ, Sattar N, Greer IA. Pre-eclampsia and cardiovascular disease: metabolic syndrome of pregnancy? Atherosclerosis 2004 Aug; 175(2): 189-202.

[275]   Wolf M, Hubel CA, Lam C, Sampson M, Ecker JL, Ness RB, et al. Preeclampsia and future cardiovascular disease: potential role of altered angiogenesis and insulin resistance. J Clin Endocrinol Metab 2004 Dec; 89(12): 6239-43.

[276]   Blaauw J, Graaff R, van Pampus MG, van Doormaal JJ, Smit AJ, Rakhorst G, et al. Abnormal endothelium-dependent microvascular reactivity in recently preeclamptic women. Obstet Gynecol 2005 Mar; 105(3): 626-32.

[277] Laufs U, Wassmann S, Czech T, Munzel T, Eisenhauer M, Bohm M, *et al.* Physical inactivity increases oxidative stress, endothelial dysfunction, and atherosclerosis. Arterioscler Thromb Vasc Biol 2005 Apr; 25(4): 809-14.

[278] Suvorava T, Lauer N, Kojda G. Physical inactivity causes endothelial dysfunction in healthy young mice. J Am Coll Cardiol 2004 Sep 15; 44(6): 1320-7.

[279] Hamburg NM, McMackin CJ, Huang AL, Shenouda SM, Widlansky ME, Schulz E, *et al.* Physical inactivity rapidly induces insulin resistance and microvascular dysfunction in healthy volunteers. Arterioscler Thromb Vasc Biol 2007 Dec; 27(12): 2650-6.

[280] Serne EH, Stehouwer CD, ter Maaten JC, ter Wee PM, Rauwerda JA, Donker AJ, *et al.* Microvascular function relates to insulin sensitivity and blood pressure in normal subjects. Circulation 1999 Feb 23; 99(7): 896-902.

Is Defective Microcirculation Responsible for Insulin Resistance?

PART 2. Insulin and Microcirculation: Physiology/ Pathophysiology

Nicolas Wiernsperger [1, 2]

[1]INSERM U870, INSA Lyon, Bat L.Pasteur, 11 avenue J.Capelle, F-69621 Villeurbanne Cedex (France)

[2]Laboratorio de Pesquisas em Microcirculaçao, Centro Medico, Universidade do Estado do Rio de Janeiro, Pav. R .Haroldo Lisboa da Cunha, Rua Sao Francisco Xavier 524, 20550-013 Rio de Janeiro (Brazil)

E Mail: nicolas.wiernsperger@free.fr

Keywords: Insulin, glucose, arterioles, capillaries, vasomotion.

1. INTRODUCTION

Although a role for blood circulation in IR has been suggested many years ago [1,2] and regularly reconsidered [3-8], possible causal and bidirectional relationships between these processes as well as recognition of the pandemic evolution of prediabetes through the world have permitted to generate data increasingly supporting this concept. Indeed IR was rather considered as being associated with factors of the IR syndrome which have an impact on large vessels, while microcirculation was completely ignored and preferentially associated with typical diabetic microangiopathy complications. A key step was the pioneering work of Baron and coworkers who suggested that insulin had vasodilating effects and that they might be involved in its metabolic effects [7]. Subsequent intensive work during the last 10-15years has then shown that this effect was mainly microvascular within the physiological range of plasma insulin variations; from this several groups proposed that primary defects in microcirculation could impair the metabolic action of insulin [9-12]. That microvascular disturbances can be instrumental to IR is a very new concept, however, which also requires that proof be provided that defective microvascular reactivity or in nutritive flow distribution can precede IR.

Although only limited direct data are presently available, due to the very novel nature of this concept, the following examples show that microvascular disorders can indeed precede -and thus be a potential cause of- IR. In mice a high fat diet for up to 14weeks showed that inflammation and IR developed in the vasculature well before such changes could be observed in muscle, liver or adipose tissues [13]; in fructose-fed rats, both IR and ED appeared before HT [14]. In humans the concept of 'intrinsic endotheliopathy' was proposed 10years ago, stating that ED antedated diabetes [15, 16]. Many findings described above have not only demonstrated that microvascular dysfunction and IR occur concomitantly but many of them strongly are in line with the notion that there exist microvascular disturbances which precede IR. Because ED can be substantially different from microvascular reactivity, however, intensive research is still needed to definitively assess this hypothesis. In the following, the implication of insulin in microvascular physiology and the mechanisms whereby microcirculation could lead to impairments in glucose homeostasis and CVD are developed.

2. BLOOD FLOW AND ITS LINK WITH GLUCOSE UPTAKE

A main critical question is if, and to what extent, glucose uptake (GU) is governed by blood flow (BF). Here again it must be stated that BF is generally considered as the amount of blood flowing through a tissue in a given period of time. This is only a global estimate; not considering nutritive vs non nutritive perfusion; thus, elevated bulk flow does not mean that more blood supplies muscle fibers and, conversely, microflow distribution may experience drastic distribution changes which are not reflected in bulk flow measurements. In other terms, absolute flow [as determined by most techniques], especially in basal states, may be increased or decreased without metabolic consequences [17]. Therefore dissociations between BF and GU, as reported [18-20] have limited meanings if nutritive flow is not investigated. Moreover BF can increase simply secondarily to activation of metabolism in perivascular tissues, due to the coupling between both parameters [21].

That BF may be important is suggested by the large difference in insulin sensitivity between tissues investigated either in situ or ex vivo; muscle or adipocyte insulin sensitivity is drastically lowered in excised tissues and, although other factors such as nervous control or manipulation may contribute, this strongly suggests that tissue perfusion and oxygenation are key determinants of physiological metabolism. Unfortunately few studies have dealt with this cardinal question but they show that GU is indeed much higher in perfused skeletal muscle [22, 23]. In athletes basal BF was associated with higher glycogen synthase fractional activity despite similar capillary density to non athletes [24]. Increasing perfusion rate in rat hindlimbs increased glucose uptake [25, 26] and energy metabolism [27]. That delivery of glucose is part of muscle GU was also shown in humans [28]. Conversely, decreasing BF by injections of 15µm microspheres had no effect on basal BF but hampered insulin-mediated GU [29]. In an apparent paradox, some vasoconstrictors increase muscle oxygen consumption as a consequence of microflow redistribution [30]. Such data demonstrate that, ultimately, the key factor is not how much blood flows but where it flows.

3. MACRO vs MICROCIRCULATION

The link between large and small vessel behaviour is a complicated question because, while their physiology and functions are very different [E.Bouskela, this book], they are anatomically linked and therefore under reciprocal influence. Macrovessels are conduit arteries which propagate flow and pressure downstream to smaller resistance arteries and finally microvessels. For various reasons, however, the microvascular bed functions with a low blood pressure, meaning that control mechanisms must operate to ensure this pressure gradient. One major mechanism is the myogenic response. Defects in these protective mechanisms will consequently impair microflow.

Conversely microcirculation is the site of tissue nutrient supply and, as such, largely determines normal metabolic homeostasis as well as postischemic tissue survival. For example the role of microcirculation in CV mortality and morbidity has been clearly demonstrated [31-35]. The enormous surface of microvascular endothelium in the body is the main source of inflammation, oxidative stress and fibrinolysis, all factors which act in a deleterious fashion of large vessels and underlie atherosclerosis.

Finally, it must be realized that changes in microcirculation are not necessarily structural but that functional abnormalities (reactivity) as well as qualitative distribution of microflow (spatial heterogeneity) are extremely important factors which are hardly measurable.

4. VASCULAR EFFECTS OF GLUCOSE

Physiologically, insulin rises in response to elevations in blood glucose either after meals or after endogenous glucose production by the liver in particular. It is therefore important to know if hyperglycemia has vascular effects in the absence of concomitant hyperinsulinemia. Data must be analyzed with caution, however, because handling of glucose by the body also depends on the way of glucose administration. Thus iv glucose with concomitant blockade of pancreatic insulin secretion did not affect coronary vasodilating function [36]. In human tissue BF was unchanged under hyperglycaemic clamp conditions performed at basal insulin levels [37]. In human forearm systemic hyperglycemia without hyperinsulinemia caused sympathetic neural activation and vasodilation, but the latter was essentially attributed to osmolar stress [38]. In diabetes the same approach induced reductions in endothelial function [39]. A very interesting comparison was made in humans, comparing normo- and hyperglycaemic clamps with mixed meal: calf BF increased after hyperinsulinemia and mixed meal while hyperglycemia increased peripheral vascular resistance [40]. A study using local intrarterial glucose injection reported impairments in endothelium-dependent VD [41], while another reported VD [42]. A 24h local hyperglycemia did not change forearm BF, neither in muscle nor in skin [43].

In the mesenteric microcirculation infusion of glucose decreased leucocyte rolling and increased their adhesion to the vessel walls [44]. Again this effect was largely attributed to osmolarity. In perfused rat hearts, acute hyperglycemia induced vasoconstriction [45]. Intraperitoneal glucose administration induced reduction in cerebral BF in rats, also possibly due to osmolarity [46]. Thus, it appears that, in particular in animals, acute transient hyperglycaemic episodes are rather constrictive and impair NIO-dependent VD. In fact glucose reduces NO synthesis [47, 48] and is shown to directly scavenge NO [49].

5. VASODILATING EFFECTS OF INSULIN AND ITS MECHANISMS

Hemodynamic effects of insulin are known for long time. Insulin has direct vasodilating as well as anticonstrictor properties. Many reviews have appeared describing and discussing the significance of this effect [50-52]. Indeed most studies have used supraphysiological hormone concentrations and all showed vasodilatation, which were frequently long-lasting [53]. In other studies it was reported that vasodilatation appeared long after starting infusion [54, 55]. This effect is not compatible with direct vasomotor effects and may be attributed to secondary phenomena linked to either metabolic effects of insulin or activation of other systems; in addition to its dilating effects, insulin also acts as an anticonstrictor against several agonists [56, 57].

Numerous studies showed that insulin increases NO synthesis and stimulates eNOS genes [58, 59] and that the vascular (and the metabolic?) effects of insulin can be largely attenuated by NO blockade. It was also shown that insulin increased the availability of tetrahydrobiopterin, a co-factor of NO [60]. This dilating effect is partly counterbalanced by a constrictor effect in arterioles [61] which can be revealed by blocking the NO pathway or using very high insulin concentrations. It has even been reported that insulin can acutely induce ED [62]. The production of NO by insulin in vascular cells is mediated by the same pathway as for glucose uptake, i.e. PI3kinase and Akt [58, 63]. In vivo the PI3 kinase inhibitor wortmannin inhibited insulin effects completely in the liver and partially in skeletal muscle [64].

At low, physiological concentrations insulin does not increase the bulk flow; this might be explained by the fact that small arterioles depend on EDHF much more than on NO [65]. Loss of EDHF has been reported during insulin resistance in small arterioles of rats fed with high fructose [66].

In addition to NO, adenosine [67, 68], cholinergic muscarinic receptors with variable impact according to muscle type [69] and the sodium/potassium pump [70] also appear to be involved.

Whether these vasodilating effects are relevant for its metabolic action is a highly debated question [71, 72]; indeed quite unphysiological conditions have been used for most studies [clamp], in particular the hormone concentrations, raising the question of whether the observed vasodilatations were due to direct vasomotor effects or were mediated through activation of the sympathetic nervous system. In dogs, infusion of insulin activated the sympathetic system but without influencing skeletal muscle blood flow [73]. In humans it was found that both low and high insulin doses induced vasodilatation despite the increases in muscle sympathetic nervous activity and plasma norepinephrine [74]. Another study showed that modest hyperinsulinemia [25 µU/ml] increased sympathetic activity without concomitant changes in vascular resistance [75], also showing that vasodilatation of large vessels by insulin requires relatively high concentrations. Other reported no changes in plasma epinephrine and norepinephrine [76]. Hyperinsulinemia induced by oral carbohydrate intake also produced both sympathetic activation and a 47% increase in calf BF [77]. Others showed that the nervous system was not necessary to increase BF in human legs [78].

A cardinal question is which flow is increased and where. As stated elsewhere, most BF measurements only reflect bulk flow and cannot reveal flow distribution changes in the microvasculature. Thus local vasodilatation can increase GU or not, according to the procedure used [79]. Several reports exist showing that skin and subcutaneous fat can substantially contribute to limb BF measurements [80]. A study in humans showed that under euglycemic clamp conditions calf and forearm BF increased but not in these limb's skeletal muscles [81]. In addition, it appears that sex differences exist, women showing larger flow increases than men [82]. These data nicely demonstrate that increasing flow means little by itself and that the key factor is where blood is flowing [tissue, vessel type]. It also possibly explains why provoked BF increases do not necessarily lead to parallel increases in GU [83]. Furthermore there are reports showing no vasoactive effect of insulin after local injection [84, 85], in contrast to systemic insulin [85, 86]. Also the increase in adipose tissue BF after oral glucose was higher than after iv infusion of similar glucose and insulin concentrations, suggesting that additional factors possibly originating in the digestive tract may be involved in daily life.

Finally it must be recalled that high does of insulin also stimulate IGF-1 receptors and that, like insulin, IGF-1 is able to provoke vasodilatation but not to increase GU [87,88]. IGF-1 receptors are more numerous than insulin receptors on human macro- and microvascular endothelial cells [89]. Most of the insulin receptors in endothelial cells are in fact hybrid IGF-1/insulin receptors [. As it was also shown that the vasodilatation induced by IGF-1 is not blocked by NO blockade [90], these clearcut differences with insulin could mean that it is the endothelium rather than flow increase as such which links insulin to GU; this concept would also explain why increases in organ BF do not necessarily correlate with tissue GU if high insulin concentrations, stimulating IGF-1 receptors, have been used. The eminent role of the endothelium is corroborated by experiments using NO inhibitors but since these agents also interfere with GU, results must be interpreted with caution.

6. MICROVASCULAR EFFECTS OF INSULIN

When administered alone insulin also dilates small muscle arterioles: superfusion of EDL muscles with basal insulin concentrations dilated 3 and A4 arterioles, while higher concentrations (200μU/ml) also dilated larger A2 arterioles, in agreement with in vivo studies showing flow increases with very high or supraphysiological hormone levels [91,92]. The same was found in muscle arterioles after sc administration of insulin [93, 94]. No effect was found, however, by superfusing mesenteric arterioles [95] or investigating isolated renal arterioles [96]. Sustained hyperglycemia for 5 days increased blood flow in skeletal muscle but not in other tissues [97]. The latter results suggest that microvascular reaction may differ according to the tissue and that possible skeletal muscle microvessels have a preferential sensitivity to insulin in view of the prominent role played by skeletal muscle in glucose homeostasis.

Recent work showed that more physiological doses of the hormone were increasing microflow and particularly the recruitment of blood perfused capillaries. Several sophisticated techniques have been used in animals and humans which, together, clearly demonstrate higher capillary perfusion with quite low insulin concentrations. This is mediated through dilation of precapillary arterioles, provided only insulin alone is used [98-101]: this effect occurs with hormone levels as low as 2-3fold basal plasma levels. As will be discussed later, this physiological situation corresponds to the cephalic phase of insulin secretion and to the very early postprandial phase. At these concentrations bulk organ blood flow was unchanged.

	Time to reach half-maximal response in vivo (min)
Arterial [INS]	2
Capillary recruitment	15
Glucose Disposal rate	20
Lymph [INS]	28
Receptor activation	31
Total blood flow	>30< ?

As summarized in Table 1 (modified from 102), a time-dependent logical physiological progression of physiological processes can be observed in vivo, and where capillary recruitment occurs very rapidly, is followed much later by insulin receptor stimulation and finally increases in organ blood flow. The latter is likely linked to increased tissue metabolism (lactate, others) secondarily increasing blood flow due to the intimate coupling between flow and metabolism. Very importantly capillary recruitment is accompanied by increased tissue GU [102]. The capillary recruiting effect of low insulin was also observed in postischemic situations [103] and insulin may act protectively during postischemic periods. Our own experiments in rats suggest that this process continues during the period corresponding to postprandial glucose and insulin levels, albeit by engaging different mechanisms [see below]. In humans it was shown that systemic hyperinsulinemia also increased capillary recruitment in skin and activated vasomotion [104-106]. Insulin-induced increase in microflow was also reported in human myocardium [107]. Conversely free fatty acids, glucosamine or endothelin 1 block capillary recruitment and, as expected, GU [108-110]. Blunting of capillary recruitment was also observed in human hypertension [111] and truncal subcutaneous adiposity reduced capillary recruitment in skin via inflammatory factors liberated by fat [112].

In human clamp studies, partly contradictory effects were reported: no increase in inulin distribution volume was seen at 70µU/ml insulin [113] and another study failed to observe vasodilation at physiological insulin levels, but the variation coefficient was 22% [114]. Other studies, however, reported an increase in microvascular blood volume at 2 hours and a 15% dilation of leg blood flow which correlated with capillary density [115].

Very interestingly C-peptide is also able to increase microflow [116-118], capillary surface area [119] as well as red cell deformability [120]. This is important because it could mean that it is C-peptide may add to insulin for actions on microvessels and might further provide an explanation for the less convincing results obtained under clamp conditions using external insulin.

7. GLUCOSE + INSULIN: EFFECTS ON BLOOD FLOW

Physiologically insulin increases after plasma glucose rises, because the role of the hormone in this phase is to push glucose entry into skeletal muscle and store is as glycogen. Therefore only studies on oral glucose ingestion or experimental simultaneous increases in glucose and insulin are really relevant to solve the question of causality of flow changes in glucose homeostasis. The vasodilating effects of the hormone is largely due to increased nitric oxide (NO) production by the endothelium but, as shown above, the trend of glucose is rather opposite, raising the possibility that either the net effect is neutral or shifted into the one or other direction.

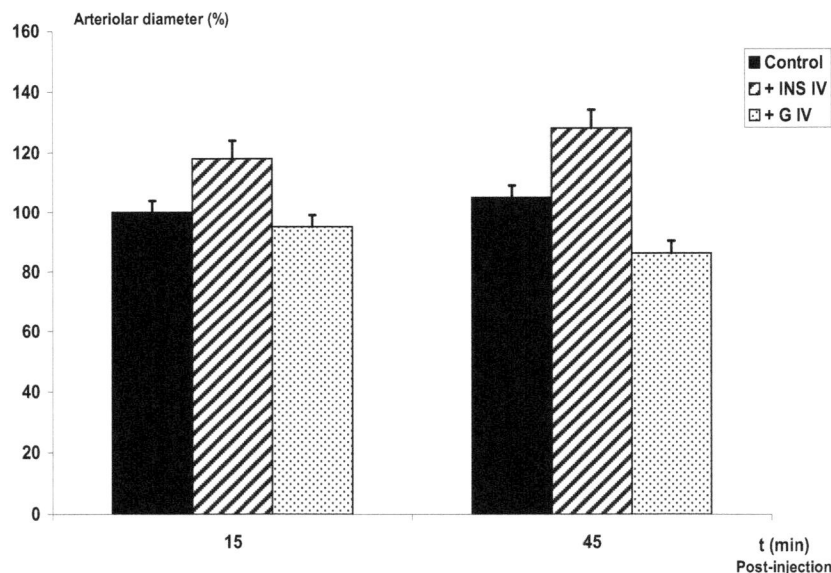

Figure 1: Changes in muscle arteriolar diameter induced by similar levels of plasma insulin, after subcutaneous injection of insulin (normoglycemia, hatched bars) or after intravenous glucose (black bars).

In cultured endothelial cells high glucose blunted the NO generation by insulin [121]. Studies using the OGTT have shown attenuated myogenic constriction, possibly explaining the postprandial hypotension [122]. Other studies showed attenuation of endothelium-dependent vasodilation [123-125]. Another study reported no changes in global forearm BF but skeletal muscle BF was reduced by 30% while subcutaneous flow increased and skin showed a biphasic response [126]. However it must be noted that noradrenaline and adrenaline strongly increased, which could explain this important constriction in muscle, since arterioles are richly innervated with beta receptors [127] and sympathetic stimulation constricts arterioles [128]. Interestingly glucose did not increase sympathetic nervous activity if administered by iv route [129]. In humans OGTT impaired coronary microcirculation [130]. OGTT increased skin microflow as well as the reactivity to acetylcholine [131]. In human skeletal muscle, calf blood flow was increased by 47% [77] and the permeability surface for glucose was increased by OGTT, suggesting increased capillary opening [132]. Still OGTT is a test procedure and not physiological and the most relevant data are found in studies using mixed meals. An ordinary mixed meal impaired endothelium-dependent vasodilation but this effect may have been ascribed to the fat content. Hypertriglyceridemia alone had no effect on calf BF, in contrast to the mixed meal [40,133,134]. In another study leg BF was increased by about 20% after a mixed meal, whether taken as bolus or in frequent small feedings [135]. Forearm BF increased almost 2fold in another investigation and it was found that BF contributed to 41% of the GU [54]. Local injection of a mixture of glucose and insulin in humans increased forearm blood flow by 30%, an effect shown to be a significant predictor of insulin-mediated GU [8].

At the microvascular level very few data have been obtained under such conditions. In rats we have visualized skeletal muscle microcirculation under 2 situations resulting in comparable insulin levels: one by subcutaneous insulin injection, the other induced by iv glucose such as to reach comparable plasma insulin concentrations [94]. It can be seen Fig. (**1**) that insulin alone dilated precapillary arterioles and abolished spontaneous arteriolar vasomotion; this effect was completely different in the presence of concomitant hyperglycemia: arterioles tended to constrict and vasomotion was activated Fig. (**2**). Microflow in these muscles showed no major modification under these circumstances [94], suggesting that dynamic modifications and flow redistribution were taking place rather than a real increase in flow

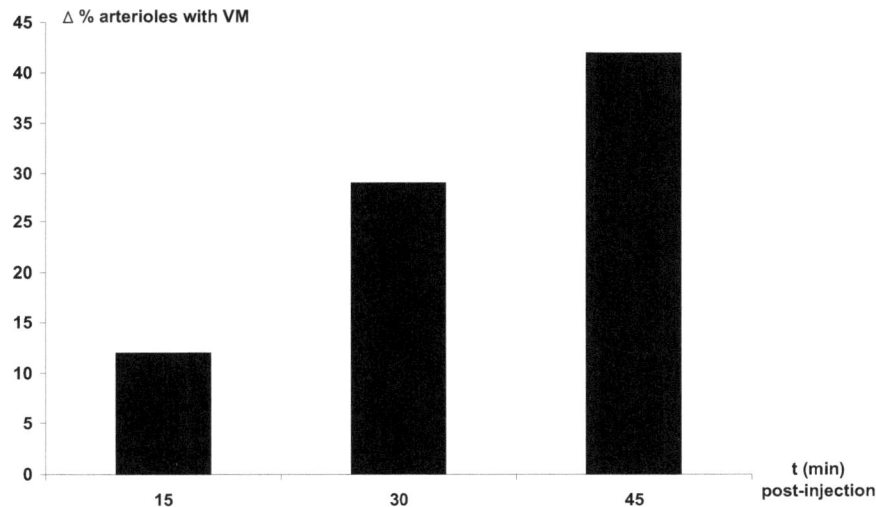

Figure 2: Increased arteriolar vasomotion induced by intravenous glucose infusion; no vasomotion was seen with insulin alone.

These data also confirm that a physiological elevation of glucose has a net microvascular effect blunting the vasodilating effect of insulin in muscle arterioles. The opposite effects between glucose and insulin + glucose fit with in vitro findings on NO production in endothelial cells [136]. Microflow was measured by using desmethylimipramine, a marker with high specificity for the microvessels. With insulin alone microflow at the end of the experiment was doubled. After acute glucose infusion, however, microflow was not significantly increased (1,25fold, ns). Nevertheless the data with insulin alone do not mean that capillaries have been recruited since the 2fold increase may simply reflect the arteriolar dilation.

In the combined administration, plasma glucose and insulin normalized relatively rapidly, so that microflow determination at the end of the experiment was made under close to normal conditions of prevailing substrates. Since postprandial states are relatively long-lasting, we studied the microvascular effects of glucose and insulin at plateau levels corresponding to physiological postprandial levels (G=9mM, INS=100-120μU/ml). Again the arteriolar vasodilation induced by insulin alone was blunted when moderate hyperglycemia was present Fig. (**3**) (C. Renaudin and N. Wiernsperger, unpublished results). However, under these conditions, microflow was increased 1,7fold, suggesting that the absence of precapillary dilatation was compensated for by capillary recruitment.

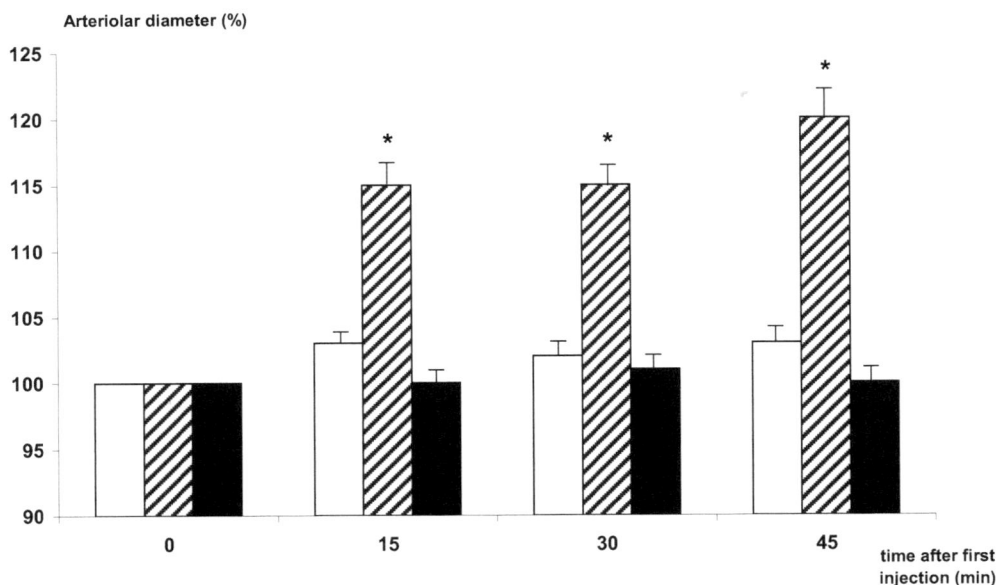

Figure 3: Muscle arteriolar diameter changes induced by a plateau of insulin at 100-120µU/ml alone (hatched bars) or with concomitant mild hyperglycemia (black bars).

These direct in situ observations of the muscle microcirculation are in agreement with the findings of other groups stating that physiological increments of insulin increase capillary perfusion without augmenting bulk BF [102].

We have suggested in 1998 that arteriolar vasomotion might be the mechanism whereby microflow could increase through more perfused capillaries without a significant augmentation of global blood volume [94]. In our hands vasomotion was always activated by arteriolar constriction, while arteriolar dilation was always seen to abolish this phenomenon. Experiments using the antidiabetic metformin,a drug with some unique direct microcirculatory effects have also shown that small arteriolar contraction in muscle or hamster cheek pouch were accompanied by stimulated vasomotion and this effect improved nutritive flow and postischemic recovery under pathological conditions [82]. Its microvascular protective effect may be a major reason for the improvements in IR observed in human prediabetics and diabetics with metformin.

Although our mechanistic concepts of vasomotion diverge from others who found activation of vasomotion by insulin alone in skin [106], we both agree that vasomotion may be the key process whereby insulin recruits the capillary bed at low concentrations [9].

8. PHYSIOLOGICAL SIGNIFICANCE OF MICROFLOW FOR GLUCOSE UPTAKE

Our data showed that microvascular modifications occurred during prevailing mild hyperglycemia such as they exist after meal. Comparison of our experimental groups suggests that the increase in microflow participates in muscle glucose uptake. If this concept is verified, it then represents an extremely important phenomenon which, if defective, would be a potential cause of tissular IR by interfering with substrate delivery and glucose storage.

Many pharmacological approaches have been used to try to better check the links between flow changes and GU induced by insulin. However one must be aware that almost without exceptions the drugs used have in fact effects on both parameters by lack of selectivity. Thus pertinent conclusions from these experiments can not be drawn. Examples of such compounds include β-adrenergic agonists [137,138], α1-drenergic drugs [139,140], dopamine [141,142], angiotensin II [143-145], endothelin 1 [146-148], adenosine [149,150], bradykinin [151-153], ACE inhibitors [154]. Because nitric oxide [NO] was considered to largely underlie insulin-induced vasodilation, stimulation or blockade of NO production has been widely tested. Thus administration of the NO-donor SNP increased leg BF to the same extent as verapamil, yet its effect on GU was greater [155], while NO blockade by L-NMMA decreased GU but not BF during exercise [156]. Disruption of eNOS and nNOS rendered mice insulin resistant [157]. While NO is a main –but not unique- player in endothelium-dependent dilatation, it is also involved in insulin signalling to GU, which strongly limits any firm conclusions on results using various NO inhibitors.

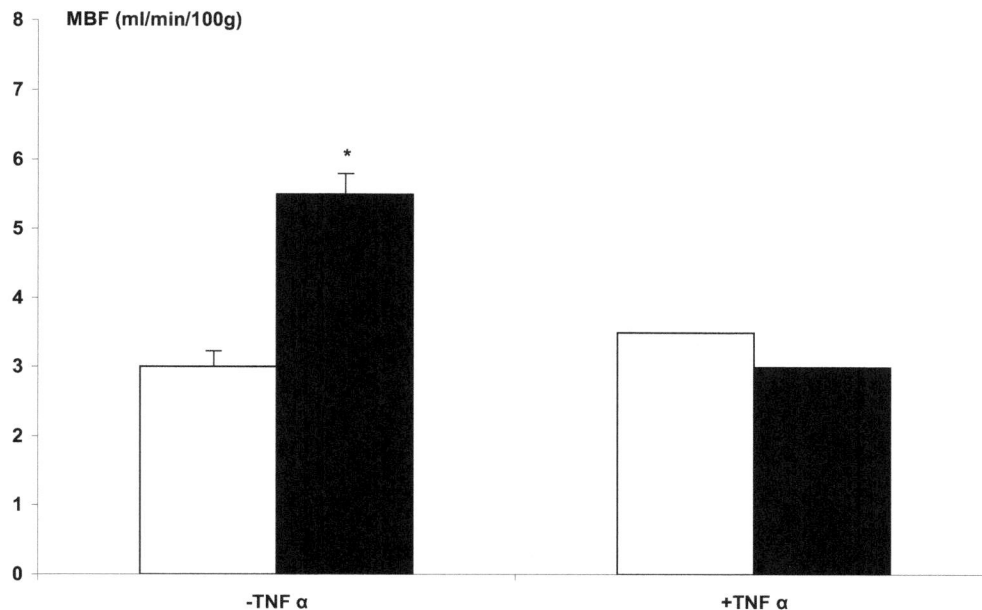

Figure 4: Muscle microflow changes after insulin in the absence (left columns) or presence (right columns) of TNFα.

An alternative might be tumor necrosis factor α (TNFα) since this cytokine is known to induce IR in vivo [158], while having no direct effect on insulin-stimulated tissue GU, at least when added acutely in vitro [159,160]. When TNFα was injected for 2h, videomicroscopic quantification in rat spinotrapezius muscle showed that, as expected, arteriolar dilatation and muscle BF elevation by insulin were blunted Fig. (**4**). Skeletal muscle GU was reduced by 40-50% Fig. (**5**), which agrees with similar findings of other groups who reported a participation of about 40% of the microflow in muscle GU (54).

One can thus conclude that microflow is indeed involved in glucose delivery to target tissues and that it represents a substantial part of peripheral muscle GU within the normal physiological range of glucose/insulin levels. It was repeatedly found that capillary recruitment occurred with insulin concentrations as low as some additional µU/ml above the basal, plasma insulin level. Thus, in addition to postprandial states, one may envisage the implication of this insulin effect very early in prandial physiology, i.e. during the so-called 'cephalic phase' of insulin secretion. In contrast to the plasma insulin elevations induced by glucose which are relatively important, the secretion during the cephalic phase, which is due to emotional, nervous and taste -related factors is quite low; nevertheless, as suggested long ago by Rasio, insulin may 'open its own way' by recruiting capillaries through such small signals in order to prepare the muscle mass to receive the excess in glucose entering circulation after meals. Eating is a conditioned situation in which daily habits and immediate psychological aspects as well as food taste represent factors leading to pancreatic secretion starting within minutes. Conditioned feeding [161] as well as sham feeding experiments in rats revealed increases in plasma insulin in the absence of food [162,163]. Even in humans it could be shown that insulin oscillations took place at the normal time of a lunch meal [164]. Insulinemia can start to rise as early as 1-4 min after meal onset [164], i.e. long before glycemia starts to rise. There is clearly a temporal organization of insulin secretion and optimal hormone secretion is dependent on periodic rather than continuous exposure to extracellular signals [165]. Further, palatability also determines insulin peaks since plasma insulin can rise up to 65µU/ml in rats if food tastes sweet [166].

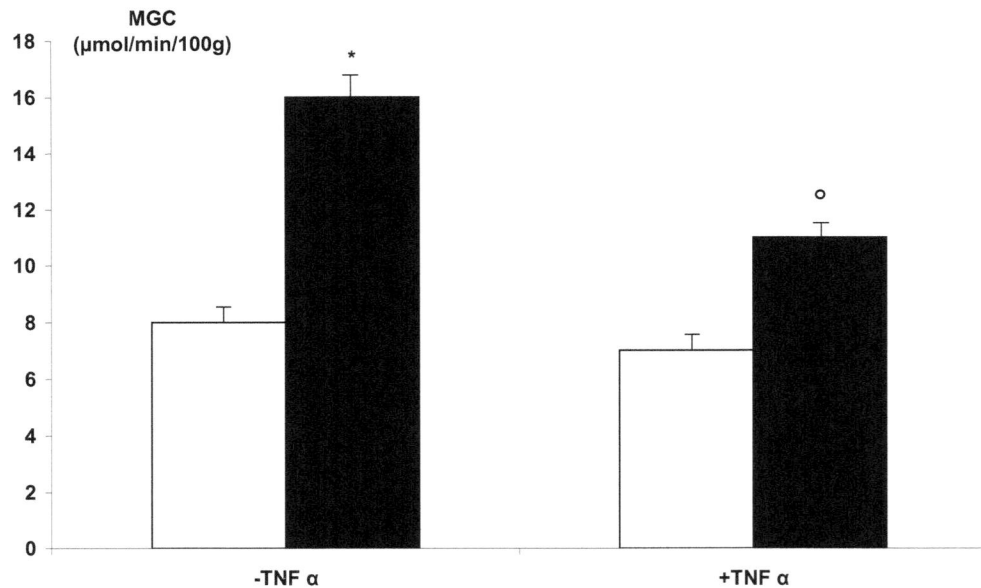

Figure 5: Changes in muscle glucose consumption induced by insulin in the absence (left columns) or presence (right columns) of TNFα.

It is thus extremely likely that these early peaks of plasma insulin which proceed postprandial the glucose and insulin elevations in blood may open the microvascular bed to a maximum such that the muscle mass can exert its role to store maximally excessive glucose. However this exciting hypothesis has to be confirmed by appropriate kinetic experiments for which technology is now available.

9. TRANSENDOTHELIAL INSULIN TRANSPORT

To reach its target cells insulin must cross the wall of microvessels; while this is easy in the fenestrated microvessels of the liver it is more difficult in skeletal muscle, where endothelium is much tighter. It was shown that insulin stimulates its own transport across endothelial cells [167] but how this is done is still a matter of debate: vesicular transport, receptor-mediated processes or paracellular passage have all been proposed [168-173]. It is also very interesting to recall an old observation showing that endothelium was able to store insulin, possibly allowing thereby the hormone to be very rapidly liberated into interstitial fluid [174]. It was demonstrated by direct sampling of lymph or interstitial fluid that 1] there exists an important gradient between plasma and interstitial insulin concentrations [175,176] and 2] that muscle GU was correlated with interstitial rather than plasma insulin [177].

Therefore, impairment of any step in transendothelial access of the hormone to its target cells is a rate-limiting one and, as such, a potential cause of IR [178]. This concept has been raised long time ago [179,180]. In animals it was shown that insulin can be delayed substantially either by artificial means [181] or by using obese insulin resistant rats [182] in which the transfer time was doubled. Similar findings were obtained in obese dogs [183]. Few data exits in humans: this defect was suspected in acromegalics to explain their IR [179] and reported in hypertensive subjects [184]. In obese subjects, delivery of insulin to muscle interstitial fluid was delayed after OGTT [185]. More information on these exciting topics can be found in some recent reviews on these various aspects [186-188].

10. REFERENCES

[1]   Ganrot PO, Curman B, Kron B. Type 2 diabetes. Primary vascular disorder with metabolic symptoms? Med Hypotheses 1987 Sep; 24(1): 77-86.
[2]   Egan BM. Neurohumoral, hemodynamic and microvascular changes as mechanisms of insulin resistance in hypertension: a provocative but partial picture. Int J Obes 1991 Sep; 15 Suppl 2: 133-9.
[3]   Wiernsperger N. Vascular defects in the aetiology of peripheral insulin resistance in diabetes. A critical review of hypotheses and facts. Diabetes Metab Rev 1994 Oct; 10(3): 287-307.

[4]   Pinkney JH, Stehouwer CD, Coppack SW, Yudkin JS. Endothelial dysfunction: cause of the insulin resistance syndrome. Diabetes 1997 Sep; 46 Suppl 2: S9-13.

[5]   Shoemaker JK, Bonen A. Vascular actions of insulin in health and disease. Can J Appl Physiol 1995 Jun; 20(2): 127-54.

[6]   Tooke J. The association between insulin resistance and endotheliopathy. Diabetes Obes Metab 1999 May; 1 Suppl 1: S17-22.

[7]   Baron AD. Insulin and the vasculature--old actors, new roles. J Investig Med 1996 Oct; 44(8): 406-12.

[8]   Cleland SJ, Petrie JR, Ueda S, Elliott HL, Connell JM. Insulin as a vascular hormone: implications for the pathophysiology of cardiovascular disease. Clin Exp Pharmacol Physiol 1998 Mar-Apr; 25(3-4): 175-84.

[9]   Clark MG. Impaired microvascular perfusion: a consequence of vascular dysfunction and a potential cause of insulin resistance in muscle. Am J Physiol Endocrinol Metab 2008 Oct; 295(4): E732-50.

[10]   Bakker W, Eringa EC, Sipkema P, van Hinsbergh VW. Endothelial dysfunction and diabetes: roles of hyperglycemia, impaired insulin signaling and obesity. Cell Tissue Res 2009 Jan; 335(1): 165-89.

[11]   Wiernsperger NF, Bouskela E. Microcirculation in insulin resistance and diabetes: more than just a complication. Diabetes Metab 2003 Sep; 29(4 Pt 2): 6S77-87.

[12]   Wiernsperger N, Nivoit P, De Aguiar LG, Bouskela E. Microcirculation and the metabolic syndrome. Microcirculation 2007 Jun-Jul; 14(4-5): 403-38.

[13]   Kim F, Pham M, Maloney E, Rizzo NO, Morton GJ, Wisse BE, *et al.* Vascular inflammation, insulin resistance, and reduced nitric oxide production precede the onset of peripheral insulin resistance. Arterioscler Thromb Vasc Biol 2008 Nov; 28(11): 1982-8.

[14]   Katakam PV, Ujhelyi MR, Hoenig ME, Miller AW. Endothelial dysfunction precedes hypertension in diet-induced insulin resistance. Am J Physiol 1998 Sep; 275(3 Pt 2): R788-92.

[15]   Gopaul NK, Manraj MD, Hebe A, Lee Kwai Yan S, Johnston A, Carrier MJ, *et al.* Oxidative stress could precede endothelial dysfunction and insulin resistance in Indian Mauritians with impaired glucose metabolism. Diabetologia 2001 Jun; 44(6): 706-12.

[16]   Tooke JE, Goh KL. Endotheliopathy precedes type 2 diabetes. Diabetes Care 1998 Dec; 21(12): 2047-9.

[17]   Ronnemaa EM, Ronnemaa T, Utriainen T, Raitakari M, Laine H, Takala T, *et al.* Decreased blood flow but unaltered insulin sensitivity of glucose uptake in skeletal muscle of chronic smokers. Metabolism 1999 Feb; 48(2): 239-44.

[18]   Andersson P, Lind L, Berne C, Berglund L, Lithell HO. Insulin-mediated vasodilation and glucose uptake are independently related to fasting serum nonesterified fatty acids in elderly men. J Intern Med 1999 Dec; 246(6): 529-37.

[19]   Raitakari M, Nuutila P, Ruotsalainen U, Laine H, Teras M, Iida H, *et al.* Evidence for dissociation of insulin stimulation of blood flow and glucose uptake in human skeletal muscle: studies using [15O]H2O, [18F]fluoro-2-deoxy-D-glucose, and positron emission tomography. Diabetes 1996 Nov; 45(11): 1471-7.

[20]   Utriainen T, Makimattila S, Virkamaki A, Bergholm R, Yki-Jarvinen H. Dissociation between insulin sensitivity of glucose uptake and endothelial function in normal subjects. Diabetologia 1996 Dec; 39(12): 1477-82.

[21]   Mather K, Laakso M, Edelman S, Hook G, Baron A. Evidence for physiological coupling of insulin-mediated glucose metabolism and limb blood flow. Am J Physiol Endocrinol Metab 2000 Dec; 279(6): E1264-70.

[22]   Kern M, Tapscott EB, Snider RD, Dohm GL. Differences in glucose transport rates between perfused and in vitro incubated muscles. Horm Metab Res 1990 Jul; 22(7): 366-8.

[23]   Wallis MG, Smith ME, Kolka CM, Zhang L, Richards SM, Rattigan S, *et al.* Acute glucosamine-induced insulin resistance in muscle in vivo is associated with impaired capillary recruitment. Diabetologia 2005 Oct; 48(10): 2131-9.

[24]   Ebeling P, Bourey R, Koranyi L, Tuominen JA, Groop LC, Henriksson J, *et al.* Mechanism of enhanced insulin sensitivity in athletes. Increased blood flow, muscle glucose transport protein (GLUT-4) concentration, and glycogen synthase activity. J Clin Invest 1993 Oct; 92(4): 1623-31.

[25]   Grubb B, Snarr JF. Effect of flow rate and glucose concentration on glucose uptake rate by the rat limb. Proc Soc Exp Biol Med 1977 Jan; 154(1): 33-6.

[26]   Schultz TA, Lewis SB, Westbie DK, Wallin JD, Gerich JE. Glucose delivery: a modulator of glucose uptake in contracting skeletal muscle. Am J Physiol 1977 Dec; 233(6): E514-8.

[27]   Stefl B, Zurmanova J. Effects of the perfusion flow rate on skeletal muscle energy metabolism and a possible role of second messengers in this process. Physiol Res 2006; 55(1): 79-88.

[28]   Bertoldo A, Pencek RR, Azuma K, Price JC, Kelley C, Cobelli C, *et al.* Interactions between delivery, transport, and phosphorylation of glucose in governing uptake into human skeletal muscle. Diabetes 2006 Nov; 55(11): 3028-37.

[29]   Vollus GC, Bradley EA, Roberts MK, Newman JM, Richards SM, Rattigan S, *et al.* Graded occlusion of perfused rat muscle vasculature decreases insulin action. Clin Sci (Lond) 2007 Apr; 112(8): 457-66.

[30]   Clark MG, Colquhoun EQ, Rattigan S, Dora KA, Eldershaw TP, Hall JL, *et al.* Vascular and endocrine control of muscle metabolism. Am J Physiol 1995 May; 268(5 Pt 1): E797-812.

[31]   Camici PG. From microcirculation to cardiac event: protection with Preterax. J Hypertens 2008 Jun; 26 Suppl 2: S8-S10.

[32]   Lockhart CJ, Hamilton PK, Quinn CE, McVeigh GE. End-organ dysfunction and cardiovascular outcomes: the role of the microcirculation. Clin Sci (Lond) 2009 Feb; 116(3): 175-90.

[33]   Lerman A, Holmes DR, Herrmann J, Gersh BJ. Microcirculatory dysfunction in ST-elevation myocardial infarction: cause, consequence, or both? Eur Heart J 2007 Apr; 28(7): 788-97.

[34]   Abularrage CJ, Sidawy AN, Aidinian G, Singh N, Weiswasser JM, Arora S. Evaluation of the microcirculation in vascular disease. J Vasc Surg 2005 Sep; 42(3): 574-81.

[35]   Strain WD, Chaturvedi N, Bulpitt CJ, Rajkumar C, Shore AC. Albumin excretion rate and cardiovascular risk: could the association be explained by early microvascular dysfunction? Diabetes 2005 Jun; 54(6): 1816-22.

[36]   Capaldo B, Galderisi M, Turco AA, D'Errico A, Turco S, Rivellese AA, *et al.* Acute hyperglycemia does not affect the reactivity of coronary microcirculation in humans. J Clin Endocrinol Metab 2005 Jul; 90(7): 3871-6.

[37]   Henry S, Schneiter P, Jequier E, Tappy L. Effects of hyperinsulinemia and hyperglycemia on lactate release and local blood flow in subcutaneous adipose tissue of healthy humans. J Clin Endocrinol Metab 1996 Aug; 81(8): 2891-5.

[38]   Hoffman RP, Hausberg M, Sinkey CA, Anderson EA. Hyperglycemia without hyperinsulinemia produces both sympathetic neural activation and vasodilation in normal humans. J Diabetes Complications 1999 Jan-Feb; 13(1): 17-22.

[39]   Kim SH, Park KW, Kim YS, Oh S, Chae IH, Kim HS, *et al.* Effects of acute hyperglycemia on endothelium-dependent vasodilation in patients with diabetes mellitus or impaired glucose metabolism. Endothelium 2003; 10(2): 65-70.

[40]   Fugmann A, Millgard J, Sarabi M, Berne C, Lind L. Central and peripheral haemodynamic effects of hyperglycaemia, hyperinsulinaemia, hyperlipidaemia or a mixed meal. Clin Sci (Lond) 2003 Dec; 105(6): 715-21.

[41]   Williams SB, Goldfine AB, Timimi FK, Ting HH, Roddy MA, Simonson DC, *et al.* Acute hyperglycemia attenuates endothelium-dependent vasodilation in humans in vivo. Circulation 1998 May 5; 97(17): 1695-701.

[42]   van Veen S, Frolich M, Chang PC. Acute hyperglycaemia in the forearm induces vasodilation that is not modified by hyperinsulinaemia. J Hum Hypertens 1999 Apr; 13(4): 263-8.

[43]   Houben AJ, Schaper NC, de Haan CH, Huvers FC, Slaaf DW, de Leeuw PW, *et al.* Local 24-h hyperglycemia does not affect endothelium-dependent or -independent vasoreactivity in humans. Am J Physiol 1996 Jun; 270(6 Pt 2): H2014-20.

[44]   Schaffler A, Arndt H, Scholmerich J, Palitzsch K. Acute hyperglycaemia causes severe disturbances of mesenteric microcirculation in an in vivo rat model. Eur J Clin Invest 1998 Nov; 28(11): 886-93.

[45]   Ward BJ, al-Haboubi HA. Structural changes in the cardiac microvasculature of the rat in response to acute high glucose levels: a comparison with diabetes. Microcirculation 1997 Dec; 4(4): 429-37.

[46]   Duckrow RB, Beard DC, Brennan RW. Regional cerebral blood flow decreases during hyperglycemia. Ann Neurol 1985 Mar; 17(3): 267-72.

[47]   Noyman I, Marikovsky M, Sasson S, Stark AH, Bernath K, Seger R, *et al.* Hyperglycemia reduces nitric oxide synthase and glycogen synthase activity in endothelial cells. Nitric Oxide 2002 Nov; 7(3): 187-93.

[48]   Salt IP, Morrow VA, Brandie FM, Connell JM, Petrie JR. High glucose inhibits insulin-stimulated nitric oxide production without reducing endothelial nitric-oxide synthase Ser1177 phosphorylation in human aortic endothelial cells. J Biol Chem 2003 May 23; 278(21): 18791-7.

[49]   Brodsky SV, Morrishow AM, Dharia N, Gross SS, Goligorsky MS. Glucose scavenging of nitric oxide. Am J Physiol Renal Physiol 2001 Mar; 280(3): F480-6.

[50]   Ganrot PO. Insulin resistance syndrome: possible key role of blood flow in resting muscle. Diabetologia 1993 Sep; 36(9): 876-9.

[51]   Baron AD. Insulin resistance and vascular function. J Diabetes Complications 2002 Jan-Feb; 16(1): 92-102.

[52]   Mather K, Anderson TJ, Verma S. Insulin action in the vasculature: physiology and pathophysiology. J Vasc Res 2001 Sep-Oct; 38(5): 415-22.

[53]   Raitakari M, Knuuti MJ, Ruotsalainen U, Laine H, Makea P, Teras M, *et al.* Insulin increases blood volume in human skeletal muscle: studies using [15O]CO and positron emission tomography. Am J Physiol 1995 Dec; 269(6 Pt 1): E1000-5.

[54]   Fugmann A, Lind L, Andersson PE, Millgard J, Hanni A, Berne C, *et al.* The effect of euglucaemic hyperinsulinaemia on forearm blood flow and glucose uptake in the human forearm. Acta Diabetol 1998 Dec; 35(4): 203-6.

[55]   Hermann TS, Ihlemann N, Dominguez H, Rask-Madsen C, Kober L, Torp-Pedersen C. Prolonged local forearm hyperinsulinemia induces sustained enhancement of nitric oxide-dependent vasodilation in healthy subjects. Endothelium 2004 Sep-Dec; 11(5-6): 231-9.

[56]   McNally PG, Lawrence IG, Watt PA, Hillier C, Burden AC, Thurston H. The effect of insulin on the vascular reactivity of isolated resistance arteries taken from healthy volunteers. Diabetologia 1995 Apr; 38(4): 467-73.

[57]   Wambach GK, Liu D. Insulin attenuates vasoconstriction by noradrenaline, serotonin and potassium chloride in rat mesenteric arterioles. Clin Exp Hypertens A 1992; 14(4): 733-40.

[58]   Zeng G, Nystrom FH, Ravichandran LV, Cong LN, Kirby M, Mostowski H, *et al.* Roles for insulin receptor, PI3-kinase, and Akt in insulin-signaling pathways related to production of nitric oxide in human vascular endothelial cells. Circulation 2000 Apr 4; 101(13): 1539-45.

[59]   Kuboki K, Jiang ZY, Takahara N, Ha SW, Igarashi M, Yamauchi T, *et al.* Regulation of endothelial constitutive nitric oxide synthase gene expression in endothelial cells and in vivo : a specific vascular action of insulin. Circulation 2000 Feb 15; 101(6): 676-81.

[60]   Ishii M, Shimizu S, Nagai T, Shiota K, Kiuchi Y, Yamamoto T. Stimulation of tetrahydrobiopterin synthesis induced by insulin: possible involvement of phosphatidylinositol 3-kinase. Int J Biochem Cell Biol 2001 Jan; 33(1): 65-73.

[61]   Schroeder CA, Jr., Chen YL, Messina EJ. Inhibition of NO synthesis or endothelium removal reveals a vasoconstrictor effect of insulin on isolated arterioles. Am J Physiol 1999 Mar; 276(3 Pt 2): H815-20.

[62]   Arcaro G, Cretti A, Balzano S, Lechi A, Muggeo M, Bonora E, *et al.* Insulin causes endothelial dysfunction in humans: sites and mechanisms. Circulation 2002 Feb 5; 105(5): 576-82.

[63]   Zeng G, Quon MJ. Insulin-stimulated production of nitric oxide is inhibited by wortmannin. Direct measurement in vascular endothelial cells. J Clin Invest 1996 Aug 15; 98(4): 894-8.

[64]   Bradley EA, Clark MG, Rattigan S. Acute effects of wortmannin on insulin's hemodynamic and metabolic actions in vivo. Am J Physiol Endocrinol Metab 2007 Mar; 292(3): E779-87.

[65]   de Wit C, Wolfle SE. EDHF and gap junctions: important regulators of vascular tone within the microcirculation. Curr Pharm Biotechnol 2007 Feb; 8(1): 11-25.

[66]   Miller AW, Hoenig ME, Ujhelyi MR. Mechanisms of Impaired Endothelial Function Associated With Insulin Resistance. J Cardiovasc Pharmacol Ther 1998 Apr; 3(2): 125-34.

[67]   Abbink-Zandbergen EJ, Vervoort G, Tack CJ, Lutterman JA, Schaper NC, Smits P. The role of adenosine in insulin-induced vasodilation. J Cardiovasc Pharmacol 1999 Sep; 34(3): 374-80.

[68]   Vergauwen L, Hespel P, Richter EA. Adenosine receptors mediate synergistic stimulation of glucose uptake and transport by insulin and by contractions in rat skeletal muscle. J Clin Invest 1994 Mar; 93(3): 974-81.

[69]   Levesque M, Santure M, Pitre M, Nadeau A, Bachelard H. Cholinergic involvement in vascular and glucoregulatory actions of insulin in rats. Diabetes 2006 Feb; 55(2): 398-404.

[70]   Tack CJ, Lutterman JA, Vervoort G, Thien T, Smits P. Activation of the sodium-potassium pump contributes to insulin-induced vasodilation in humans. Hypertension 1996 Sep; 28(3): 426-32.

[71]   Yki-Jarvinen H, Utriainen T. Insulin-induced vasodilatation: physiology or pharmacology? Diabetologia 1998 Apr; 41(4): 369-79.

[72]   Utriainen T, Malmstrom R, Makimattila S, Yki-Jarvinen H. Methodological aspects, dose-response characteristics and causes of interindividual variation in insulin stimulation of limb blood flow in normal subjects. Diabetologia 1995 May; 38(5): 555-64.

[73]   Liang C, Doherty JU, Faillace R, Maekawa K, Arnold S, Gavras H, *et al.* Insulin infusion in conscious dogs. Effects on systemic and coronary hemodynamics, regional blood flows, and plasma catecholamines. J Clin Invest 1982 Jun; 69(6): 1321-36.

[74]   Anderson EA, Hoffman RP, Balon TW, Sinkey CA, Mark AL. Hyperinsulinemia produces both sympathetic neural activation and vasodilation in normal humans. J Clin Invest 1991 Jun; 87(6): 2246-52.

[75]   Hausberg M, Mark AL, Hoffman RP, Sinkey CA, Anderson EA. Dissociation of sympathoexcitatory and vasodilator actions of modestly elevated plasma insulin levels. J Hypertens 1995 Sep; 13(9): 1015-21.

[76]   Mitrakou A, Mokan M, Bolli G, Veneman T, Jenssen T, Cryer P, *et al.* Evidence against the hypothesis that hyperinsulinemia increases sympathetic nervous system activity in man. Metabolism 1992 Feb; 41(2): 198-200.

[77]   Scott EM, Greenwood JP, Vacca G, Stoker JB, Gilbey SG, Mary DA. Carbohydrate ingestion, with transient endogenous insulinaemia, produces both sympathetic activation and vasodilatation in normal humans. Clin Sci (Lond) 2002 May; 102(5): 523-9.

[78]   Dela F, Stallknecht B, Biering-Sorensen F. An intact central nervous system is not necessary for insulin-mediated increases in leg blood flow in humans. Pflugers Arch 2000 Dec; 441(2-3): 241-50.

[79]   Sarabi M, Lind L, Millgard J, Hanni A, Hagg A, Berne C, *et al.* Local vasodilatation with metacholine, but not with nitroprusside, increases forearm glucose uptake. Physiol Res 1999; 48(4): 291-5.

[80]   Blaak EE, van Baak MA, Kemerink GJ, Pakbiers MT, Heidendal GA, Saris WH. Total forearm blood flow as an indicator of skeletal muscle blood flow: effect of subcutaneous adipose tissue blood flow. Clin Sci (Lond) 1994 Nov; 87(5): 559-66.

[81]   Rosdahl H, Lind L, Millgard J, Lithell H, Ungerstedt U, Henriksson J. Effect of physiological hyperinsulinemia on blood flow and interstitial glucose concentration in human skeletal muscle and adipose tissue studied by microdialysis. Diabetes 1998 Aug; 47(8): 1296-301.

[82]   Polderman KH, Stehouwer CD, van Kamp GJ, Gooren LJ. Effects of insulin infusion on endothelium-derived vasoactive substances. Diabetologia 1996 Nov; 39(11): 1284-92.

[83]   Laine H, Yki-Jarvinen H, Kirvela O, Tolvanen T, Raitakari M, Solin O, *et al.* Insulin resistance of glucose uptake in skeletal muscle cannot be ameliorated by enhancing endothelium-dependent blood flow in obesity. J Clin Invest 1998 Mar 1; 101(5): 1156-62.

[84]   Natali A, Buzzigoli G, Taddei S, Santoro D, Cerri M, Pedrinelli R, *et al.* Effects of insulin on hemodynamics and metabolism in human forearm. Diabetes 1990 Apr; 39(4): 490-500.

[85]   Cardillo C, Kilcoyne CM, Nambi SS, Cannon RO, 3rd, Quon MJ, Panza JA. Vasodilator response to systemic but not to local hyperinsulinemia in the human forearm. Hypertension 1998 Oct; 32(4): 740-5.

[86]   Randin D, Vollenweider P, Tappy L, Jequier E, Nicod P, Scherrer U. Effects of adrenergic and cholinergic blockade on insulin-induced stimulation of calf blood flow in humans. Am J Physiol 1994 Mar; 266(3 Pt 2): R809-16.

[87]   Pendergrass M, Fazioni E, Collins D, DeFronzo RA. IGF-I increases forearm blood flow without increasing forearm glucose uptake. Am J Physiol 1998 Aug; 275(2 Pt 1): E345-50.

[88]   Arnqvist HJ. The role of IGF-system in vascular insulin resistance. Horm Metab Res 2008 Sep; 40(9): 588-92.

[89]   Chisalita SI, Arnqvist HJ. Insulin-like growth factor I receptors are more abundant than insulin receptors in human micro- and macrovascular endothelial cells. Am J Physiol Endocrinol Metab 2004 Jun; 286(6): E896-901.

[90]   Fryburg DA. NG-monomethyl-L-arginine inhibits the blood flow but not the insulin-like response of forearm muscle to IGF- I: possible role of nitric oxide in muscle protein synthesis. J Clin Invest 1996 Mar 1; 97(5): 13 19-28.

[91]   McKay MK, Hester RL. Role of nitric oxide, adenosine, and ATP-sensitive potassium channels in insulin-induced vasodilation. Hypertension 1996 Aug; 28(2): 202-8.

[92]   Wehrens XH, van Breda E, van Velzen JS, oude Egbrink MG, Slaaf DW. Use of an intact mouse skeletal muscle preparation for endocrine vascular studies: evaluation of the model. Horm Metab Res 2000 Sep; 32(9): 378-80.

[93]   Iwashita S, Yanagi K, Ohshima N, Suzuki M. Insulin increases blood flow rate in the microvasculature of cremaster muscle of the anesthetized rats. In Vivo 2001 Jan-Feb; 15(1): 11-5.

[94]   Renaudin C, Michoud E, Rapin JR, Lagarde M, Wiernsperger N. Hyperglycaemia modifies the reaction of microvessels to insulin in rat skeletal muscle. Diabetologia 1998 Jan; 41(1): 26-33.

[95]   Fortes ZB, Garcia Leme J, Scivoletto R. Vascular reactivity in diabetes mellitus: possible role of insulin on the endothelial cell. Br J Pharmacol 1984 Nov; 83(3): 635-43.

[96]   Juncos LA, Ito S. Disparate effects of insulin on isolated rabbit afferent and efferent arterioles. J Clin Invest 1993 Oct; 92(4): 1981-5.

[97]   Hilzenrat N, Arish A, Yaari A, Sikuler E. Systemic and splanchnic hemodynamics following hemorrhage and volume restitution with Haemaccel in portal hypertensive rats: the effect of propranolol. J Gastroenterol Hepatol 2001 Jul; 16(7): 796-800.

[98]   Clerk LH, Vincent MA, Lindner JR, Clark MG, Rattigan S, Barrett EJ. The vasodilatory actions of insulin on resistance and terminal arterioles and their impact on muscle glucose uptake. Diabetes Metab Res Rev 2004 Jan-Feb; 20(1): 3-12.

[99]   Coggins M, Lindner J, Rattigan S, Jahn L, Fasy E, Kaul S, et al. Physiologic hyperinsulinemia enhances human skeletal muscle perfusion by capillary recruitment. Diabetes 2001 Dec; 50(12): 2682-90.

[100]   Dawson D, Vincent MA, Barrett EJ, Kaul S, Clark A, Leong-Poi H, et al. Vascular recruitment in skeletal muscle during exercise and hyperinsulinemia assessed by contrast ultrasound. Am J Physiol Endocrinol Metab 2002 Mar; 282(3): E714-20.

[101]   Zhang L, Vincent MA, Richards SM, Clerk LH, Rattigan S, Clark MG, et al. Insulin sensitivity of muscle capillary recruitment in vivo. Diabetes 2004 Feb; 53(2): 447-53.

[102]   Vincent MA, Clerk LH, Rattigan S, Clark MG, Barrett EJ. Active role for the vasculature in the delivery of insulin to skeletal muscle. Clin Exp Pharmacol Physiol 2005 Apr; 32(4): 302-7.

[103]   Colantuoni A, Lapi D, Paterni M, Marchiafava PL. Protective effects of insulin during ischemia-reperfusion injury in hamster cheek pouch microcirculation. J Vasc Res 2005 Jan-Feb; 42(1): 55-66.

[104]   de Jongh RT, Clark AD, RG IJ, Serne EH, de Vries G, Stehouwer CD. Physiological hyperinsulinaemia increases intramuscular microvascular reactive hyperaemia and vasomotion in healthy volunteers. Diabetologia 2004 Jun; 47(6): 978-86.

[105]   Rossi M, Maurizio S, Carpi A. Skin blood flowmotion response to insulin iontophoresis in normal subjects. Microvasc Res 2005 Jul; 70(1-2): 17-22.

[106]   Serne EH, RG IJ, Gans RO, Nijveldt R, De Vries G, Evertz R, et al. Direct evidence for insulin-induced capillary recruitment in skin of healthy subjects during physiological hyperinsulinemia. Diabetes 2002 May; 51(5): 1515-22.

[107]   Liu Z. Insulin at physiological concentrations increases microvascular perfusion in human myocardium. Am J Physiol Endocrinol Metab 2007 Nov; 293(5): E1250-5.

[108]   Clerk LH, Rattigan S, Clark MG. Lipid infusion impairs physiologic insulin-mediated capillary recruitment and muscle glucose uptake in vivo. Diabetes 2002 Apr; 51(4): 1138-45.

[109]   Ross RM, Kolka CM, Rattigan S, Clark MG. Acute blockade by endothelin-1 of haemodynamic insulin action in rats. Diabetologia 2007 Feb; 50(2): 443-51.

[110]   Holmang A, Nilsson C, Niklasson M, Larsson BM, Lonroth P. Induction of insulin resistance by glucosamine reduces blood flow but not interstitial levels of either glucose or insulin. Diabetes 1999 Jan; 48(1): 106-11.

[111]   Serne EH, Gans RO, ter Maaten JC, ter Wee PM, Donker AJ, Stehouwer CD. Capillary recruitment is impaired in essential hypertension and relates to insulin's metabolic and vascular actions. Cardiovasc Res 2001 Jan; 49(1): 161-8.

[112]   de Jongh RT, Ijzerman RG, Serne EH, Voordouw JJ, Yudkin JS, de Waal HA, et al. Visceral and truncal subcutaneous adipose tissue are associated with impaired capillary recruitment in healthy individuals. J Clin Endocrinol Metab 2006 Dec; 91(12): 5100-6.

[113]   Weinhandl H, Pachler C, Mader JK, Ikeoka D, Mautner A, Falk A, et al. Physiological hyperinsulinemia has no detectable effect on access of macromolecules to insulin-sensitive tissues in healthy humans. Diabetes 2007 Sep; 56(9): 2213-7.

[114] Bonadonna RC, Saccomani MP, Del Prato S, Bonora E, DeFronzo RA, Cobelli C. Role of tissue-specific blood flow and tissue recruitment in insulin-mediated glucose uptake of human skeletal muscle. Circulation 1998 Jul 21; 98(3): 234-41.

[115] Hedman A, Andersson PE, Reneland R, Lithell HO. Insulin-mediated changes in leg blood flow are coupled to capillary density in skeletal muscle in healthy 70-year-old men. Metabolism 2001 Sep; 50(9): 1078-82.

[116] Forst T, De La Tour DD, Kunt T, Pfutzner A, Goitom K, Pohlmann T, et al. Effects of proinsulin C-peptide on nitric oxide, microvascular blood flow and erythrocyte Na+,K+-ATPase activity in diabetes mellitus type I. Clin Sci (Lond) 2000 Mar; 98(3): 283-90.

[117] Forst T, Kunt T, Wilhelm B, Weber MM, Pfutzner A. Role of C-Peptide in the regulation of microvascular blood flow. Exp Diabetes Res 2008; 2008: 176245.

[118] Delaney C, Shaw J, Day T. Acute, local effects of iontophoresed insulin and C-peptide on cutaneous microvascular function in Type 1 diabetes mellitus. Diabet Med 2004 May; 21(5): 428-33.

[119] Lindstrom K, Johansson C, Johnsson E, Haraldsson B. Acute effects of C-peptide on the microvasculature of isolated perfused skeletal muscles and kidneys in rat. Acta Physiol Scand 1996 Jan; 156(1): 19-25.

[120] Hach T, Forst T, Kunt T, Ekberg K, Pfutzner A, Wahren J. C-peptide and its C-terminal fragments improve erythrocyte deformability in type 1 diabetes patients. Exp Diabetes Res 2008; 2008: 730594.

[121] Schnyder B, Pittet M, Durand J, Schnyder-Candrian S. Rapid effects of glucose on the insulin signaling of endothelial NO generation and epithelial Na transport. Am J Physiol Endocrinol Metab 2002 Jan; 282(1): E87-94.

[122] Lott ME, Hogeman C, Herr M, Gabbay R, Sinoway LI. Effects of an oral glucose tolerance test on the myogenic response in healthy individuals. Am J Physiol Heart Circ Physiol 2007 Jan; 292(1): H304-10.

[123] Kawano H, Motoyama T, Hirashima O, Hirai N, Miyao Y, Sakamoto T, et al. Hyperglycemia rapidly suppresses flow-mediated endothelium-dependent vasodilation of brachial artery. J Am Coll Cardiol 1999 Jul; 34(1): 146-54.

[124] Akbari CM, Saouaf R, Barnhill DF, Newman PA, LoGerfo FW, Veves A. Endothelium-dependent vasodilatation is impaired in both microcirculation and macrocirculation during acute hyperglycemia. J Vasc Surg 1998 Oct; 28(4): 687-94.

[125] Title LM, Cummings PM, Giddens K, Nassar BA. Oral glucose loading acutely attenuates endothelium-dependent vasodilation in healthy adults without diabetes: an effect prevented by vitamins C and E. J Am Coll Cardiol 2000 Dec; 36(7): 2185-91.

[126] Bulow J, Astrup A, Christensen NJ, Kastrup J. Blood flow in skin, subcutaneous adipose tissue and skeletal muscle in the forearm of normal man during an oral glucose load. Acta Physiol Scand 1987 Aug; 130(4): 657-61.

[127] Martin WH, 3rd, Murphree SS, Saffitz JE. Beta-adrenergic receptor distribution among muscle fiber types and resistance arterioles of white, red, and intermediate skeletal muscle. Circ Res 1989 Jun; 64(6): 1096-105.

[128] Marshall JM. The influence of the sympathetic nervous system on individual vessels of the microcirculation of skeletal muscle of the rat. J Physiol 1982 Nov; 332: 169-86.

[129] Rowe JW, Young JB, Minaker KL, Stevens AL, Pallotta J, Landsberg L. Effect of insulin and glucose infusions on sympathetic nervous system activity in normal man. Diabetes 1981 Mar; 30(3): 2 19-25.

[130] Fujimoto K, Hozumi T, Watanabe H, Tokai K, Shimada K, Yoshiyama M, et al. Acute hyperglycemia induced by oral glucose loading suppresses coronary microcirculation on transthoracic Doppler echocardiography in healthy young adults. Echocardiography 2006 Nov; 23(10): 829-34.

[131] Forst T, Kunt T, Pohlmann T, Goitom K, Lobig M, Engelbach M, et al. Microvascular skin blood flow following the ingestion of 75 g glucose in healthy individuals. Exp Clin Endocrinol Diabetes 1998; 106(6): 454-9.

[132] Gudbjornsdottir S, Sjostrand M, Strindberg L, Wahren J, Lonnroth P. Direct measurements of the permeability surface area for insulin and glucose in human skeletal muscle. J Clin Endocrinol Metab 2003 Oct; 88(10): 4559-64.

[133] Sarabi M, Fugmann A, Karlstrom B, Berne C, Lithell H, Lind L. An ordinary mixed meal transiently impairs endothelium-dependent vasodilation in healthy subjects. Acta Physiol Scand 2001 Jun; 172(2): 107-13.

[134] Steer P, Sarabi DM, Karlstrom B, Basu S, Berne C, Vessby B, et al. The effect of a mixed meal on endothelium-dependent vasodilation is dependent on fat content in healthy humans. Clin Sci (Lond) 2003 Jul; 105(1): 81-7.

[135] Hernandez Mijares A, Jensen MD. Contribution of blood flow to leg glucose uptake during a mixed meal. Diabetes 1995 Oct; 44(10): 1165-9.

[136] Ding Y, Vaziri ND, Coulson R, Kamanna VS, Roh DD. Effects of simulated hyperglycemia, insulin, and glucagon on endothelial nitric oxide synthase expression. Am J Physiol Endocrinol Metab 2000 Jul; 279(1): E11-7.

[137] Yang YT, McElligott MA. Multiple actions of beta-adrenergic agonists on skeletal muscle and adipose tissue. Biochem J 1989 Jul 1; 261(1): 1-10.

[138] Liu CY, Mills SE. Decreased insulin binding to porcine adipocytes in vitro by beta-adrenergic agonists. J Anim Sci 1990 Jun; 68(6): 1603-8.

[139] Faintrenie G, Geloen A. Alpha-1 adrenergic stimulation of glucose uptake in rat white adipocytes. J Pharmacol Exp Ther 1998 Aug; 286(2): 607-10.

[140]   Nolte LA, Gulve EA, Holloszy JO. Epinephrine-induced in vivo muscle glycogen depletion enhances insulin sensitivity of glucose transport. J Appl Physiol 1994 May; 76(5): 2054-8.

[141]   Chiarenza A, Scarselli M, Novi F, Lempereur L, Bernardini R, Corsini GU, *et al.* Apomorphine, dopamine and phenylethylamine reduce the proportion of phosphorylated insulin receptor substrate 1. Eur J Pharmacol 2001 Dec 14; 433(1): 47-54.

[142]   Sandyk R. Dopamine and insulin interact to modulate in vitro glucose transport in rat adipocytes. Int J Neurosci 1988 Nov; 43(1-2): 9-14.

[143]   Patiag D, Qu X, Gray S, Idris I, Wilkes M, Seale JP, *et al.* Possible interactions between angiotensin II and insulin: effects on glucose and lipid metabolism in vivo and in vitro. J Endocrinol 2000 Dec; 167(3): 525-31.

[144]   Fukuda N, Satoh C, Hu WY, Nakayama M, Kishioka H, Kanmatsuse K. Endogenous angiotensin II suppresses insulin signaling in vascular smooth muscle cells from spontaneously hypertensive rats. J Hypertens 2001 Sep; 19(9): 1651-8.

[145]   Elbaz N, Bedecs K, Masson M, Sutren M, Strosberg AD, Nahmias C. Functional trans-inactivation of insulin receptor kinase by growth-inhibitory angiotensin II AT2 receptor. Mol Endocrinol 2000 Jun; 14(6): 795-804.

[146]   Idris I, Patiag D, Gray S, Donnelly R. Tissue- and time-dependent effects of endothelin-1 on insulin-stimulated glucose uptake. Biochem Pharmacol 2001 Dec 15; 62(12): 1705-8.

[147]   Wu-Wong JR, Berg CE, Wang J, Chiou WJ, Fissel B. Endothelin stimulates glucose uptake and GLUT4 translocation via activation of endothelin ETA receptor in 3T3-L1 adipocytes. J Biol Chem 1999 Mar 19; 274(12): 8103-10.

[148]   Ottosson-Seeberger A, Lundberg JM, Alvestrand A, Ahlborg G. Exogenous endothelin-1 causes peripheral insulin resistance in healthy humans. Acta Physiol Scand 1997 Oct; 161(2): 211-20.

[149]   Heseltine L, Webster JM, Taylor R. Adenosine effects upon insulin action on lipolysis and glucose transport in human adipocytes. Mol Cell Biochem 1995 Mar 23; 144(2): 147-51.

[150]   Bush P, Souness JE, Chagoya de Sanchez V. Effect of age and day time on the adenosine modulation of basal and insulin-stimulated glucose transport in rat adipocytes. Int J Biochem 1988; 20(3): 279-83.

[151]   Kishi K, Muromoto N, Nakaya Y, Miyata I, Hagi A, Hayashi H, *et al.* Bradykinin directly triggers GLUT4 translocation via an insulin-independent pathway. Diabetes 1998 Apr; 47(4): 550-8.

[152]   Motoshima H, Araki E, Nishiyama T, Taguchi T, Kaneko K, Hirashima Y, *et al.* Bradykinin enhances insulin receptor tyrosine kinase in 32D cells reconstituted with bradykinin and insulin signaling pathways. Diabetes Res Clin Pract 2000 Jun; 48(3): 155-70.

[153]   Taguchi T, Kishikawa H, Motoshima H, Sakai K, Nishiyama T, Yoshizato K, *et al.* Involvement of bradykinin in acute exercise-induced increase of glucose uptake and GLUT-4 translocation in skeletal muscle: studies in normal and diabetic humans and rats. Metabolism 2000 Jul; 49(7): 920-30.

[154]   Carvalho CR, Thirone AC, Gontijo JA, Velloso LA, Saad MJ. Effect of captopril, losartan, and bradykinin on early steps of insulin action. Diabetes 1997 Dec; 46(12): 1950-7.

[155]   Henstridge DC, Kingwell BA, Formosa MF, Drew BG, McConell GK, Duffy SJ. Effects of the nitric oxide donor, sodium nitroprusside, on resting leg glucose uptake in patients with type 2 diabetes. Diabetologia 2005 Dec; 48(12): 2602-8.

[156]   Bradley SJ, Kingwell BA, McConell GK. Nitric oxide synthase inhibition reduces leg glucose uptake but not blood flow during dynamic exercise in humans. Diabetes 1999 Sep; 48(9): 1815-21.

[157]   Shankar RR, Wu Y, Shen HQ, Zhu JS, Baron AD. Mice with gene disruption of both endothelial and neuronal nitric oxide synthase exhibit insulin resistance. Diabetes 2000 May; 49(5): 684-7.

[158]   Young ME, Radda GK, Leighton B. Nitric oxide stimulates glucose transport and metabolism in rat skeletal muscle in vitro. Biochem J 1997 Feb 15; 322 (Pt 1): 223-8.

[159]   Nolte LA, Hansen PA, Chen MM, Schluter JM, Gulve EA, Holloszy JO. Short-term exposure to tumor necrosis factor-alpha does not affect insulin-stimulated glucose uptake in skeletal muscle. Diabetes 1998 May; 47(5): 721-6.

[160]   Byrne CD. Does tumour necrosis factor alpha influence insulin sensitivity in skeletal muscle? Clin Sci (Lond) 2000 Oct; 99(4): 329-30.

[161]   Woods SC, Vasselli JR, Kaestner E, Szakmary GA, Milburn P, Vitiello MV. Conditioned insulin secretion and meal feeding in rats. J Comp Physiol Psychol 1977 Feb; 91(1): 128-33.

[162]   Strubbe JH. Parasympathetic involvement in rapid meal-associated conditioned insulin secretion in the rat. Am J Physiol 1992 Sep; 263(3 Pt 2): R615-8.

[163]   Berthoud HR, Jeanrenaud B. Sham feeding-induced cephalic phase insulin release in the rat. Am J Physiol 1982 Apr; 242(4): E280-5.

[164]   Bellisle F, Louis-Sylvestre J, Demozay F, Blazy D, Le Magnen J. Cephalic phase of insulin secretion and food stimulation in humans: a new perspective. Am J Physiol 1985 Dec; 249(6 Pt 1): E639-45.

[165]   Rasmussen H, Zawalich KC, Ganesan S, Calle R, Zawalich WS. Physiology and pathophysiology of insulin secretion. Diabetes Care 1990 Jun; 13(6): 655-66.

[166]   Louis-Sylvestre J, Le Magnen J. Palatability and preabsorptive insulin release. Neurosci Biobehav Rev 1980; 4 Suppl 1: 43-6.

[167]   Wang H, Wang AX, Liu Z, Barrett EJ. Insulin signaling stimulates insulin transport by bovine aortic endothelial cells. Diabetes 2008 Mar; 57(3): 540-7.

[168]   Rippe B, Rosengren BI, Carlsson O, Venturoli D. Transendothelial transport: the vesicle controversy. J Vasc Res 2002 Sep-Oct; 39(5): 375-90.

[169] Hamilton-Wessler M, Ader M, Dea MK, Moore D, Loftager M, Markussen J, *et al.* Mode of transcapillary transport of insulin and insulin analog NN304 in dog hindlimb: evidence for passive diffusion. Diabetes 2002 Mar; 51(3): 574-82.

[170] Eggleston EM, Jahn LA, Barrett EJ. Hyperinsulinemia rapidly increases human muscle microvascular perfusion but fails to increase muscle insulin clearance: evidence that a saturable process mediates muscle insulin uptake. Diabetes 2007 Dec; 56(12): 2958-63.

[171] Miles PD, Levisetti M, Reichart D, Khoursheed M, Moossa AR, Olefsky JM. Kinetics of insulin action in vivo. Identification of rate-limiting steps. Diabetes 1995 Aug; 44(8): 947-53.

[172] Salvetti F, Cecchetti P, Janigro D, Lucacchini A, Benzi L, Martini C. Insulin permeability across an in vitro dynamic model of endothelium. Pharm Res 2002 Apr; 19(4): 445-50.

[173] Bendayan M, Rasio EA. Transport of insulin and albumin by the microvascular endothelium of the rete mirabile. J Cell Sci 1996 Jul; 109 (Pt 7): 1857-64.

[174] Rasio EA. The displacement of insulin from blood capillaries. Diabetologia 1969 Dec; 5(6): 416-9.

[175] Bergman RN. Pathogenesis and prediction of diabetes mellitus: lessons from integrative physiology. Mt Sinai J Med 2002 Oct; 69(5): 280-90.

[176] Herkner H, Klein N, Joukhadar C, Lackner E, Langenberger H, Frossard M, *et al.* Transcapillary insulin transfer in human skeletal muscle. Eur J Clin Invest 2003 Feb; 33(2): 141-6.

[177] Castillo C, Bogardus C, Bergman R, Thuillez P, Lillioja S. Interstitial insulin concentrations determine glucose uptake rates but not insulin resistance in lean and obese men. J Clin Invest 1994 Jan; 93(1): 10-6.

[178] Chiu JD, Richey JM, Harrison LN, Zuniga E, Kolka CM, Kirkman E, *et al.* Direct administration of insulin into skeletal muscle reveals that the transport of insulin across the capillary endothelium limits the time course of insulin to activate glucose disposal. Diabetes 2008 Apr; 57(4): 828-35.

[179] Butterfield WJ, Garratt,C.J., Whichelow M.J. Peripheral hormone action: studies on the clearance and effect of [131I] iodo-insulin in the peripheral tissues of normal, acromegalic and diabetic subjects. Clin Sci 1963; 24: 331-41.

[180] Rasio EA, Mack E, Egdahl RH, Herrera MG. Passage of insulin and inulin across vascular membranes in the dog. Diabetes 1968 Nov; 17(11): 668-72.

[181] Holmang A, Niklasson M, Rippe B, Lonnroth P. Insulin insensitivity and delayed transcapillary delivery of insulin in oophorectomized rats treated with testosterone. Acta Physiol Scand 2001 Apr; 171(4): 427-38.

[182] Wascher TC, Wolkart G, Russell JC, Brunner F. Delayed insulin transport across endothelium in insulin-resistant JCR: LA-cp rats. Diabetes 2000 May; 49(5): 803-9.

[183] Ellmerer M, Hamilton-Wessler M, Kim SP, Huecking K, Kirkman E, Chiu J, *et al.* Reduced access to insulin-sensitive tissues in dogs with obesity secondary to increased fat intake. Diabetes 2006 Jun; 55(6): 1769-75.

[184] Olsen MH, Andersen UB, Wachtell K, Ibsen H, Dige-Petersen H. A possible link between endothelial dysfunction and insulin resistance in hypertension. A LIFE substudy. Losartan Intervention For Endpoint-Reduction in Hypertension. Blood Press 2000; 9(2-3): 132-9.

[185] Sjostrand M, Gudbjornsdottir S, Strindberg L, Lonnroth P. Delayed transcapillary delivery of insulin to muscle interstitial fluid after oral glucose load in obese subjects. Diabetes 2005 Jul; 54(7): 2266.

[186] Tuma PL, Hubbard AL. Transcytosis: crossing cellular barriers. Physiol Rev 2003 Jul; 83(3): 871-932.

[187] Frank PG, Pavlides S, Lisanti MP. Caveolae and transcytosis in endothelial cells: role in atherosclerosis. Cell Tissue Res 2009 Jan; 335(1): 41-7.

[188] Barrett EJ, Eggleston EM, Inyard AC, Wang H, Li G, Chai W, *et al.* The vascular actions of insulin control its delivery to muscle and regulate the rate-limiting step in skeletal muscle insulin action. Diabetologia 2009 May; 52(5): 752-64.

CHAPTER 11

Is Defective Microcirculation Responsible for Insulin Resistance?

PART 3. Microvascular Defects Potentially Leading to Insulin Resistance

Nicolas Wiernsperger[1, 2]

[1]*INSERM U870, INSA Lyon, Bat L.Pasteur, 11 avenue J.Capelle, F-69621 Villeurbanne Cedex (France)*

[2]*Laboratorio de Pesquisas em Microcirculaçao, Centro Medico, Universidade do Estado do Rio de Janeiro, Pav. R. Haroldo Lisboa da Cunha, Rua Sao Francisco Xavier 524, 20550-013 Rio de Janeiro (Brazil)*
E Mail : *nicolas.wiernsperger@free.fr*

Keywords: Microflow, endothelium, caveolae, glycocalyx, shear stress.

1. INTRODUCTION

Peripheral insulin resistance is mainly seen as a deficiency in the capacity of insulin to store excessive glucose in the skeletal muscle mass after meals. Since glucose and insulin supply depend on nutritive capillary blood flow, it is clear that any impairment (single or in combination) of microflow regulation or operation represents, by definition, a potential cause of tissue insulin resistance. The consequent question, then, is whether there is evidence that not only can such disturbances appear concomitantly with IR but if they can precede and cause IR and, if so, how this may be achieved. Although the very final proof still requires appropriate experimentation, we describe in the following what can be learned from situations known to be both associated with the development of insulin resistance/metabolic syndrome and exhibit very early microvascular disturbances. In other words, let us see if some reasonable scheme emerges from pathophysiological situations where important confounding factors such as overweight/obesity, dyslipidemia, hypertension or impaired glucose homeostasis are not or very little present. These situations are, notably, first degree relatives of parents affected by various diseases with metabolic or cardiovascular problems, fetal growth retardation, postgestational diabetes, sleep apnea, short term physical inactivity or rheumatoid arthritis.

2. ARTERIOLES AND BLOOD FLOW

There are two major categories of mechanisms susceptible to impair flow: a] those affecting arteriolar vasomotor reactions and b] those affecting more specifically capillaries.

2.1. Arteriolar Hemodynamics

Arterioles play a central role in blood pressure and flow regulation since they must ensure the large pressure gradient between arteries and the capillary bed. They react to pressure changes by the intrinsic myogenic response (contractions) and to flow changes by vasodilation (at least within limits) [1]. Consequently defects in either sensing or effector mechanisms impair arteriolar dilatation or constriction. Because microcirculation is under combined control by the nervous system, local mechanisms (myogenic responses, vasomotion, etc) and local metabolites, this represents a quite important number of candidates. Interestingly, however, some common denominators can be found, of which the most interesting is the structural and functional colocalization of sensors and effectors in membrane microdomains, which led some to ask if IR might be a microdomain disorder [2].

2.1.1. Caveolae/ Mechanotransduction/ Vasomotricity

Microdomains are composed of caveolae and lipid rafts, but particularly caveolae have been considered to be a key structure in our mechanistic search, since they contain all 3 main players of the story:

caveolins, eNOS and insulin receptors. Moreover, they are connected to the cytoskeleton. Caveolae are signalling platforms which are involved in both signalling processes and transcytosis [3, 4]. They are highly present in ECs where they are implicated in sensing wall stretch and exert a cargo function by ensuring transcytosis. They are mainly located in the plasma membrane but can move into the cytosol, whereby they could be linked to CVD without modifications of their absolute number [5, 6]. Caveolae contain proteins termed caveolins, which act as scaffolds for multiple signalling molecules; consequently their dysfunction is linked to diseases [7]. In ECs the main protein is caveolin-1 which is cdistributed with eNOS [8]. With decreasing diameter, the microvessels increasingly depend on EDHF rather than NO [9, 10]; it is thus interesting to note that mediators of EDHF relaxation [cation channels, connexins] are effectively located in caveolae [11]. Caveolae are indeed a prerequisite for EDHF formation [12]. The neck of the caveolae concentrates insulin receptors [13] and it is of note that insulin signalling depends on interactions between the insulin receptor and caveolin-1 [14]. The insulin receptor contains a binding motif for caveolin [15] and phosphorylates caveolin-1 [16]. The colocalization of eNOS, insulin receptors and caveolin makes the membrane microdomain an exquisite candidate for our purpose. Possibly this is the basis of what some call "vascular insulin resistance [17]. Caveolin-1 is necessary for Akt-dependent signalling [18] and several groups suggested that in contrast to the MAPK pathway, the PI3kinase pathway, involved in NO formation by insulin, is selectively impaired [17]. Caveolin-1 is also involved in muscle glucose uptake [19]. Insulin signalling pathways in ECs appear to be obviously similar to those described in fat or muscle cells. In fa/fa rats, postreceptor insulin signalling and Akt phosphorylation are reduced in microvessels [20]. This pathway is also downregulated in cultured ECs exposed to chronically elevated insulin levels [21].

One major role of caveolae in ECs is to sense deformations of the plasma membrane induced by physical forces and to initiate the appropriate vasomotor reaction of arterioles. Indeed flowing blood imposes a so-called shear stress (SStr) which depends on pressure as well as on blood viscosity [9, 23] among other factors [24]. Thus caveolae are involved in the mechanotransduction, the process translating SSTr into vessel calibre changes [25-28]. Other structures such as ion channels [29] or integrins [30-32] are also involved, however. While ECs cultured under static conditions express little caveolae, cells preconditioned by laminar flow [such as in vivo] show a 5fold increase in caveolae. Imposing SStr to such cells increases phosphotyrosine signals 7fold, caveolin-1 tyrosine phosphorylation 6fold and eNOS phosphorylation 3,3fold [33]. Sensing appears to be mediated by purinergic P2X4 receptors [34] but the ATP sensitivity is heterogeneous among ECs [35]. Signals generated by caveolae following changes in SStr are then transmitted to the cytoskeleton for vasoregulation and vessel remodelling [36]. Interestingly one major signal from caveolae is intracellular, mitochondrial oxidative stress, which induced vasodilatation in arterioles [37-40]. It was shown that at least one form of EDHF is precisely H_2O_2 [41] and that under pathological conditions such as coronary artery disease, H_2O_2 can replace NO in arterioles [42]. It is of note that H_2O_2 is also involved in insulin signalling [43]. There are examples of positive integration of oxidative stress in regulatory physiology, which is in permanent equilibrium with the deleterious effects of external oxidative stress [44, 45]. Thus oxidative stress provoked by a pathological situation such as sleep apnea [46], CHF [47, 48] and many other states of IR, induces dissociation of eNOS from caveolin [49]. We may therefore envisage defects in the activation of the EC insulin receptor signal [vascular IR] as well as defects in more distal mechanisms leading to arteriolar dilatation, i.e. phosphorylation of caveolin-1, generation of NO within caveolae [50] or absence of normal sensing of SStr elevation induced upstream by insulin in larger arterioles. There are thus various potential sites on the way from SStr sensing to vasodilatation [51] which could impair insulin-induced dilatation of arterioles at low concentrations.

Although it seems paradoxical, vasoconstriction can also be a prominent physiological feature in the regulation of microflow. Three processes are particularly concerned: the myogenic response to transmural pressure changes, the initiation of low-frequency precapillary vasomotion and the closure of non-nutritive microvessels for flow redistribution. The myogenic response is a cardinal protective mechanism, which mainly operates during postural changes (upright positioning), known as veno-arteriolar reflex [52-54] whose disturbances would permit excessive blood inflow into the nutritive bed and provoke capillary hypertension [55]. The myogenic response is most prominent in smallest arterioles [56] but its precise mechanisms are still elusive [57, 58]. Myogenic response is defective in older persons [59] as well as in diabetics [60-65]. Unfortunately information is scarce because very few studies have dealt with microvascular constriction in pathological situations except diabetes: defective vasoconstriction is described in obesity [66], in peripheral arterial diseases [67, 68], in CHF patients [69] as well as after OGTT [70].. The obvious existence of non-nutritive,shunting channels in the muscle microcirculation [71,72], suggests that under some physiological need situations they must close and favour passage of blood into the nutritive channels, as has been elegantly shown by use of various kinds of vasoconstrictors [73]; thus, defects in this process can be thought of, but concrete mechanistic data in insulin resistant situations are actually lacking. However, the data obtained in vivo in rats strongly that, thanks to vasomotion, redistribution of flow based on constrictive events occurs when glycemia rises as in postprandial periods [74].

Additionally unphysiological vasoconstriction could be favoured by increases in constrictor substances like endothelin-1 or angiotensin II [75].

2.1.2. Caveolae / Transcytosis

Aside from mechanotransduction, caveolae have another function of primary importance for our present purpose since they are strongly involved in transendothelial transport [3, 76]. Caveolins trigger phosphorylations and tyrosine phosphorylation is indispensable for transcytosis [77]. That caveolae are important in CVDs has been shown in atherosclerosis [78]. Although the exact processes whereby insulin is transport across the EC are still unclear, the caveolae are most likely involved. Thus also here defects in caveolae functioning may delay insulin transcytosis, as was found in various pathological situations.

2.2. Shear Stress and Insulin Resistance States

Inappropriate arteriolar responses to SStr may originate from defective sensing and/or downstream effectors but small vessel endothelium may also be submitted to supranormal physical forces due to insufficient pulse pressure attenuation in upstream larger vessels.

It is puzzling that the clinico-pathological situations where microvascular abnormalities are clearly inherited or very early acquired are those in which a hyperdynamic circulation is found: increased heart ate, increases intima/media thickness, arterial stiffness, increased pulse wave velocity (PWV). Normally insulin opposes to aortic stiffening and this effect is blunted in IR [79, 80]. Increased intima/media thickness is seen in all these situations. This leads to exaggerated transmission of PWV to downstream located vascular beds, which will precipitate end organ damage if the autoregulatory mechanisms are defective. They may be intrinsically defective as suggested by observations in offsprings of parents presenting hyperdymanic circulation: FRDs of parents with a high cardiac index have higher BMI and waist/hip ration, diastolic blood pressure, heart rate and insulin concentrations [81]. The San Antonio Heart Study showed that in these subjects [even in lean], the odd ratio for developing NIDDM was 3, 97 [82]. PWV is increased in offpsrings of only one hypertensive parent and more if both parents are hypertensive [83]. PWV abnormalities are indeed inheritable [84]. High PWV is independently associated with MS [85-91]. Prematurity and intrauterine growth retardation are also associated with increased PWV [92, 93]. Increased aortic stiffness is associated with increased insulin concentrations in the general population [94] and with IR in non diabetic hypertensives, independently of the metabolic status [95]. In sleep apnea aortic stiffness is increased despite normal blood pressure [96], even in minimally symptomatic patients [97]. PWV and intima/media thickness are independently correlated with severity of nocturnal hypoxemia [98]. Intima/media thickness is increases in non insulin resistant, obese adolescents in which FMD is reduced [99]. Increased PWV is also reported in PCOS patients [100] and rheumatoid arthritis [101].

That elevated PWV is deleterious to the vascular system is shown by the association of ED with PWV in GDM [102], in FDRs [103] and in normal healthy humans. Even more interesting are several reports of microvascular disturbances linked to increased PWV: impaired flow reserve is associated with increased arterial stiffness and PWV even in asymptomatic subjects [104]. Increased aortic PWV is associated with structural changes in cerebral arterioles [105] and small vessel brain diseases [106]. The Framingham Heart Study showed that carotid-femoral PWV was associated with blunted microvascular reactivity, in excess of changes in conventional risk factors [107]. The anticonstrictor effect of insulin on microvessels was reduced in PCOS patients [100]. Chronic increased shear stress thus impairs the reactivity of small vessels, leading to HT, which is the likely reason why HT is the most frequent MS component [108].

Increased heart rate is found in several pathologies, likely due to sympathetic overdrive. The latter has been suggested to represent the linchpin between IR and heart rate [109] and is indeed seen in conditions defining the association between MS and CVDs [110]. It has been proposed that a decrease in parasympathetic activity shifts the balance in favour of the sympathetic nervous system, as seen in FDRs with the lowest insulin sensitivity [111]. Birth weight is also linked to elevated heart rate [112]. Importantly, it must be recalled that microvessels are richly innervated and that sympathetic stimulation decreases nutritive blood flow [113].

3. CAPILLARY BLOOD FLOW

3.1. Intravascular Processes

Flow of whole blood through tiny capillaries is a very critical process which depends on luminal diameter changes but also on biophysical properties of blood (hemorheology). Internal capillary diameter is an always changing parameter, depending both on luminal ECs dimensions and on capillary distensibility. One may therefore ask if older reports of increased capillary basement membrane in subjects genetically predisposed to diabetes may not be explained by an early adaptation to increased SStr [114,115].

Whole blood is constituted of plasma and cells, whereby blood exhibits a viscosity which can easily vary according to quantitative and qualitative changes in its composition. Viscosity is a major determinant of capillary blood flow [116-118]. It is well-known that whole blood viscosity contributes to total peripheral resistance and correlates with systolic blood pressure, triglycerides, BMI and waist/hip ratio [119]. Flow resistance is also determined by the presence and the thickness of the endothelial surface layer [120]. Therefore disturbances in blood cells or plasma can increase viscosity and thereby SStr in capillaries. Enhanced aggregation of red cells, reduced erythrocyte deformability or activation of leucocytes all impairs blood passage through capillaries. The presence of high triglycerides also modifies flow resistance in microvessels [121]. Whole blood viscosity and elevated hematocrit are associated with IR [122], indicating that slowed capillary flow has metabolic consequences. However even plasma viscosity changes are linked to IR [123]. This may for example come from increased fibrinogen plasma levels such as seen in physical inactivity [124,125], CHF [126] or sleep apnea [127]. In sleep apnea blood viscosity is independent of other CV risk factors [127] and morning plasma viscosity is inversely related with nocturnal oxygen desaturation [128,129]. Interestingly, whole blood viscosity is linked to sympathetic activity and low insulin sensitivity [122]. Finally whole blood and plasma viscosity are increased in CHF patients [130,131].

Although poorly directly investigated, microthrombosis is suggested by multiple findings of hypofibrinolysis in insulin resistant states. Indeed IR is well-known to be associated with clusterings of inflammation and coagulation factors [126,132-134]. Of particular interest is PAI-1, which is liberated from liver as well as from endothelial cells. Very interestingly, its upregulation requires caveolae [135]. Short-term physical inactivity rapidly leads to PAI-1 elevations [124,125], which are also seen in low birth weight [136], GDM [137], CHF [126] and FDRs of diabetic parents [138,139]. All these pathologies exhibit elevated PAI-1 levels despite normal glucose tolerance.

3.2. Parietal Processes

Both endothelial cells and functions may be damaged by many circulating substances. It is evident that most insulin resistance states show low-grade inflammation as well as oxidative stress [140-143]. While the latter is discussed in another chapter of this book [Roesen and Roesen], inflammation is largely related to cytokines such as TNFα, interleukin-6 and others. This is a vast topic but considering the diseases on which we concentrate here, it appears clear that CHF [144-146], sleep apnea [147], obesity [148] and physical inactivity [149] all exhibit increased TNFα levels and related oxidative stress leading to ED. It is particularly interesting to note that either too short or too long sleep duration lead to increased inflammation, by IL-6 and TNFα respectively [150]. As previously seen, TNFα is able to interfere with arteriolar vasodilation and capillary recruitment [151]. Interestingly caveolin-1 is involved in TNFα activation of ECs and closely modulated by fatty acids [152]. In inflammatory diseases, TNFα blockade improves ED and the disturbed capillary recruitment [153].

During the last decade a NO metabolite, ADMA, has been highlighted and is now considered to be involved in the development of CVDs. Like TNFα, ADMA increases NADPH oxidase, ROS production and ED [154,155]. Increased ADMA often results from the absence of degradation, due to inhibition of degrading enzymes [156]. ADMA is linked to IR, by uncoupling eNOS [157,158]. It is increased in

CHF patients [156] and GDM [159]. ADMA has also a rheological effect, by increasing red cell viscosity in HT [160]. It also inhibits dilatation to SStr [161] and impairs capillary recruitment [162]. Thus, ADMA appears to be closely related to the sensing and signalling of microvascular physical forces.

Microparticles are another recent discovery in the field of microcirculation [see Martinez, this book]. Various forms of microparticles exist, some of which are activators of ECs and procoagulant [163]. Microparticles are liberated by the activation of ECs by cytokines and participate to the decrease in NO-mediated vasodilation and to the increase in arterial stiffness [164].

Activated circulating cells and endothelium also overexpress adhesion molecules which bind monocytes. Circulating leucocytes stick to inflammatory endothelium as can be observed in situ in microvascular preparations, where leucocytes are rolling more slowly and to the vessel wall, to induce permeability but also eventually capillary obstruction. Increased level of adhesion molecules [mainly selectin-1, ICAM-1 and VCAM-1] are reported in sleep apnea [165,166], in adults and offsprings after GDM [167,168], in FDRs of diabetic patents [169,170], in SGA fetuses [171] and in CHF patients [126,144,172]. They are also frequently associated with elevated PAI-1 [168,169]

Passage of blood through very narrow capillaries can be hampered by reductions of the luminal diameter, as a consequence of endothelial swelling or modifications in the glycocalyx. The prominent role played by the glycocalyx has only recently been highlighted and is now increasingly recognized. Glycocalyx is an extremely thin [1μm] layer of essentially sugars covering the endothelial surface, which plays a prominent role in microvascular flow, especially in low-flow state conditions [120]. Changes in its properties affect shear stress distribution on ECs [173]. Its integrity is a requisite for ECs to respond to shear stress and, since the glycocalyx is itself modulated by shear stress, this forms a fragile vicious circle [174]. Evidence is now accumulating that glycocalyx is directly involved in the very first step of mechanotransduction since it is in direct contact with flowing blood [175]. Recent work showed that one of its roles is to dampen shear stress throughout the cardiac cyle [176]. Elevated shear stress modulates glycocalyx synthesis, which might become thinner [177]. Preliminary data indicate that hyperglycemia damages glycocalyx and that it can be largely reversed by treating rats with metformin [178]. It will be of high interest to see if more subtle metabolic derangements as evoked in this chapter also have a negative impact on glycocalyx structure. [179]. The beneficial effect of TNFα blockade also suggest that the glycocalyx is a target for inflammatory processes [180].

Finally, one should consider observations from a drug largely used in diabetes and recommended in prediabetes, namely metformin. This old drug has been shown in many studies to have intrinsic, glycemia-independent vascular properties which, very interestingly, are quite unique for the microcirculation. It has been demonstrated that it acts indeed on most of the disorders listed in this analysis: it has membrane stabilizing effects [181], acts against many factors involved in inflammation and [mitochondrial] oxidative stress [178,182,183], appears to protect glycocalyx [178], improves dramatically functional capillary density [rate of blood filled capillaries] in ischemic situations [178,184], improves microvascular reactivity in glucose-tolerant patients with very low metabolic syndrome [185-187] and is known to act on insulin resistance in non-diabetic subjects. In view of this large overlapping between pathophysiology and pharmacology, it is thus very tempting to put in parallel both observations in terms of causality.

4. CONCLUSION

To try to define some possible causes whereby single and combined defects in the microvasculature could underlie impaired nutritive perfusion and thereby an adequate delivery of glucose and insulin to target tissues such as skeletal muscle, this analysis has deliberately focused on some specific clinical situations exhibiting very early microvascular abnormalities as well as metabolic insulin resistance; these pathologies were selected because they are largely free of severely confounding factors such as dyslipidemia, overweight/obesity, hypertension or glycemic dysregulation. The data suggest that augmented intensity and deficient vascular compensation towards physical forces in flowing blood at the arteriolar level represent one major causative factor of nutritive flow disturbances. It appears clearly that such disturbances can be inherited or acquired by even short exposure to abnormal metabolic environment such as in GDM or fetal growth retardation [and/or subsequent catch-up growth]. Inadequate management of shear stress by the arteriolar wall is in line with the majority of tests used in human medicine to evaluate microvascular dysfunctions which are largely based on shear stress.

Modifications in flowing properties of blood as well as processes taking place in the microvascular vessel walls of arterioles and capillaries as a consequence of constant confrontation with deleterious circulating inflammatory and procoagulant substances are also prone to impair nutritive flow. They clearly represent commonalities among the diseases we have more particularly analyzed for our purpose. Very interestingly, some of these modifications share common mechanisms in both arterioles and capillaries.

The endothelial surface represents an exquisite candidate as the culprit of the very early disorders in microvascular function and related metabolic consequences as seen in most various diseases, for: 1] it is the site where glycocalyx and caveolae sense changes in physical forces of flowing blood, and 2] caveolins, eNOS and insulin receptors colocalize and interact in plasma membrane caveolae, whose function is to organize signalling and to ensure transcytosis. It is further indirectly supported by improvements afforded by metformin in these parameters. The many data presented here support the concept that inherited or early acquired defects in or close to the caveolae represent the most likely candidate to explain why microvascular dysfunction may appear concomitantly or even cause insulin resistance. While this concept is possibly not unique, it should at the least be a convincing working hypothesis for stimulating scientists to achieve the necessary appropriate investigations in order to provide the final proof.

5. REFERENCES

[1]   Safar ME, Lacolley P. Disturbance of macro- and microcirculation: relations with pulse pressure and cardiac organ damage. Am J Physiol Heart Circ Physiol 2007 Jul; 293(1): H1-7.
[2]   Inokuchi J. Insulin resistance as a membrane microdomain disorder. Biol Pharm Bull 2006 Aug; 29(8): 1532-7.
[3]   Predescu SA, Predescu DN, Malik AB. Molecular determinants of endothelial transcytosis and their role in endothelial permeability. Am J Physiol Lung Cell Mol Physiol 2007 Oct; 293(4): L823-42.
[4]   Simionescu M, Popov D, Sima A. Endothelial transcytosis in health and disease. Cell Tissue Res 2009 Jan; 335(1): 27-40.
[5]   Xu Y, Buikema H, van Gilst WH, Henning RH. Caveolae and endothelial dysfunction: filling the caves in cardiovascular disease. Eur J Pharmacol 2008 May 13; 585(2-3): 256-60.
[6]   Li XA, Everson WV, Smart EJ. Caveolae, lipid rafts, and vascular disease. Trends Cardiovasc Med 2005 Apr; 15(3): 92-6.
[7]   Schwencke C, Braun-Dullaeus RC, Wunderlich C, Strasser RH. Caveolae and caveolin in transmembrane signaling: Implications for human disease. Cardiovasc Res 2006 Apr 1; 70(1): 42-9.
[8]   Segal SS, Brett SE, Sessa WC. Codistribution of NOS and caveolin throughout peripheral vasculature and skeletal muscle of hamsters. Am J Physiol 1999 Sep; 277(3 Pt 2): H1167-77.
[9]   de Wit C, Wolfle SE. EDHF and gap junctions: important regulators of vascular tone within the microcirculation. Curr Pharm Biotechnol 2007 Feb; 8(1): 11-25.
[10]   Watanabe S, Yashiro Y, Mizuno R, Ohhashi T. Involvement of NO and EDHF in flow-induced vasodilation in isolated hamster cremasteric arterioles. J Vasc Res 2005 Mar-Apr; 42(2): 137-47.
[11]   Saliez J, Bouzin C, Rath G, Ghisdal P, Desjardins F, Rezzani R, *et al.* Role of caveolar compartmentation in endothelium-derived hyperpolarizing factor-mediated relaxation: Ca2+ signals and gap junction function are regulated by caveolin in endothelial cells. Circulation 2008 Feb 26; 117(8): 1065-74.
[12]   Graziani A, Bricko V, Carmignani M, Graier WF, Groschner K. Cholesterol- and caveolin-rich membrane domains are essential for phospholipase A2-dependent EDHF formation. Cardiovasc Res 2004 Nov 1; 64(2): 234-42.
[13]   Foti M, Porcheron G, Fournier M, Maeder C, Carpentier JL. The neck of caveolae is a distinct plasma membrane subdomain that concentrates insulin receptors in 3T3-L1 adipocytes. Proc Natl Acad Sci U S A 2007 Jan 23; 104(4): 1242-7.
[14]   Cohen AW, Combs TP, Scherer PE, Lisanti MP. Role of caveolin and caveolae in insulin signaling and diabetes. Am J Physiol Endocrinol Metab 2003 Dec; 285(6): E1151-60.
[15]   Couet J, Sargiacomo M, Lisanti MP. Interaction of a receptor tyrosine kinase, EGF-R, with caveolins. Caveolin binding negatively regulates tyrosine and serine/threonine kinase activities. J Biol Chem 1997 Nov 28; 272(48): 30429-38.
[16]   Kimura A, Mora S, Shigematsu S, Pessin JE, Saltiel AR. The insulin receptor catalyzes the tyrosine phosphorylation of caveolin-1. J Biol Chem 2002 Aug 16; 277(33): 30153-8.
[17]   Schulman IH, Zhou MS. Vascular insulin resistance: a potential link between cardiovascular and metabolic diseases. Curr Hypertens Rep 2009 Feb; 11(1): 48-55.
[18]   Albinsson S, Nordstrom I, Sward K, Hellstrand P. Differential dependence of stretch and shear stress signaling on caveolin-1 in the vascular wall. Am J Physiol Cell Physiol 2008 Jan; 294(1): C271-9.
[19]   Oh YS, Cho KA, Ryu SJ, Khil LY, Jun HS, Yoon JW, *et al.* Regulation of insulin response in skeletal muscle cell by caveolin status. J Cell Biochem 2006 Oct 15; 99(3): 747-58.

[20]   Jiang ZY, Lin YW, Clemont A, Feener EP, Hein KD, Igarashi M, *et al.* Characterization of selective resistance to insulin signaling in the vasculature of obese Zucker (fa/fa) rats. J Clin Invest 1999 Aug; 104(4): 447-57.

[21]   Madonna R, De Caterina R. Prolonged exposure to high insulin impairs the endothelial PI3-kinase/Akt/nitric oxide signalling. Thromb Haemost 2009 Feb; 101(2): 345-50.

[22]   de Wit C, Schafer C, von Bismarck P, Bolz SS, Pohl U. Elevation of plasma viscosity induces sustained NO-mediated dilation in the hamster cremaster microcirculation in vivo. Pflugers Arch 1997 Aug; 434(4): 354-61.

[23]   Koller A, Sun D, Kaley G. Role of shear stress and endothelial prostaglandins in flow- and viscosity-induced dilation of arterioles in vitro. Circ Res 1993 Jun; 72(6): 1276-84.

[24]   Resnick N, Yahav H, Shay-Salit A, Shushy M, Schubert S, Zilberman LC, *et al.* Fluid shear stress and the vascular endothelium: for better and for worse. Prog Biophys Mol Biol 2003 Apr; 81(3): 177-99.

[25]   Frank PG, Lisanti MP. Role of caveolin-1 in the regulation of the vascular shear stress response. J Clin Invest 2006 May; 116(5): 1222-5.

[26]   Davies PF. Hemodynamic shear stress and the endothelium in cardiovascular pathophysiology. Nat Clin Pract Cardiovasc Med 2009 Jan; 6(1): 16-26.

[27]   Vogel V, Sheetz M. Local force and geometry sensing regulate cell functions. Nat Rev Mol Cell Biol 2006 Apr; 7(4): 265-75.

[28]   Yu J, Bergaya S, Murata T, Alp IF, Bauer MP, Lin MI, *et al.* Direct evidence for the role of caveolin-1 and caveolae in mechanotransduction and remodeling of blood vessels. J Clin Invest 2006 May; 116(5): 1284-91.

[29]   Folgering JH, Sharif-Naeini R, Dedman A, Patel A, Delmas P, Honore E. Molecular basis of the mammalian pressure-sensitive ion channels: focus on vascular mechanotransduction. Prog Biophys Mol Biol 2008 Jun-Jul; 97(2-3): 180-95.

[30]   Frame MD, Rivers RJ, Altland O, Cameron S. Mechanisms initiating integrin-stimulated flow recruitment in arteriolar networks. J Appl Physiol 2007 Jun; 102(6): 2279-87.

[31]   Martinez-Lemus LA, Sun Z, Trache A, Trzciakowski JP, Meininger GA. Integrins and regulation of the microcirculation: from arterioles to molecular studies using atomic force microscopy. Microcirculation 2005 Jan-Feb; 12(1): 99-112.

[32]   Reneman RS, Arts T, Hoeks AP. Wall shear stress--an important determinant of endothelial cell function and structure--in the arterial system in vivo. Discrepancies with theory. J Vasc Res 2006; 43(3): 251-69.

[33]   Rizzo V, Morton C, DePaola N, Schnitzer JE, Davies PF. Recruitment of endothelial caveolae into mechanotransduction pathways by flow conditioning in vitro. Am J Physiol Heart Circ Physiol 2003 Oct; 285(4): H1720-9.

[34]   Yamamoto K, Ando J. [Shear-stress sensing via P2 purinoceptors in vascular endothelial cells]. Nippon Yakurigaku Zasshi 2004 Nov; 124(5): 3 19-28.

[35]   Hong D, Jaron D, Buerk DG, Barbee KA. Heterogeneous response of microvascular endothelial cells to shear stress. Am J Physiol Heart Circ Physiol 2006 Jun; 290(6): H2498-508.

[36]   Helmke BP, Davies PF. The cytoskeleton under external fluid mechanical forces: hemodynamic forces acting on the endothelium. Ann Biomed Eng 2002 Mar; 30(3): 284-96.

[37]   Koller A, Bagi Z. Nitric oxide and H2O2 contribute to reactive dilation of isolated coronary arterioles. Am J Physiol Heart Circ Physiol 2004 Dec; 287(6): H2461-7.

[38]   Liu Y, Li H, Bubolz AH, Zhang DX, Gutterman DD. Endothelial cytoskeletal elements are critical for flow-mediated dilation in human coronary arterioles. Med Biol Eng Comput 2008 May; 46(5): 469-78.

[39]   Ungvari Z, Wolin MS, Csiszar A. Mechanosensitive production of reactive oxygen species in endothelial and smooth muscle cells: role in microvascular remodeling? Antioxid Redox Signal 2006 Jul-Aug; 8(7-8): 1121-9.

[40]   Parat MO, Fox PL. Oxidative stress, caveolae and caveolin-1. Subcell Biochem 2004; 37: 425-41.

[41]   Shimokawa H, Matoba T. Hydrogen peroxide as an endothelium-derived hyperpolarizing factor. Pharmacol Res 2004 Jun; 49(6): 543-9.

[42]   Phillips SA, Hatoum OA, Gutterman DD. The mechanism of flow-induced dilation in human adipose arterioles involves hydrogen peroxide during CAD. Am J Physiol Heart Circ Physiol 2007 Jan; 292(1): H93-100.

[43]   Kozlovsky N, Rudich A, Potashnik R, Bashan N. Reactive oxygen species activate glucose transport in L6 myotubes. Free Radic Biol Med 1997; 23(6): 859-69.

[44]   Bashan N, Kovsan J, Kachko I, Ovadia H, Rudich A. Positive and negative regulation of insulin signaling by reactive oxygen and nitrogen species. Physiol Rev 2009 Jan; 89(1): 27-71.

[45]   Valko M, Leibfritz D, Moncol J, Cronin MT, Mazur M, Telser J. Free radicals and antioxidants in normal physiological functions and human disease. Int J Biochem Cell Biol 2007; 39(1): 44-84.

[46]   Yamauchi M, Kimura H. Oxidative stress in obstructive sleep apnea: putative pathways to the cardiovascular complications. Antioxid Redox Signal 2008 Apr; 10(4): 755-68.

[47]   de Lorgeril M, Salen P. Selenium and antioxidant defenses as major mediators in the development of chronic heart failure. Heart Fail Rev 2006 Mar; 11(1): 13-7.

[48]   Eleuteri E, Magno F, Gnemmi I, Carbone M, Colombo M, La Rocca G, *et al.* Role of oxidative and nitrosative stress biomarkers in chronic heart failure. Front Biosci 2009; 14: 2230-7.

[49]   Peterson TE, Poppa V, Ueba H, Wu A, Yan C, Berk BC. Opposing effects of reactive oxygen species and cholesterol on endothelial nitric oxide synthase and endothelial cell caveolae. Circ Res 1999 Jul 9; 85(1): 29-37.

[50]   Balligand JL, Feron O, Dessy C. eNOS activation by physical forces: from short-term regulation of contraction to chronic remodeling of cardiovascular tissues. Physiol Rev 2009 Apr; 89(2): 481-534.

[51]   Koller A, Bagi Z. On the role of mechanosensitive mechanisms eliciting reactive hyperemia. Am J Physiol Heart Circ Physiol 2002 Dec; 283(6): H2250-9.

[52]   Carlson BE, Arciero JC, Secomb TW. Theoretical model of blood flow autoregulation: roles of myogenic, shear-dependent, and metabolic responses. Am J Physiol Heart Circ Physiol 2008 Oct; 295(4): H1572-9.

[53]   Johnson PC. Landis Award Lecture. The myogenic response and the microcirculation. Microvasc Res 1977 Jan; 13(1): 1-18.

[54]   Husmann M, Willenberg T, Keo HH, Spring S, Kalodiki E, Delis KT. Integrity of venoarteriolar reflex determines level of microvascular skin flow enhancement with intermittent pneumatic compression. J Vasc Surg 2008 Dec; 48(6): 1509-13.

[55]   Loutzenhiser R, Bidani A, Chilton L. Renal myogenic response: kinetic attributes and physiological role. Circ Res 2002 Jun 28; 90(12): 1316-24.

[56]   Meininger GA, Mack CA, Fehr KL, Bohlen HG. Myogenic vasoregulation overrides local metabolic control in resting rat skeletal muscle. Circ Res 1987 Jun; 60(6): 861-70.

[57]   Hill MA, Zou H, Potocnik SJ, Meininger GA, Davis MJ. Invited review: arteriolar smooth muscle mechanotransduction: Ca(2+) signaling pathways underlying myogenic reactivity. J Appl Physiol 2001 Aug; 91(2): 973-83.

[58]   Vissing SF, Secher NH, Victor RG. Mechanisms of cutaneous vasoconstriction during upright posture. Acta Physiol Scand 1997 Feb; 159(2): 131-8.

[59]   Groothuis JT, Thijssen DH, Kooijman M, Paulus R, Hopman MT. Attenuated peripheral vasoconstriction during an orthostatic challenge in older men. Age Ageing 2008 Nov; 37(6): 680-4.

[60]   Belcaro G, Nicolaides AN. The venoarteriolar response in diabetics. Angiology 1991 Oct; 42(10): 827-35.

[61]   Cacciatori V, Dellera A, Bellavere F, Bongiovanni LG, Teatini F, Gemma ML, et al. Comparative assessment of peripheral sympathetic function by postural vasoconstriction arteriolar reflex and sympathetic skin response in NIDDM patients. Am J Med 1997 Apr; 102(4): 365-70.

[62]   Golster H, Hyllienmark L, Ledin T, Ludvigsson J, Sjoberg F. Impaired microvascular function related to poor metabolic control in young patients with diabetes. Clin Physiol Funct Imaging 2005 Mar; 25(2): 100-5.

[63]   Rai A, Riemann M, Gustafsson F, Holstein-Rathlou NH, Torp-Pedersen C. Streptozotocin-induced diabetes decreases conducted vasoconstrictor response in mouse cremaster arterioles. Horm Metab Res 2008 Sep; 40(9): 651-4.

[64]   Shore AC, Price KJ, Sandeman DD, Tripp JH, Tooke JE. Posturally induced vasoconstriction in diabetes mellitus. Arch Dis Child 1994 Jan; 70(1): 22-6.

[65]   Yu G, Zou H, Prewitt RL, Hill MA. Impaired arteriolar mechanotransduction in experimental diabetes mellitus. J Diabetes Complications 1999 Sep-Dec; 13(5-6): 235-42.

[66]   Valensi P, Smagghue O, Paries J, Velayoudon P, Lormeau B, Attali JR. Impairment of skin vasoconstrictive response to sympathetic activation in obese patients: influence of rheological disorders. Metabolism 2000 May; 49(5): 600-6.

[67]   Khiabani HZ, Anvar MD, Kroese AJ, Stranden E. The role of the veno-arteriolar reflex (VAR) in the pathogenesis of peripheral oedema in patients with chronic critical limb ischaemia (CLI). Ann Chir Gynaecol 2000; 89(2): 93-8.

[68]   Vayssairat M, Tribout L, Gouny P, Gaitz JP, Baudot N, Cheynel C, et al. Importance of cutaneous postural reflex vasoconstriction in patients with atherosclerotic occlusive disease of the lower extremities. Int Angiol 1998 Mar; 17(1): 53-7.

[69]   Chiba Y, Maehara K, Yaoita H, Yoshihisa A, Izumida J, Maruyama Y. Vasoconstrictive response in the vascular beds of the non-exercising forearm during leg exercise in patients with mild chronic heart failure. Circ J 2007 Jun; 71(6): 922-8.

[70]   Lott ME, Hogeman C, Herr M, Gabbay R, Sinoway LI. Effects of an oral glucose tolerance test on the myogenic response in healthy individuals. Am J Physiol Heart Circ Physiol 2007 Jan; 292(1): H304-10.

[71]   Barlow TE, Haigh AL, Walder DN. Evidence for two vascular pathways in skeletal muscle. Clin Sci 1961 Jun; 20: 367-85.

[72]   Newman JM, Steen JT, Clark MG. Vessels supplying septa and tendons as functional shunts in perfused rat hindlimb. Microvasc Res 1997 Jul; 54(1): 49-57.

[73]   Jamerson KA, Smith SD, Amerena JV, Grant E, Julius S. Vasoconstriction with norepinephrine causes less forearm insulin resistance than a reflex sympathetic vasoconstriction. Hypertension 1994 Jun; 23(6 Pt 2): 1006-11.

[74]   Renaudin C, Michoud E, Rapin JR, Lagarde M, Wiernsperger N. Hyperglycaemia modifies the reaction of microvessels to insulin in rat skeletal muscle. Diabetologia 1998 Jan; 41(1): 26-33.

[75]   Thijssen DH, Rongen GA, Smits P, Hopman MT. Physical (in)activity and endothelium-derived constricting factors: overlooked adaptations. J Physiol 2008 Jan 15; 586(2): 3 19-24.

[76]   Ogawa K, Imai M, Ogawa T, Tsukamoto Y, Sasaki F. Caveolar and intercellular channels provide major transport pathways of macromolecules across vascular endothelial cells. Anat Rec 2001 Sep 1; 264(1): 32-42.

[77]   Sverdlov M, Shajahan AN, Minshall RD. Tyrosine phosphorylation-dependence of caveolae-mediated endocytosis. J Cell Mol Med 2007 Nov-Dec; 11(6): 1239-50.

[78]   Frank PG, Pavlides S, Lisanti MP. Caveolae and transcytosis in endothelial cells: role in atherosclerosis. Cell Tissue Res 2009 Jan; 335(1): 41-7.

[79]   Westerbacka J, Yki-Jarvinen H. Arterial stiffness and insulin resistance. Semin Vasc Med 2002 May; 2(2): 157-64.

[80]   Yki-Jarvinen H, Westerbacka J. Insulin resistance, arterial stiffness and wave reflection. Adv Cardiol 2007; 44: 252-60.

[81]   Palatini P, Vriz O, Nesbitt S, Amerena J, Majahalme S, Valentini M, *et al.* Parental hyperdynamic circulation predicts insulin resistance in offspring: The Tecumseh Offspring Study. Hypertension 1999 Mar; 33(3): 769-74.

[82]   Stern MP, Morales PA, Haffner SM, Valdez RA. Hyperdynamic circulation and the insulin resistance syndrome ("syndrome X"). Hypertension 1992 Dec; 20(6): 802-8.

[83]   Kyvelou SM, Vyssoulis GP, Karpanou EA, Adamopoulos DN, Gialernios TP, Spanos PG, *et al.* Arterial hypertension parental burden affects arterial stiffness and wave reflection to the aorta in young offsprings. Int J Cardiol 2009 Jan 26.

[84]   Ge D, Young TW, Wang X, Kapuku GK, Treiber FA, Snieder H. Heritability of arterial stiffness in black and white American youth and young adults. Am J Hypertens 2007 Oct; 20(10): 1065-72.

[85]   Ghiadoni L, Penno G, Giannarelli C, Plantinga Y, Bernardini M, Pucci L, *et al.* Metabolic syndrome and vascular alterations in normotensive subjects at risk of diabetes mellitus. Hypertension 2008 Feb; 51(2): 440-5.

[86]   Achimastos AD, Efstathiou SP, Christoforatos T, Panagiotou TN, Stergiou GS, Mountokalakis TD. Arterial stiffness: determinants and relationship to the metabolic syndrome. Angiology 2007 Feb-Mar; 58(1): 11-20.

[87]   Lee JW, Lee DC, Im JA, Shim JY, Kim SM, Lee HR. Insulin resistance is associated with arterial stiffness independent of obesity in male adolescents. Hypertens Res 2007 Jan; 30(1): 5-11.

[88]   Kovaite M, Petrulioniene Z, Ryliskyte L, Badariene J, Dzenkeviciute V, Cypiene A, *et al.* Systemic assessment of arterial wall structure and function in metabolic syndrome. Proc West Pharmacol Soc 2007; 50: 123-30.

[89]   Kasayama S, Saito H, Mukai M, Koga M. Insulin sensitivity independently influences brachial-ankle pulse-wave velocity in non-diabetic subjects. Diabet Med 2005 Dec; 22(12): 1701-6.

[90]   Nam JS, Park JS, Cho MH, Jee SH, Lee HS, Ahn CW, *et al.* The association between pulse wave velocity and metabolic syndrome and adiponectin in patients with impaired fasting glucose: cardiovascular risks and adiponectin in IFG. Diabetes Res Clin Pract 2009 May; 84(2): 145-51.

[91]   Zhe XW, Zeng J, Tian XK, Chen W, Gu Y, Cheng LT, *et al.* Pulse wave velocity is associated with metabolic syndrome components in CAPD patients. Am J Nephrol 2008; 28(4): 641-6.

[92]   Oren A, Vos LE, Bos WJ, Safar ME, Uiterwaal CS, Gorissen WH, *et al.* Gestational age and birth weight in relation to aortic stiffness in healthy young adults: two separate mechanisms? Am J Hypertens 2003 Jan; 16(1): 76-9.

[93]   Cheung YF, Wong KY, Lam BC, Tsoi NS. Relation of arterial stiffness with gestational age and birth weight. Arch Dis Child 2004 Mar; 89(3): 217-21.

[94]   Hansen TW, Jeppesen J, Rasmussen S, Ibsen H, Torp-Pedersen C. Relation between insulin and aortic stiffness: a population-based study. J Hum Hypertens 2004 Jan; 18(1): 1-7.

[95]   Seo HS, Kang TS, Park S, Park HY, Ko YG, Choi D, *et al.* Insulin resistance is associated with arterial stiffness in nondiabetic hypertensives independent of metabolic status. Hypertens Res 2005 Dec; 28(12): 945-51.

[96]   Tomiyama H, Takata Y, Shiina K, Matsumoto C, Yamada J, Yoshida M, *et al.* Concomitant existence and interaction of cardiovascular abnormalities in obstructive sleep apnea subjects with normal clinic blood pressure. Hypertens Res 2009 Mar; 32(3): 201-6.

[97]   Kohler M, Craig S, Nicoll D, Leeson P, Davies RJ, Stradling JR. Endothelial function and arterial stiffness in minimally symptomatic obstructive sleep apnea. Am J Respir Crit Care Med 2008 Nov 1; 178(9): 984-8.

[98]   Protogerou AD, Laaban JP, Czernichow S, Kostopoulos C, Lekakis J, Safar ME, *et al.* Structural and functional arterial properties in patients with obstructive sleep apnoea syndrome and cardiovascular comorbidities. J Hum Hypertens 2008 Jun; 22(6): 415-22.

[99]   Karpoff L, Vinet A, Schuster I, Oudot C, Goret L, Dauzat M, *et al.* Abnormal vascular reactivity at rest and exercise in obese boys. Eur J Clin Invest 2009 Feb; 39(2): 94-102.

[100] Kelly CJ, Speirs A, Gould GW, Petrie JR, Lyall H, Connell JM. Altered vascular function in young women with polycystic ovary syndrome. J Clin Endocrinol Metab 2002 Feb; 87(2): 742-6.

[101] Arosio E, De Marchi S, Rigoni A, Prior M, Delva P, Lechi A. Forearm haemodynamics, arterial stiffness and microcirculatory reactivity in rheumatoid arthritis. J Hypertens 2007 Jun; 25(6): 1273-8.

[102] Hu J, Norman M, Wallensteen M, Gennser G. Increased large arterial stiffness and impaired acetylcholine induced skin vasodilatation in women with previous gestational diabetes mellitus. Br J Obstet Gynaecol 1998 Dec; 105(12): 1279-87.

[103] Scuteri A, Tesauro M, Rizza S, Iantorno M, Federici M, Lauro D, *et al.* Endothelial function and arterial stiffness in normotensive normoglycemic first-degree relatives of diabetic patients are independent of the metabolic syndrome. Nutr Metab Cardiovasc Dis 2008 Jun; 18(5): 349-56.

[104] Malik AR, Kondragunta V, Kullo IJ. Forearm vascular reactivity and arterial stiffness in asymptomatic adults from the community. Hypertension 2008 Jun; 51(6): 1512-8.

[105] Baumbach GL. Effects of increased pulse pressure on cerebral arterioles. Hypertension 1996 Feb; 27(2): 159-67.

[106] Henskens LH, Kroon AA, van Oostenbrugge RJ, Gronenschild EH, Fuss-Lejeune MM, Hofman PA, *et al.* Increased aortic pulse wave velocity is associated with silent cerebral small-vessel disease in hypertensive patients. Hypertension 2008 Dec; 52(6): 1120-6.

[107] Mitchell GF, Vita JA, Larson MG, Parise H, Keyes MJ, Warner E, *et al.* Cross-sectional relations of peripheral microvascular function, cardiovascular disease risk factors, and aortic stiffness: the Framingham Heart Study. Circulation 2005 Dec 13; 112(24): 3722-8.

[108] Fiuza M, Cortez-Dias N, Martins S, Belo A. Metabolic syndrome in Portugal: prevalence and implications for cardiovascular risk--results from the VALSIM Study. Rev Port Cardiol 2008 Dec; 27(12): 1495-529.

[109] Facchini FS, Stoohs RA, Reaven GM. Enhanced sympathetic nervous system activity. The linchpin between insulin resistance, hyperinsulinemia, and heart rate. Am J Hypertens 1996 Oct; 9(10 Pt 1): 1013-7.

[110] Grassi G, Quarti-Trevano F, Seravalle G, Dell'Oro R. Cardiovascular risk and adrenergic overdrive in the metabolic syndrome. Nutr Metab Cardiovasc Dis 2007 Jul; 17(6): 473-81.

[111] Lindmark S, Wiklund U, Bjerle P, Eriksson JW. Does the autonomic nervous system play a role in the development of insulin resistance? A study on heart rate variability in first-degree relatives of Type 2 diabetes patients and control subjects. Diabet Med 2003 May; 20(5): 399-405.

[112] Stern MP, Bartley M, Duggirala R, Bradshaw B. Birth weight and the metabolic syndrome: thrifty phenotype or thrifty genotype? Diabetes Metab Res Rev 2000 Mar-Apr; 16(2): 88-93.

[113] Hall JL, Ye JM, Clark MG, Colquhoun EQ. Sympathetic stimulation elicits increased or decreased VO2 in the perfused rat hindlimb via alpha 1-adrenoceptors. Am J Physiol 1997 May; 272(5 Pt 2): H2146-53.

[114] Feingold KR, Browner WS, Siperstein MD. Prospective studies of muscle capillary basement membrane width in prediabetics. J Clin Endocrinol Metab 1989 Oct; 69(4): 784-9.

[115] Camerini-Davalos RA, Oppermann W, Rebagliati H, Glasser M, Bloodworth JM. Muscle capillary basement membrane width in genetic prediabetes. J Clin Endocrinol Metab 1979 Feb; 48(2): 251-9.

[116] Cortinovis A, Crippa A, Cavalli R, Corti M, Cattaneo L. Capillary blood viscosity in microcirculation. Clin Hemorheol Microcirc 2006; 35(1-2): 183-92.

[117] Lipowsky HH. Microvascular rheology and hemodynamics. Microcirculation 2005 Jan-Feb; 12(1): 5-15.

[118] Pries AR, Secomb TW. Rheology of the microcirculation. Clin Hemorheol Microcirc 2003; 29(3-4): 143-

[119] Fossum E, Hoieggen A, Moan A, Rostrup M, Nordby G, Kjeldsen SE. Relationship between insulin sensitivity and maximal forearm blood flow in young men. Hypertension 1998 Nov; 32(5): 838-43.

[120] Pries AR, Secomb TW. Microvascular blood viscosity in vivo and the endothelial surface layer. Am J Physiol Heart Circ Physiol 2005 Dec; 289(6): H2657-64.

[121] Maeda N, Cicha I, Tateishi N, Suzuki Y. Triglyceride in plasma: prospective effects on microcirculatory functions. Clin Hemorheol Microcirc 2006; 34(1-2): 341-6.

[122] Reims HM, Sevre K, Hoieggen A, Fossum E, Eide I, Kjeldsen SE. Blood viscosity: effects of mental stress and relations to autonomic nervous system function and insulin sensitivity. Blood Press 2005; 14(3): 159-69.

[123] Hoieggen A, Fossum E, Moan A, Enger E, Kjeldsen SE. Whole-blood viscosity and the insulin-resistance syndrome. J Hypertens 1998 Feb; 16(2): 203-10.

[124] Abramson JL, Vaccarino V. Relationship between physical activity and inflammation among apparently healthy middle-aged and older US adults. Arch Intern Med 2002 Jun 10; 162(11): 1286-92.

[125] Nienaber C, Pieters M, Kruger SH, Stonehouse W, Vorster HH. Overfatness, stunting and physical inactivity are determinants of plasminogen activator inhibitor-1activity, fibrinogen and thrombin-antithrombin complex in African adolescents. Blood Coagul Fibrinolysis 2008 Jul; 19(5): 361-8.

[126] Cugno M, Mari D, Meroni PL, Gronda E, Vicari F, Frigerio M, *et al.* Haemostatic and inflammatory biomarkers in advanced chronic heart failure: role of oral anticoagulants and successful heart transplantation. Br J Haematol 2004 Jul; 126(1): 85-92.

[127] Steiner S, Jax T, Evers S, Hennersdorf M, Schwalen A, Strauer BE. Altered blood rheology in obstructive sleep apnea as a mediator of cardiovascular risk. Cardiology 2005; 104(2): 92-6.

[128] Nobili L, Schiavi G, Bozano E, De Carli F, Ferrillo F, Nobili F. Morning increase of whole blood viscosity in obstructive sleep apnea syndrome. Clin Hemorheol Microcirc 2000; 22(1): 21-7.

[129] Dikmenoglu N, Ciftci B, Ileri E, Guven SF, Seringec N, Aksoy Y, *et al.* Erythrocyte deformability, plasma viscosity and oxidative status in patients with severe obstructive sleep apnea syndrome. Sleep Med 2006 Apr; 7(3): 255-61.

[130] Gibbs CR, Blann AD, Watson RD, Lip GY. Abnormalities of hemorheological, endothelial, and platelet function in patients with chronic heart failure in sinus rhythm: effects of angiotensin-converting enzyme inhibitor and beta-blocker therapy. Circulation 2001 Apr 3; 103(13): 1746-51.

[131] Hoffmeister A, Hetzel J, Sander S, Kron M, Hombach V, Koenig W. Plasma viscosity and fibrinogen in relation to haemodynamic findings in chronic congestive heart failure. Eur J Heart Fail 1999 Aug; 1(3): 293-5.

[132] Sakkinen PA, Wahl P, Cushman M, Lewis MR, Tracy RP. Clustering of procoagulation, inflammation, and fibrinolysis variables with metabolic factors in insulin resistance syndrome. Am J Epidemiol 2000 Nov 15; 152(10): 897-907.

[133] Wannamethee SG, Lowe GD, Shaper AG, Rumley A, Lennon L, Whincup PH. The metabolic syndrome and insulin resistance: relationship to haemostatic and inflammatory markers in older non-diabetic men. Atherosclerosis 2005 Jul; 181(1): 101-8.

[134]   Yudkin JS. Abnormalities of coagulation and fibrinolysis in insulin resistance. Evidence for a common antecedent? Diabetes Care 1999 Apr; 22 Suppl 3: C25-30.

[135]   Venugopal J, Hanashiro K, Yang ZZ, Nagamine Y. Identification and modulation of a caveolae-dependent signal pathway that regulates plasminogen activator inhibitor-1 in insulin-resistant adipocytes. Proc Natl Acad Sci U S A 2004 Dec 7; 101(49): 17120-5.

[136]   Byberg L, McKeigue PM, Zethelius B, Lithell HO. Birth weight and the insulin resistance syndrome: association of low birth weight with truncal obesity and raised plasminogen activator inhibitor-1 but not with abdominal obesity or plasma lipid disturbances. Diabetologia 2000 Jan; 43(1): 54-60.

[137]   Heitritter SM, Solomon CG, Mitchell GF, Skali-Ounis N, Seely EW. Subclinical inflammation and vascular dysfunction in women with previous gestational diabetes mellitus. J Clin Endocrinol Metab 2005 Jul; 90(7): 3983-8.

[138]   Chen HS, Hwu CM, Kwok CF, Shih KC, Hsiao LC, Lee SH, et al. Insulin sensitivity in normotensive offspring of hypertensive parents. Horm Metab Res 2000 Mar; 32(3): 110-4.

[139]   Trifiletti A, Lasco A, Scamardi R, Cincotta M, Gaudio A, Barbera N, et al. Hemostasis and fibrinolysis factors in first-degree relatives of patients with Type 2 diabetes without hypertension. Pathophysiol Haemost Thromb 2002 May-Jun; 32(3): 127-30.

[140]   Natali A, Ferrannini E. Hypertension, insulin resistance, and the metabolic syndrome. Endocrinol Metab Clin North Am 2004 Jun; 33(2): 417-29.

[141]   Hanley AJ, Festa A, D'Agostino RB, Jr., Wagenknecht LE, Savage PJ, Tracy RP, et al. Metabolic and inflammation variable clusters and prediction of type 2 diabetes: factor analysis using directly measured insulin sensitivity. Diabetes 2004 Jul; 53(7): 1773-81.

[142]   Andersen K, Pedersen BK. The role of inflammation in vascular insulin resistance with focus on IL-6. Horm Metab Res 2008 Sep; 40(9): 635-9.

[143]   Zhang H, Park Y, Wu J, Chen X, Lee S, Yang J, et al. Role of TNF-alpha in vascular dysfunction. Clin Sci (Lond) 2009 Feb; 116(3): 2 19-30.

[144]   Anker SD, von Haehling S. Inflammatory mediators in chronic heart failure: an overview. Heart 2004 Apr; 90(4): 464-70.

[145]   Heymans S, Hirsch E, Anker SD, Aukrust P, Balligand JL, Cohen-Tervaert JW, et al. Inflammation as a therapeutic target in heart failure? A scientific statement from the Translational Research Committee of the Heart Failure Association of the European Society of Cardiology. Eur J Heart Fail 2009 Feb; 11(2): 1 19-29.

[146]   Vila V, Martinez-Sales V, Almenar L, Lazaro IS, Villa P, Reganon E. Inflammation, endothelial dysfunction and angiogenesis markers in chronic heart failure patients. Int J Cardiol 2008 Nov 12; 130(2): 276-7.

[147]   McNicholas WT. Obstructive sleep apnea and inflammation. Prog Cardiovasc Dis 2009 Mar-Apr; 51(5): 392-9.

[148]   Picchi A, Gao X, Belmadani S, Potter BJ, Focardi M, Chilian WM, et al. Tumor necrosis factor-alpha induces endothelial dysfunction in the prediabetic metabolic syndrome. Circ Res 2006 Jul 7; 99(1): 69-77.

[149]   Smith DT, Carr LJ, Dorozynski C, Gomashe C. Internet-delivered lifestyle physical activity intervention: limited inflammation and antioxidant capacity efficacy in overweight adults. J Appl Physiol 2009 Jan; 106(1): 49-56.

[150]   Patel SR, Zhu X, Storfer-Isser A, Mehra R, Jenny NS, Tracy R, et al. Sleep duration and biomarkers of inflammation. Sleep 2009 Feb 1; 32(2): 200-4.

[151]   Youd JM, Rattigan S, Clark MG. Acute impairment of insulin-mediated capillary recruitment and glucose uptake in rat skeletal muscle in vivo by TNF-alpha. Diabetes 2000 Nov; 49(11): 1904-9.

[152]   Wang L, Lim EJ, Toborek M, Hennig B. The role of fatty acids and caveolin-1 in tumor necrosis factor alpha-induced endothelial cell activation. Metabolism 2008 Oct; 57(10): 1328-39.

[153]   van Eijk IC, Peters MJ, Serne EH, van der Horst-Bruinsma IE, Dijkmans BA, Smulders YM, et al. Microvascular function is impaired in ankylosing spondylitis and improves after tumour necrosis factor alpha blockade. Ann Rheum Dis 2009 Mar; 68(3): 362-6.

[154]   Veresh Z, Racz A, Lotz G, Koller A. ADMA impairs nitric oxide-mediated arteriolar function due to increased superoxide production by angiotensin II-NAD(P)H oxidase pathway. Hypertension 2008 Nov; 52(5): 960-6.

[155]   Gao X, Belmadani S, Picchi A, Xu X, Potter BJ, Tewari-Singh N, et al. Tumor necrosis factor-alpha induces endothelial dysfunction in Lepr(db) mice. Circulation 2007 Jan 16; 115(2): 245-54.

[156]   Chen Y, Li Y, Zhang P, Traverse JH, Hou M, Xu X, et al. Dimethylarginine dimethylaminohydrolase and endothelial dysfunction in failing hearts. Am J Physiol Heart Circ Physiol 2005 Nov; 289(5): H2212-9.

[157]   Sydow K, Mondon CE, Cooke JP. Insulin resistance: potential role of the endogenous nitric oxide synthase inhibitor ADMA. Vasc Med 2005 Jul; 10 Suppl 1: S35-43.

[158]   Toutouzas K, Riga M, Stefanadi E, Stefanadis C. Asymmetric dimethylarginine (ADMA) and other endogenous nitric oxide synthase (NOS) inhibitors as an important cause of vascular insulin resistance. Horm Metab Res 2008 Sep; 40(9): 655-9.

[159]   Telejko B, Zonenberg A, Kuzmicki M, Modzelewska A, Niedziolko-Bagniuk K, Ponurkiewicz A, et al. Circulating asymmetric dimethylarginine, endothelin-1 and cell adhesion molecules in women with gestational diabetes. Acta Diabetol 2009 Jan 13.

[160]   Tsuda K, Nishio I. An association between plasma asymmetric dimethylarginine and membrane fluidity of erythrocytes in hypertensive and normotensive men: an electron paramagnetic resonance investigation. Am J Hypertens 2005 Sep; 18(9 Pt 1): 1243-8.

[161] Toth J, Racz A, Kaminski PM, Wolin MS, Bagi Z, Koller A. Asymmetrical dimethylarginine inhibits shear stress-induced nitric oxide release and dilation and elicits superoxide-mediated increase in arteriolar tone. Hypertension 2007 Mar; 49(3): 563-8.

[162] Vincent MA, Barrett EJ, Lindner JR, Clark MG, Rattigan S. Inhibiting NOS blocks microvascular recruitment and blunts muscle glucose uptake in response to insulin. Am J Physiol Endocrinol Metab 2003 Jul; 285(1): E123-9.

[163] Horstman LL, Jy W, Jimenez JJ, Bidot C, Ahn YS. New horizons in the analysis of circulating cell-derived microparticles. Keio J Med 2004 Dec; 53(4): 210-30.

[164] Chironi GN, Boulanger CM, Simon A, Dignat-George F, Freyssinet JM, Tedgui A. Endothelial microparticles in diseases. Cell Tissue Res 2009 Jan; 335(1): 143-51.

[165] Ryan S, McNicholas WT. Intermittent hypoxia and activation of inflammatory molecular pathways in OSAS. Arch Physiol Biochem 2008 Oct; 114(4): 261-6.

[166] Ursavas A, Karadag M, Rodoplu E, Yilmaztepe A, Oral HB, Gozu RO. Circulating ICAM-1 and VCAM-1 levels in patients with obstructive sleep apnea syndrome. Respiration 2007; 74(5): 525-32.

[167] Kautzky-Willer A, Fasching P, Jilma B, Waldhausl W, Wagner OF. Persistent elevation and metabolic dependence of circulating E-selectin after delivery in women with gestational diabetes mellitus. J Clin Endocrinol Metab 1997 Dec; 82(12): 4117-21.

[168] Manderson JG, Mullan B, Patterson CC, Hadden DR, Traub AI, McCance DR. Cardiovascular and metabolic abnormalities in the offspring of diabetic pregnancy. Diabetologia 2002 Jul; 45(7): 991-6.

[169] Bannan S, Mansfield MW, Grant PJ. Soluble vascular cell adhesion molecule-1 and E-selectin levels in relation to vascular risk factors and to E-selectin genotype in the first degree relatives of NIDDM patients and in NIDDM patients. Diabetologia 1998 Apr; 41(4): 460-6.

[170] Caballero AE, Arora S, Saouaf R, Lim SC, Smakowski P, Park JY, *et al.* Microvascular and macrovascular reactivity is reduced in subjects at risk for type 2 diabetes. Diabetes 1999 Sep; 48(9): 1856-62.

[171] Bretelle F, Sabatier F, Blann A, D'Ercole C, Boutiere B, Mutin M, *et al.* Maternal endothelial soluble cell adhesion molecules with isolated small for gestational age fetuses: comparison with pre-eclampsia. BJOG 2001 Dec; 108(12): 1277-82.

[172] Yin WH, Chen JW, Jen HL, Chiang MC, Huang WP, Feng AN, *et al.* The prognostic value of circulating soluble cell adhesion molecules in patients with chronic congestive heart failure. Eur J Heart Fail 2003 Aug; 5(4): 507-16.

[173] Wang W. Change in properties of the glycocalyx affects the shear rate and stress distribution on endothelial cells. J Biomech Eng 2007 Jun; 129(3): 324-9.

[174] Yao Y, Rabodzey A, Dewey CF, Jr. Glycocalyx modulates the motility and proliferative response of vascular endothelium to fluid shear stress. Am J Physiol Heart Circ Physiol 2007 Aug; 293(2): H1023-30.

[175] Tarbell JM, Pahakis MY. Mechanotransduction and the glycocalyx. J Intern Med 2006 Apr; 259(4): 339-50.

[176] Savery MD, Damiano ER. The endothelial glycocalyx is hydrodynamically relevant in arterioles throughout the cardiac cycle. Biophys J 2008 Aug; 95(3): 1439-47.

[177] Gouverneur M, Berg B, Nieuwdorp M, Stroes E, Vink H. Vasculoprotective properties of the endothelial glycocalyx: effects of fluid shear stress. J Intern Med 2006 Apr; 259(4): 393-400.

[178] Wiernsperger N. 50 years later: is metformin a vascular drug with antidiabetic properties ? Br J Diabetes Vasc Dis 2007; 7: 204-10.

[179] Broekhuizen LN, Mooij HL, Kastelein JJ, Stroes ES, Vink H, Nieuwdorp M. Endothelial glycocalyx as potential diagnostic and therapeutic target in cardiovascular disease. Curr Opin Lipidol 2009 Feb; 20(1): 57-62.

[180] Nieuwdorp M, Meuwese MC, Mooij HL, van Lieshout MH, Hayden A, Levi M, *et al.* Tumor necrosis factor-alpha inhibition protects against endotoxin-induced endothelial glycocalyx perturbation. Atherosclerosis 2009 Jan; 202(1): 296-303.

[181] Wiernsperger NF. Membrane physiology as a basis for the cellular effects of metformin in insulin resistance and diabetes. Diabetes Metab 1999 Jun; 25(2): 110-27.

[182] Rosen P, Wiernsperger NF. Metformin delays the manifestation of diabetes and vascular dysfunction in Goto-Kakizaki rats by reduction of mitochondrial oxidative stress. Diabetes Metab Res Rev 2006 Jul-Aug; 22(4): 323-30.

[183] Batandier C, Guigas B, Detaille D, El-Mir MY, Fontaine E, Rigoulet M, *et al.* The ROS production induced by a reverse-electron flux at respiratory-chain complex 1 is hampered by metformin. J Bioenerg Biomembr 2006 Feb; 38(1): 33-42.

[184] Wiernsperger NF, Bouskela E. Microcirculation in insulin resistance and diabetes: more than just a complication. Diabetes Metab 2003 Sep; 29(4 Pt 2): 6S77-87.

[185] de Aguiar LG, Bahia LR, Villela N, Laflor C, Sicuro F, Wiernsperger N, *et al.* Metformin improves endothelial vascular reactivity in first-degree relatives of type 2 diabetic patients with metabolic syndrome and normal glucose tolerance. Diabetes Care 2006 May; 29(5): 1083-9.

[186] Kraemer de Aguiar LG, Laflor CM, Bahia L, Villela NR, Wiernsperger N, Bottino DA, *et al.* Metformin improves skin capillary reactivity in normoglycaemic subjects with the metabolic syndrome. Diabet Med 2007 Mar; 24(3): 272-9.

[187] Kraemer-Aguiar LG, Laflor CM, Bouskela E. Skin microcirculatory dysfunction is already present in normoglycemic subjects with metabolic syndrome. Metabolism 2008 Dec; 57(12): 1740-6.